FOOD AND THE STATUS QUEST

FOOD AND THE STATUS QUEST
An Interdisciplinary Perspective

edited by Polly Wiessner *and* Wulf Schiefenhövel

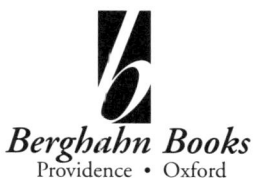

Berghahn Books
Providence • Oxford

First published in 1996 by
Berghahn Books

© Polly Wiessner and Wulf Schiefenhövel 1996, 1998

All rights reserved.
No part of this publication may be reproduced in any form or by any means without the written permission of Berghahn Books.

Library of Congress Cataloging-in-Publication Data
Food and the status quest : an interdisciplinary perspective / edited by Polly Wiessner and Wulf Schiefenhövel.
    p.   cm.
Includes bibliographical references and index.
(alk. paper)
    1. Food.   2. Food supply.   3. Food consumption.   4. Nutritional anthropology.   5. Needs, Nutritional--Developing countries.
I. Wiessner, Pauline Wilson, 1947-   .   II. Schiefenhövel, Wulf, 1943-   .
GN407.F657   1995   95-37304
363.8--dc20   CIP

ISBN 1-57181-871-5 hardback
ISBN 1-57181-123-0 paperpack

British Library Cataloguing-in-Publication Data
A catalogue record for this book is available from the British Library.

Printed in the USA on acid-free paper.

CONTENTS

Preface
Wulf Schiefenhövel — vii

1. Introduction: Food, Status, Culture, and Nature
Polly Wiessner — 1

2. The Ethological Bases of Status Hierarchies
Barbara Hold-Cavell — 19

3. The Evolution of Nurturant Dominance
Irenäus Eibl-Eibesfeldt — 33

4. Dominance Status, Food Sharing, and Reproductive Success in Chimpanzees
William C. McGrew — 39

5. Food Sharing and Status in Unprovisioned Bonobos
Gottfried Hohmann & Barbara Fruth — 47

6. Systems of Power: The Function and Evolution of Social Status
Karl Grammer — 69

7. Feasts and Commensal Politics in the Political Economy: Food, Power, and Status in Prehistoric Europe
Michael Dietler — 87

8. Feasting in Prehistoric and Traditional Societies
Brian Hayden — 127

9. **Food Production and Social Status as Documented in Proto-Cuneiform Texts**
   Peter Damerow — 149

10. **Leveling the Hunter: Constraints on the Status Quest in Foraging Societies**
    Polly Wiessner — 171

11. **Food and the Status Quest in Five African Cultures**
    Igor de Garine — 193

12. **Food, Competition, and the Status of Food in New Guinea**
    Pierre Lemonnier — 219

13. **Of Harvests and Hierarchies: Securing Staple Food and Social Position in the Trobriand Islands**
    Wulf Schiefenhövel & Ingrid Bell-Krannhals — 235

14. **Food and Household Status in Nepal**
    Catherine Panter-Brick — 253

15. **Nutritional Security and the Status Quest in Developing Countries**
    Rainer Gross & Günter Dresrüsse — 263

Notes on Contributors — 277

Index — 281

PREFACE

Wulf Schiefenhövel

Food, like sex, satisfies a primary need of humans and consequently lies at the crossroad of biology and culture. In this strategic position, it presents many interesting facets. Food and nutrition considered from the viewpoint of both social and biological sciences have been the focus of interest of the European Commission on the Anthropology of Food and Nutrition of the International Union of Anthropological and Ethnological Sciences, under the coordination of Igor de Garine of the Centre National de la Recherche Scientifique. The founding meeting was held in New Delhi, India in 1978 at the International Congress of Anthropological and Ethological Sciences. Since then sixteen other symposia have been held, each with a different topic: uncertainty in food supply; cultural and physiological aspects of fatness; food sharing; seasonality of food supply; nutritional problems of the elderly; children's food traditions; the formation of the Mediterranean diet; food preference and taste; food tradition and innovation, etc.

The present volume is the outcome of one of these symposia convened by Polly Wiessner and me at Ringberg Castle of the Max Planck Society at Lake Tegernsee in Bavaria. Together with the authors of this volume, the following colleagues contributed: Serge Bahuchet, Renate Edelhofer, Mark Eggerman, Isabel Gonzales Turmo, Geoffrey Harrison, Adel den Hartog, Helen Macbeth, Marianne Oertl, Jana Parizková, Armin Prinz, Detlev Ploog, Khosrow Saidi, Frank Salter, and Vasile Zamfirescu.

The use of food to enhance status has been the subject of excellent studies, many of which are discussed in this volume, but little has been done to put this topic into a cross-cultural and interdisciplinary perspective. However, research in human ethology, anthropology and other fields on defining and measuring status, that traces its phylogenetic roots and elucidates its evolutionary functions, have the potential to facilitate new perspectives and syntheses.

There is probably no society that does not assign some status value to different kinds of food. However, the importance of food in the quest for status seems to vary among societies, ranging from hunter-gatherer groups, in which the procurer of meat receives esteem, to India where food plays an important role in caste distinctions, to societies in eastern Melanesia and the Northwest coast of America where extravagant competitive feasts are held to impress the guests in a ritualized form of aggression. Furthermore, the use of food to display status has profound effects on development programs. Nutritious foods may be rejected simply because a negative status value is attached to them. Foods given out in relief operations may be distributed inequitably in attempts to gain or preserve status, or families may consume nutritionally poor foods in order to sell better crops to get cash and purchase status goods.

We are grateful to the Max Planck Society for supporting the meeting and to the staff of Schloß Ringberg for generously hosting us. Sabine Eggebrecht, Annette Heunemann, Sibylle Salter, Sylvia Shipp, and Susanne Töpler have helped in preparing this manuscript, and Frank Salter and Irenäus Eibl-Eibesfeldt have made valuable suggestions; to all of them we own many thanks. This book presents a new perspective on how food and status seeking are intertwined in human societies. We hope that the readers will get similar rewards reading it, just as we have gained in putting it together.

1. INTRODUCTION
FOOD, STATUS, CULTURE, AND NATURE

Polly Wiessner

Behavioral predispositions that are shared by all humans and that have an impact on the organization of society are few but significant. In addition to those that structure perception and communication, only a handful have been identified in ethology: social and spatial territoriality, possessiveness and respect for norms of possession, giving and reciprocating in a social context to create bonds, incest avoidance, the tendency of humans to form in-group and out-group identities, and the quest to seek status or high regard (Eibl-Eibesfeldt 1989). These predispositions can provide important guidelines for research in the social sciences because they operate in all contemporary societies, and they can be used to formulate questions about the past and to anticipate problems of the future. Although their roots in human phylogeny and their universality in human societies suggest a biological basis, they are not wholly determined by biology, for it is in these realms that culture experiments most creatively.

In 1988, when the European Committee for the Anthropology of Food and Nutrition met to discuss topics for future projects, we decided to take one of these universal tendencies, and to ask: how does culture guide, restrict, or elaborate a biologically-based behavior, and, in turn, how do biological predispositions channel or restrain culture? With food at the center of our interest, the status quest was a logical topic on which to concentrate. After all, it has been long accepted that the popular adage "you are what you eat" applies to our social as well as to our physical being. Participants from a number of different disciplines were invited so that in addition to biological and cultural approaches prehistoric, historic, and contemporary perspectives could be gained. In October 1991, we met at the Max Planck Society's Schloß Ringberg in Bavaria to present our ideas and findings. This volume is the product of our papers, discussion, and afterthoughts. Before turning to the individual contributions, it is important to align ethological and cultural concepts of status.

Status: Ethological and Ethnological Perspectives

Status is a word of Indo-European origin. Its root is found in old Indian languages, the Greek *histemi*, the Latin *stare*, the English *stand*, and the German *stehen*. The nouns derived from these verbs imply the notion of verticality, the physical act of being in a certain place, and the impact or impression that one makes on others from that position. Probably as old as the concept of status is the question of whether status differences and corresponding social inequalities are natural or cultural and environmental in origin, and which differences are natural or cultural. Certainly this sensitive issue has long plagued social and political scientists and philosophers (Locke 1690: second treatise; Rousseau 1755), because of the inherent moral double bind: inequalities bring oppression of the lower echelons, while achieving equality in large-scale societies requires using repressive force.

Ethological concepts of status, to which the chapters by Barbara Hold-Cavell and Karl Grammer are devoted, correspond closely to the root meaning of the word. Status seeking in ethology is regarded as part of a complex of behaviors in which individuals consciously or unconsciously strive to be in the focus of attention in order to improve their position in the rank hierarchy of a group. As these two authors discuss in detail, ethological constructs of rank order were first derived from pecking orders in birds and formulated on the basis of dominance. This criterion later proved to be inadequate for the identification of rank orders in higher primates, where prosocial behavior (organization, mediation, nurturing), as opposed to antisocial behavior (aggression), can be an important factor in rank achievements. Subsequent kindergarten studies revealed that structure of attention by group members, that is, how much a person is in the focus of attention, provided the best measure of status. The more a child is looked at by several group mates, the higher is his or her position in the rank order. Low-ranking group members look at high-ranking ones out of fear because high-ranking members are potentially dangerous or assertive, or out of attraction because high-ranking ones provide protection and are sources of information about the socioecological environment. Thus, attention structure provides information for the structuring of behavior and goals.

Ethological studies of children have shown that high rank or status is associated with display behavior, initiation and organization of group activities, conflict mediation, and widespread access to resources, among other things. Status relations are highly dependent on ability to recruit allies and to maintain them over a longer period of time. In other words, high status must be agreed upon in part by others.

Like all branches of evolutionary biology, human ethology argues that the predisposition to seek status has been selected for throughout our evolution, because higher status on the average has permitted better access to mates and resources, and has thereby increased reproductive success. The logic for the evolution of rank orders is somewhat different. In all populations individuals follow different strategies according to their own abilities. For those who do not have the strength and social competence to achieve high rank, acceptance of a lower position can have its relative rewards. Examples include avoidance of conflict, predictability of relations, protection, the benefits of organization and other factors that also can increase reproductive success. Rank orders are thus formed by the combination of different individual strategies, so they are constantly in flux. Human ethology departs from some branches of evolutionary biology in that it does not assume that status seeking or rank formation always serves to maximize reproductive success, but only that it has done so significantly more often than not in our evolutionary history. As Tooby and Cosmides (1989: 36) point out, "In short, evolutionary theory does not itself constitute a theory of human nature: instead, it is a theory of how human nature came to be, and an invaluable tool in the campaign to discover what human nature actually is." Thus, human ethology seeks only to identify status seeking and rank orders, and to elucidate their effects on an individual or group, whether this be positive or negative in evolutionary terms.

Ethnological concepts of status are more complex and ambiguous than ethological ones since culture comes into play. Cultural prescriptions structure the status quest and formation of rank orders by channeling, reducing, accentuating, or preventing competition, and by institutionalizing status competition. Linton (1936: 115), the first anthropologist to formally develop the concept of status for the discipline, divided it into ascribed status and achieved status according to how one comes to occupy a certain social position. Ascribed status is an assigned, fixed social position that is often closed to competition, such as age, gender, inherited rank or office. Although some ascribed statuses are for the most part biologically designated, like age and gender, they are usually culturally redefined: age categories are stipulated differently from culture to culture, and in some societies gender changes are permitted (Désy 1980; Robbe 1976). Linton's second category, achieved status, designates a social position attained through accomplishments (or lack of them) and/or competition: leader, specialist, friend, exchange partner, etc. Linton drew a further distinction between status, a position that people occupy with accompanying behaviors, attitudes, rights, and obligations, and the roles that they play.

Linton's work provided the basis for one meaning of status in the human sciences, that is, status as position in the social structure. It is generally neutral with respect to the concept of verticality inherent in the ethological concept, though social positions may conform to rank positions. However, status also is used in ethnology in a second sense, one synonymous with prestige or social ranking, as in Weber's (1922) three dimensions of social stratification: economic status or wealth, power, and prestige. In his critique of anthropological concepts of status, Goodenough (1965) also turned in this direction, proposing that Linton's concept of status be termed "social identity", and that status should be seen as a series of rights and duties vis-à-vis others. He constructed "status scales" using techniques developed by Guttman on the basis of duties owed to others in the society, duties being defined primarily in behavioral terms (Goodenough 1951: 113, Goodenough 1965: 13). His definition of status, methodology, and resulting tables of rank orders for specific activities and realms of life are remarkably close to those of ethology.

Although definitions of status as published by Linton and Goodenough were used primarily for descriptive purposes, the parallel between status as social rank or prestige in ethnology and status in ethology is not a superficial one and it can be carried over into theoretical underpinnings: that the pursuit of status or prestige serves to increase access to a wide range of resources. For example, Bourdieu (1977: 171-83) argues that prestige is "symbolic capital" that is readily convertible back into economic capital, and that "symbolic capital is always credit in the widest sense of the word" (Bourdieu 1977: 181). Because symbolic capital in the form of honor or prestige is costly in terms of time and material investments, it can often be accumulated only at the expense of economic capital. In compensation for its high costs, symbolic capital is the best economic guarantee in societies with severe climates, limited technical resources, and demand for collective labor, because it is readily convertible back into economic capital and/or labor when need arises. One can go further and argue that symbolic capital serves as credit for many forms of support in addition to labor and goods. It is also the best guarantee that credit will be extended in the future, for people tend to invest in the prestigious with expectation of a good return. This concept of prestige or status and the goals of prestige seeking are fully compatible with evolutionary explanations of the status quest.

Prestige is the only form of accumulation permitted in many societies with a strong egalitarian ethos; accordingly, so-called "prestige economies" develop. This is partly because the benefits of prestige accumulation filter out to others in the form of material goods distributed in exchange for status and/or the protective umbrella of a prestigious reputation, which can cover both high-ranking individuals and their fellow group members. In culture as in nature, then, not only is the tendency to seek status favored, but a certain degree of stabilization in rank orders also is favored.

Fried (1968: 252-55) has classified societies by how extensively rank orders are institutionalized by culture:

1. Egalitarian societies in which "there are as many positions of prestige in any given age-sex grade as there are persons capable of filling them" (Fried 1968: 252). This definition includes cultures with age- and sex-based status differences. Because it does not define the rights and duties of "prestigeous positions", it encompasses a very wide range of leadership styles.
2. Ranked societies, in which there are fewer positions of valued status than individuals capable of filling them, but neither exploitative economic nor genuine political power is vested in these. Here individuals may attain position by election, birth order, membership in certain lineages, and so on.
3. Stratified societies are those distinguished by "differential relationships between the members of the society and its subsistence means – some of the members of society have unimpeded access to its strategic resources while others have various impediments in their access to the same fundamental resources" (Fried 1968: 255).

The chapters in this volume concentrate on the use of food to gain status in the sense of prestige or social ranking, as the title implies. Nonetheless, status as social position will not be ignored. Every person is born into a society with a defined set of social positions that may be ascribed or attained. Culturally defined social positions stipulate who is equal and therefore eligible to compete in different activities, and which achievements confer status. They are society's way of guiding the status quest, and in human societies there can be no status quest that is not played out within the framework of such identities and values.

Food in the Status Quest

Negotiation of status relations takes place in a wide variety of settings and via different mediums. Food is prominent among these for a number of reasons. Food and corresponding evaluations of appetite/satiation, taste/distaste, and nutritious/unnutritious evoke associations of superiority or inferiority in many cultures. For example, control of hunger, an indicator of discipline and self-restraint, is often demanded when people undergo initiation to mark a change of status in the life cycle. Conversely, gluttonous consumption of food may indicate lack of restraint, or be seen as indicating a voracious appetite, vigor, and capacity. Foods that are preferred for their taste, such as those containing fat and other critical nutrients (Speth 1990) are often associated with well-being and confer superiority on those who can regularly produce, consume or distribute them. The reverse is true for inferior or famine foods; the extreme example is dehumanizing via culinary curses – "eater of shit", etc. Furthermore, certain qualities of food, such as strong taste, odor or texture, are believed to make them suitable or unsuitable for persons at different stages of life or with different areas of specialization. Finally, cooking or cuisine, the subject of major theoretical works (Douglas 1984; Douglas and Isherwood 1979; Goody 1982; Lévi-Strauss 1969) is also an active tool of the status quest.

A second and most important dimension in the relation of food to status is that it is the product of labor. Procurement or production of a more than adequate food supply is an indicator of superior skill, vitality, and/or control over the labor of others. When food distributions are financed from outside, such as in many Highland New Guinea Big-man societies, abundance of food is also an indicator of a broad network of supportive social ties. As the basis for life, food attracts attention and is highly divisible, making the distributor or host the center of attention for food sharing. Commensal occasions create, affirm or reproduce a wide variety of social relationships.

The Pursuit of Status: Repressive and Affiliative Strategies

Strategies used to gain status or rank position, whether conscious or unconscious, differ markedly between nonhuman primates and humans. Nonhuman primates mainly use aggression or repression to dominate and displace competitors, while in human societes nurturant and affiliative or "prosocial behaviour" – initiating and organizing activities, protection or sharing – plays a greater and, in the long run, a more effective role. Repressive and prosocial tactics can have similar results in terms of greater access to resources and/or decisive influence of one individual over another. Strategies for status seeking do not, however, clearly separate nonhuman primates from humans. For instance, William McGrew's chapter shows that although chimpanzee males obtain high rank by physically defeating or displacing others, they also use affiliative strategies to enlist support. Food sharing with adult males follows unwritten rules: "Don't share with competitors, but with nonchallenging males and old, influential males", both of whom can assist in the rank struggle. Gottfried Hohmann and Barbara Fruth present parallel findings for bonobos, whose social organization is similar to that of chimpanzees except that bonobos females tend to have higher rank. Their preliminary results indicate that females share food with other unrelated females, who in turn help them maintain dominance over males. Also fascinating with regard to affiliative behavior are McGrew's findings concerning chimpanzee status, health, food sharing, and reproduction. While alpha (dominant) males gain reproductive advantage through physically displacing competitors, those lower down in the rank hierarchy find their own paths to reproduction. Such males, who are not as occupied as alphas in holding their rank positions, entice fertile females through affiliative behavior, like grooming and food sharing, to temporarily leave the group on consortships, during which an estimated 50 percent of impregnations take place. In view of the success of affiliative strategies in achieving status and reproductive success, it is not surprising that prosocial behavior became integrated into the status seeking repertoire in humans.

Just as nonhuman primates do not use aggressive strategies alone to strive for rank, humans by no means restrict their struggles to prosocial tactics, as our history and daily life attest. It is nonetheless the initiator, organizer, generous or protective leader who is the ideal of most cultures, not the bully or the despot. Irenäus Eibl-Eibesfeldt traces the roots of such behavior strategies to the evolution of parental care in birds and mammals. Prosocial behavior in humans, when expressed via food distribution, can involve truly "free gifts" in socioeconomic terms, though these often imply status differences between the nurturant and nurtured. This is distinguished from reciprocity, a relationship between equals in which each gift compels a counter gift (Mauss 1950), which also may have roots in parental care but has a more complex evolutionary history (Trivers 1971). Nurturant or prosocial behavior can be simultaneously a true expression of affection and a subtle technique to exert influence; thus it is used primarily among close kin or familiars. As relations move from familiarity to anonymity, nurturant strategies to obtain influence are eclipsed by repressive dominance, as can be seen in institutionalized status relations in stratified societies (Salter 1994).

True to its roots in parental care, the preparation and distribution of food – in the form of family meals, lavish hosting of esteemed visitors, celebratory feasts or generous redistributions of food and wealth – is often a nurturant affair. Let there be no doubt, though, that all such occasions include subtle relations of influence or even dominance on the part of the nurturant. With the family in the grip of a well-prepared meal, women may make their opinions heard, a visitor may be put in a position of gratitude by the hospitality of his host, and those who are generous in times of feasting may later call in their debts. Furthermore, commensal occasions, through their intrinsically nurturant connotations, provide camouflage behind which prestige politics can unfold. As Michael Dietler's chapter illustrates, a wide range of social and political relations can be negotiated or reproduced through feasting: entrepreneurial feasts can be used to accumulate symbolic capital in the form of prestige; patron-role or redistributive feasts legitimize or reiterate relations of unequal social/political power; and diacritical feasts, through differentiated cuisine and styles of consumption, naturalize or reify concepts of ranked differences in social status. In his fascinating analysis of archaeological materials from the Iron Age of western Europe, Dietler demonstrates how drinking and feasting ware and their contents were introduced during colonial interaction with Mediterranean states and thereafter used as new tools in existing political struggles. Of particular importance in Iron Age politics was the use of alcoholic beverages, as indicated by the large numbers and/or spectacular appearance of vessels for wine consumption found in archaeological sites. No doubt the psychoactive properties of alcohol facilitated the commensal politics of Iron Age Europe as they do in many contemporary societies.

Brian Hayden's chapter outlines the political moves that can be executed by ambitious individuals through feasting. He proposes that through the lure of feasts, with their free meals, delicacies, dances, exciting entertainment, and ambitious organizers, "triple A" personalities, draw others into contractual agreements that generate debts and thereby confer social leverage. In other words, through competitive feasts, surpluses are produced and converted into wealth and power by enterprising individuals, creating social inequalities. He then takes a step back in time and proposes that during the upper Paleolithic and Mesolithic periods in resource-rich environments, triple A individuals manipulated relationships through competitive feasting in such a way as to dodge the leveling hammer of egalitarian ethos. This leads him to the proposal, supported by compelling evidence (Hayden 1990), that the need for larger amounts of certain rare delicacies for competitive feasts may have been a significant factor in the domestication of certain plants and animals, and thus may have given impetus to early agriculture.

While the two papers described above are oriented more to individual strategies and internal politics, Pierre Lemonnier's work on New Guinea societies shows how feasting enters into intergroup competition. Feasting in the context of peacemaking can simultaneously involve affiliative overtures, like the giving of pigs as a substitution for lives lost and/or an overture for renewal of bonds, and aggressive ones, like the demonstration of productive capacity, extent of social networks, and strength of leadership, to arrive at a balance of power between groups. This brings to the fore a point concerning the status quest mentioned earlier: rank orders are in part agreed upon. Status imparted to feast organizers is a product of both their own social engineering and permission by group members for them to rise in status, because their "name" and actions benefit the group as a whole.

As Douglas (1990) has pointed out, free gifts or charity wound, for they contradict the principle of reciprocity and imply status imbalance. Thus, nurturant giving when carried to an extreme can become a tool for repressive dominance. The greater the competition expressed through food, the more likely it is that feasting will shed its camouflage of nurturant behavior and will be used outrightly to displace others, whether physically or symbolically. At the extreme, some societies literally "fight with food" (Codere 1950; Rosman and Rubel 1971; Young 1971). For instance among the Kwakuitl, one host may try to place his rivals "in the shadow of his name", turning a predominantly prosocial strategy into an outrightly aggressive one (Boas 1966).

The Cultural Factor

The wide array of cultural elaborations on the theme of status seeking and the formation of rank orders needs little discussion because it is so evident in the chapters to come. Societies such as the Massa of Cameroon described by Igor de Garine pour over 13,000 kilocalories a day into young men for periods of two months to prestigiously (and painfully) fatten them in *guru walla* consumption sessions. By contrast, Buddhist monks or Western fashion models starve themselves to achieve renown within their own areas of specialization. Among many foragers of the world, food and feasting is handled with utmost care to preserve egalitarian relations, while some hunter and gatherers in rich maritime environments distribute food and wealth in quantities so great as to bury the recipients in shame. Culture sometimes accentuates food-related practices conspicuously for extreme or even outrageous eating behavior, as the food section of the *Guinness Book of World Records* attests. This behavior can serve to put a person or group in the center of attention, to confer a "name": Michel Lolito of France stands in the eating hall of fame for having consumed ten bicycles, a supermarket cart, seven TV sets, six chandeliers, a Cessna light weight aircraft, and a coffin, handle and all, the only example in history of the coffin ending up inside the man (Guinness Book of World Records 1989: 323).

Extreme status seeking behavior can be destructive and the resulting dominance that is gained can be repressive. Accordingly, most societies guide or restrict it in some fashion through norms, ideologies, and/or the ascription of statuses that define who can compete with whom, such as cultural classification by age and gender. For instance, among the Koma described by de Garine, men improve their status and progress up an intricate age grade system to become high-ranking initiates and respected policymakers by slaughtering cattle on ritual occasions. However, a man can progress only when the community acknowledges that he has achieved the rank to which he aspires both economically and in his daily behavior. Influence gained at each step is culturally prescribed and limited. All men who are capable can follow the same steps.

This is also true for the Trobriand Islanders portrayed in the contribution of Wulf Schiefenhövel and Ingrid Bell-Krannhals. Although it is a ranked society, it is also a true meritocracy because men and women who work and give generously are granted status. Vital men with acute social and mental skills work their way up the social ladder by above-average performance in gardening and by organizing *kayasa* feasts and *kula* exchanges. When they arrive near the top, their kin and community build them a *liku* house in which to display yams. The building of a *liku* marks public recognition of their achievements, and from this point on they are principal receivers of harvest gifts. Having attained a position that affords them an important role in community politics, the pressure to produce and compete is usually reduced. To a lesser extent, women also use competitive exchange to rise in status via *sagali* post-mortuary distributions, in which traditionally great numbers of skirts from banana fibers, and, today, modern fabric, ready-made dresses, and money change hands. The competition in *kayasa* exchange, as in many forms of competitive exchange, results in overproduction, and with it a storage economy that can prove most beneficial during a bad harvest (Eibl-Eibesfeldt 1989: 308-9).

Symbolic values attributed to food, food production, and food exchange may also direct the status quest. Lemonnier makes this point by analyzing three "social logics" associated with ceremonial exchange and feasting held by different clusters of societies in New Guinea and their implications for leadership. He concentrates on three attributes of pigs that are culturally exploited or valued in some of these social logics but not others: (1) their relation to women's labor, (2) their inherent ability to reproduce and thereby to facilitate the finance of ceremonial exchange, and (3) their symbolic value as a substitute for life in bridewealth and compensation exchanges. Comparison of how these dimensions are embodied with cultural values and how they are developed and linked in the three social logics appears to be closely related to the roles and status of leaders. Only in Big-man societies of the New Guinea Highlands, where pigs are fully domesticated, represent female labor, and are used as all-purpose currencies and substitutes for life, can authority or influence in many areas of life be consolidated in one powerful personage, the Big man. The Big man, who can assemble many pigs, and plan and orchestrate ceremonial exchange, provides many more benefits to his group than do the leaders in societies with the other two social logics, who have tools that are symbolically and economically poorer. In return, he receives prestige that can be translated into labor and influence over many areas of life.

Culture not only channels the status quest, but it also severely curtails the quest through ideological and social means, as Polly Wiessner's chapter demonstrates for hunting and meat distribution in foraging societies. In ten out of twenty-five societies that were considered, meat (and food in general) was removed from the status quest by ideological means, that is, success in hunting was seen as the result of the benevolence of forest spirits or the willingness of the animal to give itself over to the hunter, not as a result of the merits of the hunter(s). For the remaining fifteen societies, measures to take the hunter out of the focus of attention during the meat distribution and/or leveling mechanisms applied by group members greatly circumscribed the amount of status that could be achieved by the hunter. The extreme repression of rank order formation found among foragers is unusual for human societies and can be related to a combination of conditions: the requirements of social security networks for pooling risk; the lack of intergroup competition that would require organization and leadership; and the current integration of foragers into the larger socioeconomic framework of neighboring societies.

The Biological Factor

Culture thus has the power to produce extraordinary variations on a biological theme through elaboration and social or ideological controls. This begs the question, "Does biology similarly restrict culture or does culture run unbounded?" A number of the chapters in this volume indicate that influence runs both ways, even though biological effect is more difficult to demonstrate than cultural effect. Perhaps the most salient result that comes out of all contributions regarding the role of biology is that culture can channel and repress the status quest, but it cannot completely eradicate it. Even in forager societies where ideology and social mechanisms for leveling status differences are pervasive, status striving constantly crops up. The strength of ideologies and sanctions needed to repress the status quest are perhaps the strongest testimony to its existence.

A number of contributions suggest further biological influences on status seeking behavior. The most obvious of these is the impact of the physiological effects of alcoholic drink on participants, which induce merriment, relaxation, and the breakdown of inhibitions when used in the appropriate context, as well as enhanced jockeying for power (Heath 1987; Douglas 1987). Both Dietler's evidence for the consumption of great quantities of drink during feasts in the Iron Age of Western Europe and de Garine's observations of negative effects of drink in West African cultures emphasize the importance of further research in this area.

Our biological heritage also may have some impact on age and sex components of the status quest. As Grammer points out, the pursuit of attention and reputation is most energetic at certain critical stages of the life cycle. Although babies have features that attract attention (Lorenz 1943; Eibl-Eibesfeldt 1989), studies of kindergarteners show that active status seeking begins between the ages of about four and six, the critical post-weaning period during which young children have to replace parental investment lost to a younger sibling and to enter a peer group. The giving and sharing of food and objects, among other things, is an important strategy used at this age, and status gained is associated with reliable and reciprocal peer relations. The next pronounced stage of status seeking occurs just prior to marriage and is most accentuated in young men who compete for female partners. Food often plays a role; for instance, in hunter-gatherer societies young men hunt vigorously at this time and thereby prove that they can provide meat for their prospective bride's family. However, status is more frequently attained by more prominent displays, prowess in fighting or competence in contests of strength. In many Western countries, the tendency of young adults and young men in particular to flaunt their strength is often demonstrated behind the wheel of a car, with unfortunate outcomes. Finally vigorous attempts to gain status are made between the ages of forty and sixty, often in the context of benevolent or competitive food distribution. This period correlates with the time when mature men and women are contemplating or arranging the marriages of their children and are attempting to advertise the strength of their families to attract suitable partners. It is also an age at which men may seek additional wives.

Biological predictions for sex-specific strategies over the life cycle also may direct the status quest. From an evolutionary perspective one would expect men to have been selected to pursue status vigorously until old age, for they have much to gain by doing so, such as the attraction of more wives to increase their reproductive success and the possibility of winning resources or exploiting the labor of others to better support their families. By contrast, women after marriage increase their reproductive success by investing as much as possible in their children or grandchildren and by trying to secure their husbands' efforts as well. Therefore they would not be expected to squander as many resources in the pursuit of renown. Although both men and women engage in the status quest, the strong male bias indicated by the contributions in this volume and the picture portrayed in the anthropological and ethological literature is indeed borne out on a statistical basis. Among kindergarten children, boys engage in more overt displays than girls. Among the Massa of Cameroun, it is young men, not women, who fatten themselves for marriage, and it is Big men and Great men of New Guinea who play the most prominent roles in ceremonial exchange. On the Trobriand Islands, men monopolize two out of three of the large status seeking events, the *kula* and *kayasa* exchanges, though in this matrilineal society women also have their turn during the post-mortuary *sagali* distributions (Weiner 1976). In other words, both men and women have the capacity to compete for status when the motivations are present; the different biological interests of men and women in reproduction mentioned above, as well as gender roles, give men more reasons to do so.

The ultimate question that always emerges during discussions beween ethnologists and evolutionary biologists – how extensively cultural practices follow biological "laws" and serve to increase our inclusive fitness – incited heated debate after a number of the papers were delivered at the Ringberg symposium. Discussion ran aground without resolution because of the difficulties of drawing and testing hypotheses from evolutionary theory in small-scale human societies.

When asking if a cultural practice is adaptive, it is first necessary to pose the question "for whom?". If a Massa man attends the *guru* fattening cure, it may be detrimental for younger siblings and other household members but beneficial for him; if a young man of exceptional skill is forced to gain status through an age grade system controlled by community elders, it may be of less than optimal benefit to him but of value to other members of the society; if an exceptional hunter is stripped of the products and status of his accomplishments, it may benefit the community more than him, but be a necessary sacrifice for his long-term survival. Even if it is clear who should stand to gain, it is often hard to define gains; studies of pure energy input and expenditure leave one with a socially impoverished picture, for social factors can be highly significant for a person's long-term survival and reproduction. What counts and therefore should be counted? The number of children fathered by a man is a difficult figure to obtain with accuracy. Even if certain cultural practices suggest a negative balance with regard to individual reproductive "fitness" after a year of meticulous study, what about the outcome over the life cycle or after one to two generations?

Though none of the contributions in this volume provide sufficient evidence to answer this question for a single case, some generalities can be drawn. The material presented by Grammer supports the proposition that high status increases survival and reproductive success. In more or less egalitarian societies considered in this volume, foragers, New Guinea societies, and the Massa, Koma, Mussey, Tassa, and Mvae described by de Garine, status achievements for the most part benefit both the individuals concerned and the group as a whole, simply because group members keep leaders in check. Through the status quest, individuals increase their chances for polygamy, and win prestige that they can later translate into labor, access to resources or an increased support base. Group members, in turn, profit from an increase in production propelled by competition, the resulting surplus that is widely distributed and/or stored for adverse times, peace-making, the protective umbrella of a strong leader, and membership in a wealthy group, among other things.

For stratified societies with institutionalized rank orders, the overall picture is somewhat different, because those in the lower position have little opportunity to exert control. Cultural practices in stratified class societies may confer strong advantage to certain strata, as the chapters by Peter Damerow and Catherine Panter-Brick's chapters show. Centuries may pass before those in the lower echelons of the rank order find new stategies to get around the system and to achieve greater access to resources.

Although biological selection pressures may ultimately guide the status quest, in the short run culture does experiment, and many experiments can misfire or run amok. This is partly because the world of today is changing so rapidly, and partly because the status quest, unlike that for food or sex, is not turned off with fulfillment though a consummatory act (Eibl-Eibesfeldt 1989). In Hobbesian terms it is a struggle for "power after power". Inter-individual competition can accelerate to the point where it is no longer of benefit for the individual or group. De Garine suggests this is so for the Massa *guru* fattening cure, aspects of Mussey magico-religious life, Koma consumption of sorghum via badly distilled alcohol, and the Yassa and Mvae's status seeking through the consumption of manufactured alcoholic beverages as part of the Westernization process.

Status, Food, and Contemporary Problems

Just as food is used as a tool in the status quest, status has its impact on the food quest, with negative consequences for many. The oldest written records of humankind record a major problem of today: the impact of social status on nutritional status. Damerow's chapter looks at this issue in Mesopotamia of 3000 B.C. via analysis of proto-cuneiform and proto-elamite texts. The great majority of these documents recorded administrative transactions and concerned the allocation of human labor and the distribution of its products, particularly basic means of subsistence. From these fascinating records, it is possible to gain some understanding of how food production was organized and distributed by centralized institutions. What emerges is a picture of a highly stratified society with extreme exploitation of human labor and enormous differences in access to resources, particularly the food supply. A small strata on the top profited immensely, and those on the bottom were locked into a system in which they could do little to improve their life conditions.

Panter-Brick brings the problem of the impact of social status on the food quest and nutritional status down to the household level some 5000 years later on the subcontinent of India. Here, systems of ascribing status and supporting such distinctions through food are among the most elaborate in human societies. With a focus on household status and food-related behaviors, she demonstrates how status affects food distribution within the household, mother-child relationships, feeding patterns, strategies to overcome food shortages, and nutrition. Although social status generally has a positive correlation with nutritional status, exceptions do exist: heavy work loads for higher-caste mothers allow them less time and energy to invest in nourishing their children than is the case for women of lower castes. Families preferentially put children first on the serving list due to perceived need regardless of status or anticipated future status. Perhaps the most significant of Panter-Brick's findings is that status relations have real impacts on small scale and intimate human relationships.

Implicit in most of the contributions in this volume is the fact that if food is a tool of the status quest, then social status will set the pace for food-related practices. Rainer Gross and Gunther Dresrüsse take up this issue for food intervention programs in developing countries today, and give a number of pertinent examples of status-related factors that affect food use. Through the process of invasion and colonization, foreign influence altered the food production and consumption patterns of many societies, either through imitation of the new rulers or because colonial regimes imposed new production programs. In the process, traditional nutritious foods were sometimes relegated low status or replaced by foods that appeared to confer economic advantage, but were nutritionally inferior or environmentally detrimental. Added to this is the urban factor, through which city dwellers of high status become trend-setters for populations. The decline and later partial resurgence in breast-feeding by people mimicking the practices of the affluent in both the West and developing countries provides one classic example. Traditional foodways are further disrupted by an "international" factor, the marketing of processed "designer foods and beverages" like infant formula, coke, cheeze pops, and fast foods via aggressive advertising campaigns that associate such nutritionally poor products with an affluent "new generation". Gross and Dresrüsse emphasizes the need to actively accommodate social as well as nutritional needs in development programs. Examples would be to avoid burdening the beneficiaries of feeding programs with low-status food and to elevate the status of nutritious indigenous foods through their association with high-ranking members of society. As the example of breast-feeding shows all too clearly, images of social status have a significant impact on food habits and nutritional status, for better or for worse.

Conclusion

When we adjourned the colloquium most participants agreed that tackling the problem of food and the status quest through a multidisciplinary approach had been valuable. The contributions of the primatologists gave an idea of just how deep status seeking and rank formation is in our phylogeny and laid down a baseline from which to measure the effects of human culture. The archaeological papers put the status quest as expressed through food in a temporal perspective, underlining its effect on the production of food and drink, and its importance in propelling the evolution of ever more complex societies. Had we met only with evolutionary biologists, we might have felt confidence in the power of biological theory and models. Had we met only with ethnologists, we might have reveled in the seemingly unbounded possibilities of culture. Without the input of those working with development problems, the issues would have remained academic, with no window on the world of today. As it was, we departed with some grasp of the universality of the status quest, the multiplicity of ways it is expressed through food, the role that it has played in our history, and the many ways it has been transformed and directed by culture. Perhaps most important, though, is the appreciation we gained for this predisposition, which can provide a healthy motor for society if it is kept within bounds, but which has no "off switch" and can run out of control. It is a current that has carried us through our past and will continue into the future. For this it must be understood and respected.

References

Boas, F. 1966. *Kwakiutl Ethnography*, ed. H. Codere. Chicago: Univer. of Chicago Press.

Bourdieu, P. 1977. *Outline of a Theory of Practice*. Cambridge: Cambridge Univer. Press.

Codere, H. 1950. *Fighting with Property*. Locust Valley, N.Y.: J.J. Augustin.

Désy, P. 1980. Comment peut-on être femme: le paradoxe du berdache. Paper presented at the Second International Conference on Hunting and Gathering Societies, Quebec City.

Douglas, M. 1971. Deciphering a meal. In *Myth, Symbol and Culture*, ed. C. Geertz. New York.

Douglas, M., ed. 1987. *Constructive Drinking*. Cambridge: Cambridge Univer. Press.

Douglas, M. 1984. *Food and the Social Order*. New York: Russell Sage Foundation.

Douglas, M. 1990. Foreword: No free gifts. In *The Gift*, ed. M. Mauss, trans. W.D. Halls. London: Routledge.

Douglas, M. and B. Isherwood. 1979. *The World of Goods: Towards an Anthropology of Consumption*. London: Basic Books.

Eibl-Eibesfeldt, I. 1989. *Human Ethology*. New York: Aldine.

Fried, M. 1968. On the evolution of social stratification. In *Theory in Anthropology*, ed. R.A. Manners and D. Kaplan, 251-259. London: Routledge and Kegan.

Goodenough, W. 1951. *Property, Kin, and Community on Truk.* New Haven: Yale Univer. Press.

Goodenough, W. 1965. Rethinking 'status' and 'role': Toward a general model of the cultural organization of social relationships. In *The Relevance of Models for Social Anthropology*, 1-24. New York: Praeger.

Goody, J. 1982. *Cooking, Cuisine and Class.* Cambridge: Cambridge Univer. Press.

Guinness Book of World Records. 1989. New York: Sterling Publishing Co.

Hayden, B. 1990. Nimrods, piscators, pluckers and planters: The emergence of food production. *Journal of Anthropological Archaeology* 9:31-69.

Heath, D. 1987. A decade of development in the anthropological study of alcohol use, 1970-1980. In *Constructive Drinking*, ed. M. Douglas, 16-69. Cambridge: Cambridge Univer. Press.

Lévi-Strauss, C. 1969. *The Raw and the Cooked,* trans. J. Weightman and D. Weightman. New York: Harper and Row.

Linton, R. 1936. *The Study of Man.* New York: D. Appleton-Century Co.

Locke, J. 1947 (orig. 1690). *Two Treatises of Government.* New York: Hafner.

Lorenz, K. 1943. Die angeborenen Formen möglicher Erfahrung. *Z. Tierpsychologie* 5: 235-409.

Mauss, M. 1950. *Essai sur le Don.* Paris: Presses Universitaires de France.

Robbe, B. 1976. Tradition et changement du rôle et des activitiés des Femmes de Chasseur dans un village de la côte est du Groenland. Actes du 42ème Congrés International des Américanistes, Paris.

Rosman, A. and P. Rubel. 1971. *Feasting with Mine Enemy.* New York: Columbia Univer. Press.

Rousseau, J. 1974 (orig.1755). Discourse on the origin and basis of inequality among men. In *The Essential Rousseau*, trans. L. Bair, 125-201. New York: New American Library.

Salter, F. 1995. *Emotions in Command. A Naturalistic Study of Institutional Dominance.* Oxford: Oxford Univer. Press.

Speth, J. 1990. Seasonality, resource stress, and food sharing in so-called "egalitarian" foraging societies. *Journal of Anthropological Archaeology* 9: 148-88.

Trivers, R. 1971. The evolution of reciprocal altruism. *Quarterly Review of Biology* 46: 35-57.

Tooby, J. and L. Cosmides. 1989. Evolutionary psychology and the generation of culture, part 1. *Ethology and Sociobiology* 10: 29-49.

Weber, M. 1968 (Orig. 1922). *Economy and society,* trans. E. Fischoff et al. New York: Bedminster Press.

Weiner, A. 1976. *Women of Value, Men of Renown.* Austin: Univ. of Texas Press.

Young, M. 1971. *Fighting with Food: Leadership Values and Social Control in a Massim Society.* Cambridge: Cambridge Univer. Press.

2. THE ETHOLOGICAL BASES OF STATUS HIERARCHIES

Barbara Hold-Cavell

Status and power relations play an important role in human life. In Western culture we try to demonstrate our status through material symbols, and a great many industrial products serve this goal alone. Food and feasting often are part of the quest for status, too. How did this motivation to seek status develop? This chapter will review the history of ethological concepts concerning status seeking and accompanying rank order formation in animal studies. The chapter will then discuss how these were revised from "rank orders", based on dominance, to "attention structures", measured by frequency of being in the center of attention, in order to be applied appropriately to higher nonhuman primates and humans. Finally, results of studies on status seeking and rank orders based on attention structure among children of different cultures are presented.

Since 1922, when Schjelderupp-Ebbe described the pecking order of domestic fowl, the rank orders of group-living species became a popular subject of investigation. The pecking order is established by a set of encounters between pairs of chickens who peck at each other in a restrained fashion when competing for food. Each encounter results in a winner and a loser. Normally, not every individual fights with every other individual in the group, because some yield to an approaching individual after having visually estimated the other's size, vigor, and signs of confidence. The highest ranking has priority of access to all resources, while the lowest ranking has to accept what is left over by the group members. The more the individuals know each other, the less frequently fights occur; they may be observed only among closely ranked group members who question the position of another.

Such a rank order, which is based on the outcomes of agonistic interactions, is called the dominance structure of a group. The order is not always a simple straight linear structure, but reversals may occur; if A dominates B and B dominates C, C could dominate A. Thus the dominance structure consists of a number of dyadic dominance relationships. The structure serves to reduce fighting and to give the strongest ones priority of access to food, mates or other resources necessary for reproduction.

Similar dominance hierarchies have been observed in many different group-living species, from invertebrates (like insects) to higher primates. In the latter, forms of ranking seem to be varied and shifting depending on, among other things, the environment: caged anubis baboons showed a linear hierarchy (Rowell 1966), while the same author found no evidence of either rank order or central hierarchy when she observed them in the forests of Uganda over a three-year period (Rowell 1967). The reason for this may lie in the inappropriate choice on the part of researchers of criteria to measure dominance, such as the direction of aggressive behavior, the outcome of competitive interactions or the order of access to food. Directed aggressive behavior, for example, may occur only when the rank position is questioned. Also, ecological factors like the food supply and resting places may account for less aggressiveness in wild animals compared to caged animals. In stable social systems, subordinates as well as dominants live peacefully most of the time, because the members avoid aggressive interactions by showing submissive gestures to the more dominant ones to signal that their higher status is recognized.

Another problem with dominance criteria for higher nonhuman primates may lie in the different characters of high-ranking individuals. Some may be very tolerant toward their group members and may even allow others to take food away. Therefore the rank often is more evident to the observer through the behavior of the other group members than through the behavior of the dominant individual. Carpenter (1964) observed very early that the area of the alpha (dominant) male or core group of dominant males is avoided by lower ranking animals. To be able to maintain a spatial relationship individuals have to inform themselves about the position and movements of the higher-ranking group members. This realization led Chance (1967) to the conclusion that the amount of attention paid to an animal by the group indicates the relative status of that animal, and that this attention is reflected in the spatial relations and head and body orientation among group members. On the basis of these observations he formulated his concept of attention structure, which will be explained later.

The concept of a dominance hierarchy suggests that superior strength is a prerequisite of high status, but the behavior of higher primates like chimpanzees indicates that the ability to coalesce against a third individual may also help to gain an alpha position, because two are stronger than one (DeWaal 1982). Furthermore, alphas avoid fights by trying to intimidate group members with charging displays or loud noises (Goodall 1986). This behavior may be directed at certain individuals or the group as a whole and is difficult to ignore. It is instrumental in ascending or maintaining a position in the dominance hierarchy (Goodall 1971).

To understand the development of status hierarchies in human beings, it is most instructive to observe the social behavior in kindergartens or day care centers, where children find themselves for the first time in a larger group. In groups of children between two to three years of age, we can observe a dominance hierarchy; conflicts over objects or space occur very frequently and the stronger one wins. At this age, children have not yet developed strategies for gaining access to desired objects other than trying to grab. This, in turn, leads to resistance and ends up in a fight in which nobody wants to give in. After a while the children recognize the winner of previous struggles and yield.

However, even at this early age some children show behavioral characteristics that differ from this pattern and can be described as those of social leaders. According to Montagner et al. (1988), "these children participate much in competitions, impose themselves in these competitions and have a frequency of linking and appeasing behaviors much higher than that of agonistic behaviors. These children communicate by varied non-aggressive and non-fearful behavioral sequences. They do not confuse threat and aggression, the frequency of threats is most often higher than the frequency of overt aggression. These children are imitated and followed the most often and for longer periods than the others. It is as if more effective attention is paid by peers to their behavior than to that of the other children." However, according to my own observations (Hold 1975), the status hierarchy at this early age has more to do with dominance than with leadership.

In groups of slightly older children (four to six years old) conflicts over dominance are much more frequently observed in boys than in girls. A dominance hierarchy is apparent among boys but not among girls (McGrew 1972), even though girls engage in as much leadership behavior as boys. Thus, dominance criteria that are restricted to a functional outcome like "preferential access to resources" omit many other characteristics of a rank order (see contribution of K. Grammer in this volume).

The Concept of Attention Structure

While studying the social structure of nonhuman primate societies, Chance (1967) became more and more dissatisfied with the most commonly used operational definitions. In his attempt to find a criterion for social structure that was not limited to only one species of primates and that reflected both social control and influence over group members, he looked at the differential spacing out of individuals within a colony. As mentioned earlier, in order to be able to maintain a certain distance from higher-ranking group members, individuals have to keep informed about their position and movements. The consequences will be different for an individual who does not react appropriately to the approach of an alpha male compared to that of a low-ranking juvenile. Thus Chance (1967) concluded that "spatial features are the outcome of subordinate behavior and of the attention to the dominant animal."

The concept was later reformulated together with Jolly (Chance and Jolly 1970) when Virgo and Waterhouse (1969) had demonstrated that in their group of rhesus monkeys two foci of attention could be differentiated. One focus was based on positive relations, such as social grooming and proximity, where dominance status is maintained through display, and the other was based on negative relations such as attack and threat. This bimodality of attention structure also was observed by other authors studying other nonhuman primate groups (Emory 1976; Waterhouse and Waterhouse 1976; Pitcairn 1976).

This raises the question: what is the significance of visual behavior in human social interaction? Looking at another person may have different meanings depending on the intensity and context, for example:

1. When sitting alone, e.g. in a restaurant, we glance or look around at regular intervals in order to collect information and to check on our environment (Wawra 1985). This is part of our "alert system" that evolved in response to predation and attacks by conspecifics.
2. Gazing or staring at another person without any reason is understood as a kind of threat, eliciting rather hostile reactions. Exline (1972) found that staring by a silent stranger was judged

by English students as one of the least pleasant interpersonal situations. Staring has a highly arousing effect. For example, Ellsworth et al. (1972) demonstrated that pedestrians staring at drivers at an intersection produced faster starts by drivers. Gaze avoidance is the common reaction of persons who feel uncomfortable being gazed at and is considered to be submissive.
3. Looking at a particular person and making eye contact signals readiness for social contact (Cary 1978; Shibasaka 1987). Reciprocal looking in conjunction with eye contact is a sign of sympathy, and in the phase of establishing attachment bonds (e.g. between mother and child or between lovers) it is an essential part of interpersonal communication.
4. Ambivalence of approach and withdrawal manifests itself clearly in coy behavior that Eibl-Eibesfeldt (1984) documented in many different cultures. It is characterized by looking and smiling, followed by a cut-off, lowering the lids and turning the face away, before looking again face to face. This fluctuation of looking and turning away and looking again together with eye contact is also part of flirtation behavior in many different cultures (Eibl-Eibesfeldt 1984).

Attention also plays an important role in cognitive processes. Selective attention is an important way of learning about the environment. When analyzing the behavior of newcomers in a kindergarten, we found that the newcomers looked at other children while not interacting with them three times more often than did the children with kindergarten experience (Hold-Cavell et al. 1986).

Visual behavior of two interacting persons can reveal much about their relative status. In a series of experiments Exline et al. (1975) found that dominant individuals were the recipients of more gazes from others, especially when speaking, while they themselves looked less often at subordinates when they were listening to them. Lower-ranking persons, by contrast, look less at dominant ones while they themselves speak, and more at the dominant person when they listen.

When looking at somebody we not only take in information about him or her, but at the same time communicate our attentiveness. Eyes give and take at the same time. Different and even contrasting motivations underlie our tendency to look at others. When we are afraid of somebody we try to maintain a safe distance. When we find somebody attractive we try to gain proximity and contact. When we see a strange or interesting person we try to get information.

High-ranking group members may thus attract the attention of the others because they are potentially frightening, popular, and/or interesting. All three aspects play an important role depending on leadership style. Some bosses may find it very important that their subordinates are afraid of them and may try to intimidate them; others may see themselves like caring fathers who are followed because they are well liked, and some are acknowledged because they are experts who know how to motivate their subordinates. In most cases different leadership styles are a mixture of these components in varying proportions. The characteristic of high-ranking persons to attract attention is expressed clearly in language; we speak of "high regard" (from Roman *wardare*, hence English *guard* and French *garder*, on a semantic spectrum between watchful attention and protection) or "respect" (from Latin *spectare* to look at, to watch), which also is found in German and French. The same concept is expressed in the German term *Ansehen* (high-regar, status) and the Swedish *anseende*. The Eipo of the West New Guinea Highlands say of a man of high rank *dildelamak*, meaning "they are looking at him" (Eibl-Eibesfeldt 1984).

In short, when looking for an index of status, attention directed toward group members is a better measure than any of the dominance indices, because it can be ascertained in every group of human beings regardless of their leadership style or political system. Such a hierarchy does not exist only in the mind of the scientific observer; group members (at least children) behave as if they recognize the status of the other person (Hold 1976).

Attention Structure in Preschool Children

High regard can be defined operationally in three ways: (1) the frequency of being looked at by single children (Abramovitch 1976; Vaughn and Waters 1980; LaFrenière and Charlesworth 1983), (2) the frequency of being looked at by three children simultaneously, that is, frequency of being the "center of attention" (Hold 1974; Grammer 1982; Kalbermatten 1979; Leupold 1979), and (3) the variance of spatial distance between every pair of children (Hudson et al. 1971).

Of these three operational definitions the "center of attention" measurement proved to be best related to leadership behavior and other dominance indices in three different cultures, Germany, Japan, and G/wi San (Hold 1974, 1976, 1980; Hold-Cavell 1992). Based on their frequency of being in the center of attention children can be grouped as high-, middle- and low-ranking. Those who receive the highest regard are most often the initiators of actions or games, and they are the most frequently imitated. They not only invent the games, but they also organize them, choose the participants, distribute the roles, and give the instructions. They accept or reject propositions of the group members and keep control over the group by interfering and solving disputes. They show self-reliance, assertiveness, and are able to integrate more children in their games than other group members. In other words they do not play only with their own friends. When they are occupied with something, they concentrate and do not look up. Group members seek their approval when showing them things that they made or when telling them about their adventures. In one of the German groups, the highest ranking individuals were more often offered little presents, mostly pieces of morning snacks, than the other children. It is quite evident that these respected group members were the authorities and the most influential.

Children who are often aggressive may be looked at frequently, but are never the highest ranking individuals. Middle-ranking children may be the leaders in small groups, but when playing with high-ranking ones they are the followers and accept any role. Children with lower or no regard imitate rather than initiate activities or they remain apart and watch other children. They are often found in vicinity of the teacher or at the edge of a play group. When they are occupied with something, they are not very concentrated, but frequently look up to see what is going on around them. They easily lose control over the group, e.g. when they are asked to distribute candies.

From the behavior of the children we can conclude that they know about one another's positions in the hierarchy. Normally in a kindergarten, children play in different yet more or less stable sub-groups that, according to the regard of its members, may be subdivided into high-, middle-, and low-ranking groups. Sometimes children shift from one group to another; low-ranking children of a high-ranking group would take on the role of leader when playing in a low-ranking group, while a leader in a middle-ranking group becomes a follower in a high-ranking group. The position in the hierarchy is largely determined by age and experience of the child and his or her social competence.

How does a child attract the attention of peers, or what kind of behavior makes children look at a particular child? We analyzed more than 500 situations in which a child was the center of attention and found that in more than 50 per cent of the cases the child was involved in aggressive interactions like threatening, physical attacks, struggles over objects or space, teasing, protesting against others, and playful aggression (for 20 percent of all situations) or was seeking attention with objects, sometimes brought from home, loud noises or voice, exaggerated body movements or by stressing his capacities (31 percent of all situations). Seeking attention from both other children and kindergarten teachers, or what we call "self-referencing behavior," seems to play an important role in becoming the center of attention and thus attaining high status (Hold-Cavell et al. 1985).

Strategies to Obtain High Regard

Rank orders are dynamic by nature; the regard of individuals may rise or fall. When new members enter the group and when others leave, the rank order has to form again. During such an unstable period children try to raise their rank in different ways. Two strategies of particular importance are: (1) Seeking the attention of the others (Hold-Cavell and Borsutzky 1986), and (2) Forming coalitions against a third party (Grammer 1982). During the course of the year every child tries more or less successfully to attract the attention of others, but the timing is also important, not just the strategy. During unstable periods, like in the beginning of the school year or after holidays, it is easier to gain high status than later, when the attention structure is more stable (see also K. Grammer's chapter).

Of all attention-seeking strategies, the manipulation of food and objects play a most prominent role. For example, Stanjek (1974) found in his studies of German kindergarten children that of forty "presents" given, twenty-one (53 percent) were candies, chocolate, fruits or snacks. These were distributed either during the morning break or during play. Friends and the highest-ranking children were offered the most, but they were also expected to be generous themselves. A child who ate his candies in a conspicuous way and did not offer some of them to group members was treated as stingy and in violation of the norm of sharing; his possessions were subject to theft by peers. Toys and food appeared to play equivalent and interchangeable roles in the strategies of kindergarten children. In addition to creating bonds through sharing, they were used in a number of strategies associated with status seeking. Food or objects were used to attract attention by displaying them, by explaining how a toy could be used, how special it was or by telling or making up stories about it. Objects thereby initiated conversation and facilitated interaction. After an aggressive encounter, the winner might give food or objects to the loser to appease. Food or objects might also be displayed with accompanying exaggerated body movements and loud commentary to attract the attention of the group.

In short, children who are successful in climbing up the hierarchy use food or objects to attract attention and make themselves interesting and attractive to other children (Hold-Cavell and Borsutzky 1986). A observation of Stanjek (1974: 61-63) vividly illustrates this:

> In May, Flori was still more often in the center of attention than Udo. This changed in July, when Udo got about the same amount of attention as Flori. What had happened? Udo had brought toys from home on two days in May and five days in July. On the tenth of July, Flori brought twenty-two American Indian figures, which he installed over a wide area. On this day, he was the undisputed leader of the play-group. On the following day Udo brought many objects from home, and on the day after that, also many Indian figures. With these he could attract as many children as Flori had before. Flori tried to interfere several times until Udo finally asked him to join. The next day Udo brought more objects from home and was again more frequently in the center of attention than Flori. The following day Flori brought a toy and asked Udo for candies, promising that he would bring candies for him the next day. And he did. (Translation by author).

To become the center of attention is apparently very important for children, because they react very aggressively when low-ranking members happen to succeed in their efforts, e.g. by bringing an interesting toy from home. The reaction of high-ranking ones is either to take possession of or to degrade the object. Attention seeking behavior leads to high regard only when a child is able to apply the attention he receives to initiating and organizing games. In such efforts objects may be of great help, because they facilitate contact with other children (Schropp 1987) and may serve to enlist the involvement of playmates or friends who are important for the second strategy, forming coalitions.

Whenever a child is involved in a struggle with another child he or she may get support from a third child. In this situation the supporting child has to make both a pro and a contra decision: whom should he or she support against whom? Grammer (1982) observed that boys interfere quite often in struggles of higher- as well as lower-ranking children, and that they can improve or at least stabilize their status when they offer support successfully against stronger and higher-ranking peers. Girls, according to Loots (1985), try to make peace when they interfere, and they only support weaker peers against stronger ones. My own observations (Hold 1975) revealed that the highest-ranking individuals are the peacemakers, while lower-ranking ones support one side against the other.

Do boys and girls behave differently concerning the status hierarchy? Both sexes are very much aware of status, but its significance for them is different. In all the groups we studied, the mean rank of boys is higher than that of girls, though girls can be in very high positions and lead a large group without difficulty. Boys stand out more, show more self-referencing behavior and seem to be much more interested in achieving a high position in the hierarchy. Playful aggression like rough-and-tumble play that serves only to determine who is stronger and more courageous is typical for them. They recognize the other's position much better than girls do, and their hierarchy is more similar to a dominance structure. Girls, by contrast, seek recognition and are less interested in competition and status symbols than boys are. They use indirect strategies, such as ignoring, when they seek a better rank. Hierarchies of boys in single-sex groups are much more stable than those of girls. In mixed-sex groups the boys stabilize the rank positions of the girls, because they recognize the position of those lower or higher in rank much more clearly than girls do. This sex difference concerning status is also observed among early and late adolescents (Savin-Williams 1987).

We may now ask: what are the cultural influences on children's behavior? To answer this question, the play behavior of children from three societies, Germany, Japan, and the G/wi San of the Kalahari was observed and compared. The latter are egalitarian foragers who aggressively discourage overt competition and self-aggrandizing behavior (Wiessner, this volume). Although their composition was more heterogeneous with regard to age (2-13 years) than the groups in Germany or Japan, the results were similar for all three in many respects (Hold 1980). Children are regarded differently in part depending on their age: older ones are more often the center of attention than younger ones. In peer groups the child with the highest regard is also the initiator and organizer of games. She or he is more often obeyed and imitated than children with low regard. Protecting and mediating functions are adopted by older children, who also often instruct the younger ones in new games and skills. Unlike in Germany and Japan, however, attempts by G/wi San children to dominate one another are not visible. They readily accept new ideas offered by low-ranking children (as long as these children are not very much younger), so roles can change quickly.

One of the dominant behaviors characteristically initiated by high-ranking German children is body contact like hugging, placing the arm around the shoulder, touching or stroking an arm, head or cheek. Among the G/wi San, rank has no influence on touching; low-ranking children touch high-ranking ones often, and vice versa. Apparently there is a cross-sexual inhibition against touching, because both boys and girls have significantly more body contact with their own sexes, following the example of the adults, where cross-sexual touch is generally avoided in public (Wiessner, personal communication; Schiefenhövel, 1994: 117). On the whole the rank order observed in the G/wi San children seems to be less rigid than in groups of German and Japanese children. Nonetheless, among San children attention is not equally distributed. Here, as in other societies, some children attract more attention than others and these are more often the initiators of games and activities. High regard in G/wi San is very much related to age and special skills or knowledge; it may lead to more influence in matters regarding these skills. This does not mean that the group members grant any privileges to the higher-status persons, but they differentiate between group members according to their regard.

In summary, cross-cultural studies among children indicate that the tendency to seek status and form rank orders is universal, and that food plays a significant role in status-related strategies. How extensively status differences are recognized, encouraged or permitted, however, depends on the social, ideological, and economic factors in any given society.

References

Abramovitch, R. 1976. The relation of attention and proximity to dominance in preschool children. In *The Social Structure of Attention*, ed. M.R.A. Chance and R.R. Larsen. London: Wiley.

Carpenter, C.R. 1964. *Naturalistic Behaviour of Non-Human Primates.* Pennsylvania: State Univer. Press.

Cary, M.S. 1978. The role of gaze in the initiation of conversation. *Social Psychology* 41, no.3: 269-71.

Chance, M.R.A. 1967. Attention-structure as the basis of primate rank orders. *Man* 2: 503-18.

Chance, M.R.A. and C. Jolly 1970. *Social Groups of Monkeys, Apes and Men.* London: Jonathan Cape.

DeWaal, F.B. 1982. *Chimpanzee Politics.* London: Jonathan Cape.

Eibl-Eibesfeldt, I. 1984. *Die Biologie des menschlichen Verhaltens. Grundriss der Humanethologie.* München: Piper.

Ellsworth, P.C., J.F. Carlsmith and A. Henson. 1972. The stare as a stimulus to flight in human subjects. *Journal of Personality and Social Psychology* 21: 302-11.

Emory, G.R. 1976. Attention-structure as a determinant of social organization in the mandril (*Mandrillus sphynx*) and the gelada baboon (*Theropithecus gelada*). In *The Social Structure of Attention*, ed. M.R.A. Chance and R.R. Larsen. London: Wiley.

Exline, R.V. 1972. Visual interaction: the glances of power and preference. In *Nebraska Symposium on Motivation*, ed. K. J. Cole, 19:162.205. Lincoln: Univer. of Nebraska Press.

Exline, R.V., S.L. Ellyson & B. Long 1975. Visual behaviour as an aspect of power role relationships. In *Nonverbal Communication of Aggression 2*, ed. P. Pliner, L. Krames, and T. Alloway, 21-51. New York: Plenum.

Goodall, J. 1971. *In the Shadow of Man*. Boston: Houghton Mifflin; London: Collins.

Goodall, J. 1986. *The Chimpanzees of Gombe. Patterns of Behaviour*. Cambridge: Cambridge Univ. Press.

Grammer, K. 1982. Wettbewerb und Kooperation: Strategien des Eingriffs in Konflikte unter Kindern einer Kindergartengruppe. Dissertation, Universität München.

Hold, B.C.L. 1974. Rangordnungsverhalten bei Vorschulkindern. *Homo* 4: 252-67.

Hold, B.C.L. 1975. Soziale Rangordnung in Kindergruppen unter besonderer Berücksichtigung der rangspezifischen Verhaltensweisen. Dissertation, Universität München.

Hold, B.C.L. 1976. Attention-structure and rank-specific behaviour in preschool children. In *The Social Structure of Attention*, ed. M.R.A. Chance and R.R. Larsen. London: Wiley.

Hold, B.C.L. 1980. Attention-structure and behaviour in G/wi San children. *Ethology and Sociobiology* 1: 275-90.

Hold-Cavell, B.C.L. 1992. Attention-structure or visual regard as measurement of social status in groups of children. *World Futures* 35: 115-39.

Hold-Cavell, B.C.L. 1985. Showing off and aggression in young children. *Aggressive Behaviour* 11: 303-314.

Hold-Cavell, B.C.L. and D. Borsutzky. 1986. Strategies to obtain high regard: a longitudinal study of a group of preschool children. *Ethology and Sociobiology* 7: 39-56.

Hudson, P.T., W.C. McGrew and P.L. McGrew. 1971. Attention-structure in a group of preschool children. In *Proceedings of the CIE Architectural Psychology Conference Kingston*, ed. B. Lorimer. Kingston Polytechnic and RiBa Publishers Ltd., No. 98.

Kalbermatten, U. 1979. Handlung – Theorie – Methode – Ergebnisse. Dissertation, Universität Bern.

LaFrenière P. and W. Charlesworth. 1983. Dominance, attention and affiliation in a preschool peer group: a nine month longitudinal study. *Ethology and Sociobiology* 4: 55-67.

Leupold, K.H. 1979. Aggression und Aggressionsbeschwichtigung im Kindergarten. Diplomarbeit, Universität München.

Loots, G.M.P. 1985. Social relationships in groups of children; an observational study. Dissertation, Universität Amsterdam.

McGrew, W.C. 1972. *An Ethological Study of Children's Behaviour*. London: Academic Press.

Montagner, H., A. Restoin, D. Rodriguez, V. Ullmann, M. Viala, D. Laurent and D. Godard. 1988. Social interactions of young children with peers and their modifications in relation to environmental factors. In *Social Fabrics of the Mind,* ed. by M.R.A. Chance. London: LEA.

Pitcairn, T.K. 1976. Attention and social structure in Makaka fascicularis. In *The Social Structure of Attention,* ed. M.R.A. Chance and L.L. Larsen. London: Wiley.

Rowell, T.E. 1966. Hierarchy in the organization of a captive baboon troop. *Anim. Behav.* 14: 430-33.

Rowell, T.E. 1967. Variability in the social organization of primates. In *Primate Ethology,* ed. D. Morris. Chicago: Aldine.

Savin-Williams, R.C. 1987. *Adolescence: An Ethological Perspective.* New York: Springer.

Schiefenhövel, W. 1994. Formen nichtsprachlicher Kommunikation. In *Zwischen Natur und Kultur. Der Mensch und seine Beziehungen,* eds.W. Schiefenhövel, Ch. Vogel, G. Vollmer, U. Opolka, 109-37. Stuttgart: Trias/Thieme.

Schjelderupp-Ebbe, T. 1922. Beiträge zur Sozialpsychologie des Haushuhns. *Zeitschrift f. Psychologie* 88: 225-52.

Schropp, G. 1987. Geben und Nehmen – humanethologische Aspekte des Objektaustausches. Dissertation, Universität München.

Stanjek, K. 1974. Vergleichende Untersuchung zur menschlichen Beziehung zu Objekten. Diplomarbeit, Univ. München.

Shibasaka, H. 1987. Children's access strategies at the entrance to the classroom. *Man-Environment Systems* 17: 17-31.

Vaughn, B. and E. Waters. 1980. Social organisation among preschool peers: dominance, attention and sociometric correlates. In *Dominance Relations: Ethological Perspectives of Human Conflict,* ed. D.T. Omark, F.F. Strayer, and D.G. Freedman. New York: Garland.

Virgo, H.B. and M.J. Waterhouse. 1969. Attention-structure among Rhesus Macaques. *Man* 4: 85-93.

Wawra, M. (1985). Aufschauverhalten und Gruppengröße beim Menschen. Diploma Thesis, University of Freiburg, Germany.

Waterhouse, M.J. and H.B. Waterhouse. 1976. The development of social organization in Rhesus monkeys (*Macaca mulatta*) – an example of attention structure. In *The Social Structure of Attention,* ed. M.R.A. Chance and R.R. Larsen. London: Wiley.

3. THE EVOLUTION OF NURTURANT DOMINANCE

Irenäus Eibl-Eibesfeldt

The evolution of nurturant parental behavior constituted a turning point in the evolution of terrestrial vertebrate behavior. Reptilian social behavior is based on repressive dominance and submission, and even their "courtship" behavior is derived from intimidation display, with females assuming submissive postures to express their readiness to copulate.

With the evolution of nurturant parental care, caretaking, corresponding motivations, and individualized bonding came into the world, along with the reciprocal motivation in offspring to seek care and protection and to send signals to trigger nurturant responses. This, of course came hand-in-hand with the capacity of parents to recognize their offspring and vice versa. For animals of the precocial type, this sometimes involves an imprinting-like learning process restricted to a short period after birth or hatching.

Thus, the reptilian heritage was overlaid by new structures in the brain responsible for prosocial behaviors. However, the older structures did not disappear, and in humans they constitute a structure as large as a fist in the brain stem that is still, among many other functions, related to aggression (Bailey 1987; Eibl-Eibesfeldt 1989, 1990). As a result, even human sexual behavior has dominance and submission components. The remaining link between male sexuality and repressive dominance is demonstrated by the fact that the achievement of dominance, e.g. winning a tennis match, is accompanied by a rise of blood testosterone levels in the winner and a corresponding drop in the loser (Mazur and Lamb 1980).

Once parental care and infantile expectations were available, they served as pre-adaptations for the development of prosocial behavior among adults. Nurturant courtship patterns replaced to a significant degree the old dominance-submission patterns. Consequently, many of the courtship patterns in birds and mammals are clearly derived from parental behaviors, such as social grooming, protective and comforting behaviors, feeding and the like. They also serve a bonding and appeasing function in the daily interactions of birds and mammals living in pairs or groups. For example, infantile behavior patterns are often used as appeals to buffer aggression. Thus, wolves who approach a high-ranking member of a pack may push their snout against the corner of the high-ranking animal's mouth, a gesture used by puppies when they beg for food. A wolf under attack may surrender to a high-ranking individual by rolling on its back and exposing its belly to the victor, a behavior pattern puppies use to solicit licking by their mothers. A victor may indeed lick the defeated, and what began as an aggressive encounter end in a friendly, playful interaction.

Human Prosocial Behaviors and Rules of Food Transfer

Human prosocial behaviors also can be traced back to the mother-child repertoire (Eibl-Eibesfeldt 1972, 1989). Two principle types of nurturant food sharing can be observed in the parent-child relationship. The first of these is kiss-feeding, a typical maternal behavior by which premasticated food is given to the baby via mouth-to-mouth contact. The mother presents food with protruding lips whereupon the baby responds with open and slightly protruded lips. The baby opens his or her mouth upon lip contact and accepts the food with sucking movements, while the mother pushes it into the baby's mouth with the help of her tongue.

Kissing derived from this pattern of kiss-feeding is thus an expression and signal of tender affection. Parents often kiss and kiss-feed their babies just to comfort or amuse them. Food may or may not be transferred; sometimes only saliva is passed on. Furthermore, kissing may occur with lip-to-lip contact or just by touching another part of the child's body with the lips. It seems that certain areas, such as the baby's cheeks, are preferred. This form of kissing is practiced in cultures all over the world and it may be considered universal.

Kiss-feeding and kissing have also been observed among chimpanzees as maternal behavior, and chimpanzees who are on friendly terms may embrace and kiss with lip contact at occasions of reunion (Goodall 1986). In humans, too, kissing occurs among adults. In the context of courtship, it often involves movement patterns which suggest that it is derived from the nurturant maternal feeding. Kissing is elaborated into a wide variety of cultural rituals: men may kiss the hand of a lady, people may embrace and kiss each other when they greet, as in Russia or the Mediterranean region, and sacred objects may be kissed in religious rituals.

The second principle type of nurturant food-sharing is hand-to-hand transfer of food. In man as well as in chimpanzees, mothers hand out food to their children, and children beg food from their mothers with extended hand and open palm. This is a very characteristic pattern that also occurs when children beg food from each other. The transfer of both food and objects is regulated by a basic rule: respect of possession. When children or adults want to be given something, they must behave in such a way as to indicate that they respect the right of ownership. Attempts to simply grab or snatch the desired morsel are regularly met with withdrawal, to make the transgressors aware that there has been a breach of etiquette. For example, Wiessner (1984) compared food sharing in four cultures and found that even though frequency of offering, begging, and teasing varied significantly by culture, in all four cultures a violation of respect of possession by grabbing was met with aggression (Figure 3.1). When reprimanded, children may then return the stolen morsel and correct their behavior by requesting it in an appropriate way. The formula of verbal requests is stipulated culturally, but the principle of respect remains.

As nuturant behavior derived from parental relationships, food giving and sharing departs from the principle of reciprocity first described by Mauss (1924/1954), who wrote that humans feel a threefold moral obligation to give, receive, and reciprocate, in which social and economic factors are closely intertwined. Reciprocity may indeed have somewhat different roots and certainly a more complex evolutionary history (Trivers 1971) that is not yet fully understood. Parental feeding of young does not require reciprocity, for the nurturant activities are self-rewarding, as are many other instinctual activities. The reward is the performance itself, "the consummatory act" and/or the reaching of a "consummatory situation" (see Eibl-Eibesfeldt 1989, 1989). The inequality inherent in nurturant behavior raises the question of nurturant dominance.

Nurturant Dominance

The parental behavior of the mother described above implies a nurturant dominance over the child. Just as young birds fly from the nest

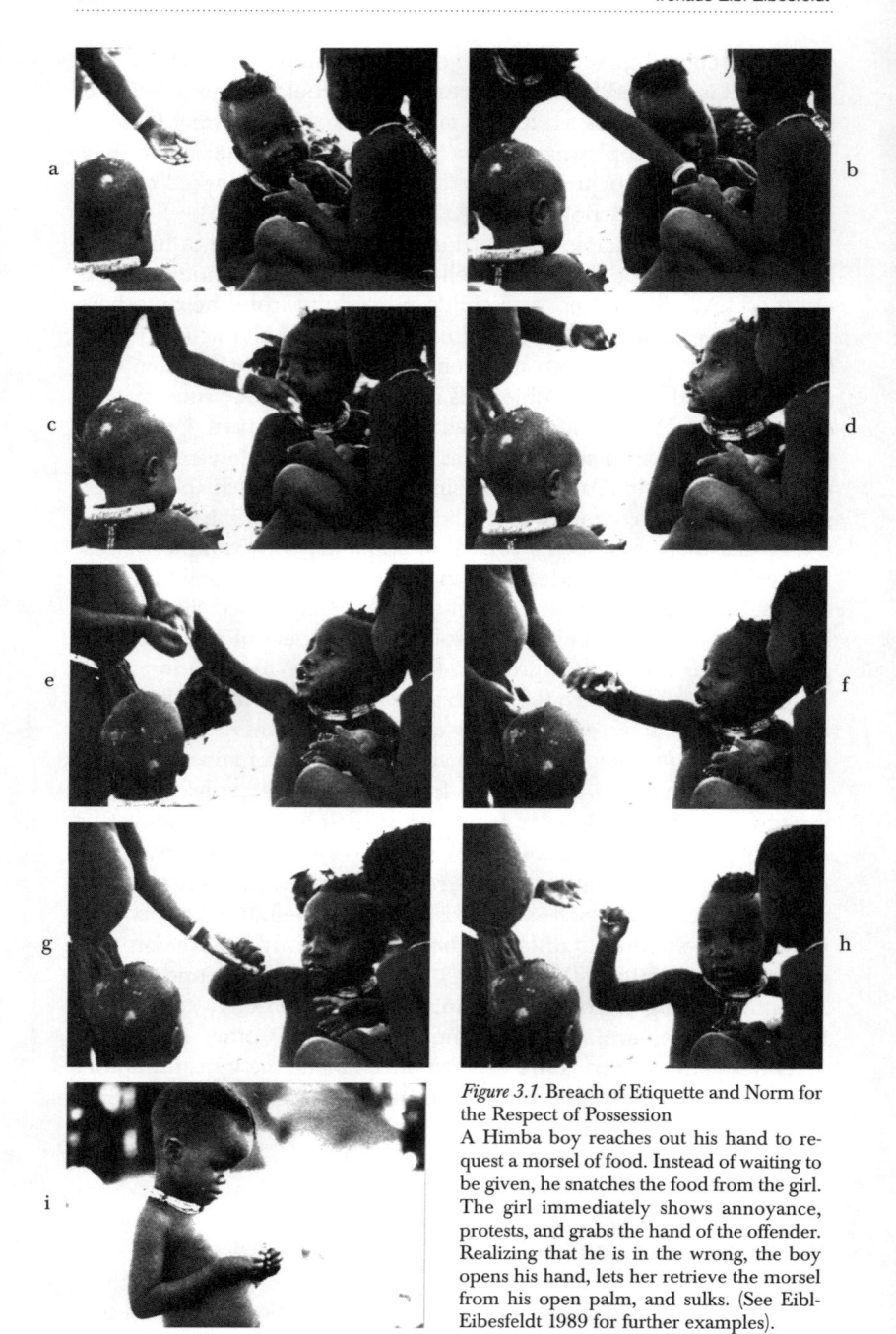

Figure 3.1. Breach of Etiquette and Norm for the Respect of Possession

A Himba boy reaches out his hand to request a morsel of food. Instead of waiting to be given, he snatches the food from the girl. The girl immediately shows annoyance, protests, and grabs the hand of the offender. Realizing that he is in the wrong, the boy opens his hand, lets her retrieve the morsel from his open palm, and sulks. (See Eibl-Eibesfeldt 1989 for further examples).

(From a 16mm film taken by the author.)

never to return, the child is not expected to pay back. He or she is dependent and accepts this status during childhood. However, children struggle for independence and equality, and as they mature they enter more and more into relationships of reciprocity.

The sharing of food occurs not only as parental feeding, but is incorporated in many aspects of daily life and finds expression in elaborate rituals of hosting, sharing, and gift exchange. These allow humans to transform friendly nurturant acts into strategies by which nurturant dominance is achieved. Finally, nurturant dominance may even blend into a repressive one, which is no longer so nurturant. If a host exaggerates his friendship by offering too much, we do not feel comfortable. Either we must play the infantile role and merely receive, or we must reciprocate. We want to reciprocate, but do not want to get involved in a competition of reciprocal hosting.

In some societies, however, such competitive giving is part of the traditional management of encounters between hosts and guests. The Trobrianders, for example, display impressive amounts of food arranged, according to the number of recipients, in different locations on the village ground; they then aggressively announce who should pick it up. The announcer shouts at the top of his voice. The ritualized aggression of this custom is sometimes enhanced by literally throwing highly valued betelnut on the ground in front of the guests, with shouted remarks that add to the atmosphere of demonstrative dominance.

In most situations people resist outright nurturant dominance when they can provide for themselves. Even a well-off person will accept hospitality, but as a friendly act for which there will be an opportunity to reciprocate. However, there are also situations where nurturant dominance is not only accepted, but is actively sought when people feel that they cannot (or are made to feel that they cannot) get along without assistance. For example, in New Guinea Highland Big-man societies (Lemonnier, this volume), war refugees or men who are physically or mentally disadvantaged attach themselves as "helpers" to the households of big men in return for support and/or protection.

As its origins indicate, nurturant dominance is a strategy primarily used by those who are intimate or familiar with one another, for example those within the family, a close circle of kin or a small camp or village. As kinship distance increases, nurturant behavior decreases and balanced reciprocity, a relationship of equality between two social entities, prevails (Sahlins 1972). With strangers, repressive dominance tends to persist. For traditional kin-based societies in which people know each other and where face-to-face interactions are the rule, hierarchies are based on prosocial abilities and rank orders are nurturant. Individuals who protect, comfort, share, and have the skills to intervene in quarrels, keep peace, heal, speak for the group, lead in war, and the like are chosen as leaders. Group members consult them and seek their advice and protection. In more complex societies, leaders even receive tribute to be able to fulfill their social integrative function by sharing and distributing gifts. Humans are prepared to accept rank orders built upon prosocial abilities if those at the bottom benefit from the nurturant dominance of those at the top. For children it is part of the natural process of maturation to start as a toddler in a mixed age play group, to be guided, protected and nurtured, and to gradually take over the role of nurturing smaller ones. Nonetheless, since individuals have different abilities, some remain in a more dependent position than others.

Nurturant dominance is characteristic for those who are acquainted, but with strangers the tendency to exploit signs of weakness and to subjugate through repressive dominance prevails with strangers. Today in our anonymous society, one sees a resurgence of strategies involving repressive dominance in many areas of life, as people seek to establish for themselves a place amid strangers.

References

Bailey, K. 1987. *Human Paleopsychology Applications to Aggression and Pathological Processes*. London: Lawrence Erlbaum Ass.
Eibl-Eibesfeldt, I. 1972. *Love and Hate. The Natural History of Behavior Patterns*. New York: Holt, Rinehart and Winston.
Eibl-Eibesfeldt, I. 1982. Warfare, Man's Indoctrinability and Group Selection. Z.f. Tierpsychologie 60: 177-98. Berlin, Hamburg: Paul Parey.
Eibl-Eibesfeldt, I. 1989. *Human Ethology*. New York: Aldine.
Eibl-Eibesfeldt, I. 1990. Dominance, Submission and Love: Sexual Pathologies from the Perspective of Ethology. In *Pedophilia-Biosocial Dimensions*, ed. J. Feierman, 150-75. New York: Springer.
Goodall, J. 1986. *The Chimpanzees of Gombe, Patterns of Behavior*. Cambridge, Mass./London: Belknap Press of Harvard Univer. Press.
Mauss, M. 1924/1954. *The Gift*, Transl. Ian Cunnison. London: Cohen and West.
Mazur, A. and Th.A. Lamb. 1980. Testosterone, status and mood in human males. *Hormones Behavior* 14: 236-46.
Sahlins, M. 1972. *Stone Age Economics*. Chicago: Aldine.
Trivers, R. 1971. The evolution of reciprocal altruism. *Quarterly Review of Biology* 46: 35-57.
Wiessner, P. 1994. Food sharing among children in four cultures. Paper presented at Reimer's Foundation Conference on Food Sharing. Bad Homburg, Germany.

4. DOMINANCE STATUS, FOOD SHARING, AND REPRODUCTIVE SUCCESS IN CHIMPANZEES

William C. McGrew

Social status in nonhuman primates (apes, monkeys and prosimians) varies as much as their social organization, and by mammalian standards, primate social structure is diverse (Dunbar 1988). For solitary species, from aye-aye *(Daubentonia madagascarensis)* to orangutan *(Pongo pygmaeus)*, status beyond that of being a territory-holder is unclear and probably unnecessary. Even when neighbors meet in passing, they need not ascribe status to one another in order to interact. For family-living species, from titi monkeys (*Callicebus* spp.) to gibbons (*Hylobates* spp.) status seems to reflect reproductive division of labor (or role?) and even sexual dimorphism. In many prosimian species (e.g. *Indri indri*), the female is bigger than and dominates her mate (Pollock 1979). In marmosets and tamarins (Callitrichidae), the breeding female in the group, who may have more than one mate, and therefore be polyandrous, may reproductively suppress all other females, dominating them both behaviorally and physiologically (Epple and Katz 1984).

The most complex social status in nonhuman primates, in terms of both attainment and maintenance, occurs in group-living forms that lack exclusive or lasting pair bonds. These are best known in the troop-living monkeys of the Old (Cercopithecidae) and New (Cebidae) worlds (Smuts et al. 1987). Here, social status seems to reflect sex differences in patterns of dispersal or philopatry: the sex that stays in the natal group takes part in the most complicated competition for status. For example, in baboons (*Papio* spp.) a female lives her whole life in the troop in which she is born, and so the persisting core of the troop comprises multigenerational lines of maternal kinship. She normally inherits the rank of her mother, indicating the marked stability of the status system. Males migrate to other troops, sometimes transferring more than once, and each such move means a new struggle for high rank in the unstable hierarchy of male dominance. Humankind's nearest relations, chimpanzees (*Pan troglodytes*) and pygmy chimpanzees (*P. paniscus*) fall into this pattern, but their "fission-fusion" societies present special problems of status.

Chimpanzees

The social lives of wild chimpanzees have been studied for more than thirty years. The longest and most detailed study is that of Jane Goodall and her colleagues in the Gombe National Park, Tanzania (Goodall 1986). Because great apes are such long-lived and intelligent creatures, we can appreciate the complexity of their societies only by looking at their subsistence, social, and reproductive strategies in a life-history perspective.

The aim of this chapter is to illuminate the interface between food, sex, and status, in both proximate and ultimate ways. Proximate analysis will focus on the sharing of food, and ultimate analysis on reproductive success. Throughout, the contrasting viewpoints of the two sexes (or genders) will be stressed. Most of the data come from Gombe, but these will be supplemented by the two other field studies for which enough behavioral data are available. These are from the chimpanzees of the Mahale Mountains, Tanzania (Nishida 1990) and of the Tai Forest, Ivory Coast (Boesch and Boesch 1989).

Food and Foraging

Chimpanzees are omnivores, but most of their calories come from fruit. Most foraging and consumption is individualistic, even when done in groups. However, sex (or gender) differences emerge when the prey is of high nutritional or caloric quality. Data at Gombe are from Goodall (1968, 1986) and Wrangham (1975). In seeking animal prey, males predominate in hunting and subduing mammals, especially agile and mobile prey such as monkeys. Females predominate in gathering social insect prey such as ants and termites, by making use of extractive techniques. Both sexes engage in both types of food-getting, but each sex predominates in one sphere. Data from Gombe come from Teleki (1973) and McGrew (1979); for Mahale, see Uehara (1986); and for Tai see Boesch and Boesch (1989).

When high-calorie, artificial foods such as bananas or sugar cane are provided, both sexes are keen to consume them. Competition is acute, and males regularly gain and control access to these localized, limited resources. This is an exaggerated form of what occurs rarely with some natural plant foods, such as *Perinari* fruits, and in crop-raiding. For data on the effects of provisioning, see Wrangham (1974); for similar competition over nuts in an unprovisioned population, see Boesch and Boesch (1984).

Social Status

Wild chimpanzees live in groups termed communities or unit groups, which show territoriality and xenophobia. However, for an individual in daily life, much time is spent alone or in small parties of fluctuating composition (hence the fission-fusion social structure). Males are philopatric, while females disperse, either temporarily or permanently. Males patrol together, thus cooperating to defend the group's territory, and so they must balance collaboration and competition. Females range less widely, often accompanied only by their dependent offspring, and rarely cooperate with one another. Not surprisingly, males show an approximately linear hierarchy of social dominance, while females do not. On agonistic criteria, all adult males dominate all adult females, at least in one-to-one encounters. The clearest signal of social rank is one of submission: who pant-grunts to whom. This is consistently one-sided, unlike the more spectacular displays and loud vocalizations, which are situationally specific.

The key status role is that of alpha male. Tenure may last for years, and its proximate benefits are clear in terms of access to resources and to sexually receptive females. Successful alpha males forge and maintain agonistic alliances, often with matrilineal kin, especially a brother, or with post-prime but apparently unrelated males. For data on dominance, see Goodall (1986), Nishida (1983), Riss and Goodall (1977).

Mating System

Chimpanzees mate promiscuously, in the sense that there are no lasting pair-bonds between the sexes. However they do not mate indiscriminately, and conceptions are highly nonrandom. Although most copulations occur opportunistically in parties in which several males may mate successively with a single female in estrus, most conceptions result from restrictive mating practices. These are instances of possessiveness by an adult male or consortship, in which a male and female collude in order to seclude themselves in a temporary pair bond. Though possessiveness can be imposed upon a female by a more dominant male, consortship entails female choice, in that she cannot be sequestered from the group against her will. (To resist, all she or any accompanying dependent offspring needs to do is to call out, thereby attracting other suitors).

At Gombe, although almost 75 percent of copulations are opportunistic and only 2 percent are in consortships, at least half of the conceptions occur during consortships. This indicates that female choice of impregnator is important, and that most copulations likely occur when the female is not fertile or is pregnant. Females choose males for consorting on grounds unrelated to rank; males who are successful in this strategy do so by persuasion, not intimidation. An alpha male probably can ill-afford to spend long periods consorting away from the center of social life, without risking being usurped. For details, see Tutin (1979).

At Mahale, opportunistic mating is similar, but big party sizes make consortship impossible for logistic reasons. There, possessiveness is the strategy of high-ranking males, and male participation in mating is positively correlated with the number of females in estrus at one time. For details, see Hasegawa and Hiraiwa-Hasegawa (1983).

Thus, in terms of mating strategies, female choice is expressed by acquiescing in consortships, and her consort can be chosen on any criteria, none of which needs to be related to dominance. For males, only the alpha male can indulge in unconstrained possessiveness, since any lower-ranking male can always be displaced by one of higher rank. Thus consorting is the preferred strategy for other males, which puts a premium on their relative attractiveness or persuasiveness to females. For some unattractive males, opportunistic copulations may be their only, slim chance of reproductive success.

Food Sharing

Chimpanzees share both plant and animal foods, but frequent sharing is limited to high-quality foods that are scarce (bananas), large-sized and thus divisible (meat), or hard to process (nuts). Patterns of sharing differ according to food type. Bananas (Gombe) or sugar cane (Mahale) are available to all intermittently; acquisition is not related to social status. Most are shared along matrilineal kinship lines, primarily from mother to immature offspring. Of non-kin sharing, about three-quarters of distribution events are from adult males to adult females. Note that neither of these patterns can be coercive, since offspring are subordinate to parents, and females are subordinate to males. For details, see McGrew (1975) for Gombe, and Nishida (1970) for Mahale.

Meat is initially available to successful hunters, mostly cooperating males, and hunting success is not correlated with social status in either sex. At both Gombe and Tai, adult males share meat mostly with other adults of both sexes. Initial possession, combined with preferred sharing with allies, and competitive dominance means that males end up consuming more meat than females. When females do have meat, most of their sharing is with immature offspring. For details, see Boesch and Boesch (1989).

Meat-sharing may be highly political. The alpha male in Mahale's M-group distributes meat as if he were following these rules: (1) Do not share with potential challengers to status, i.e. younger males, (2) Do not share with the beta male, i.e. the closest rival, (3) Do share with non-challenging males; i.e. weak peers, (4) Do share with old and influential males, and (5) Do share with your mother, with your past and present consorts, and with old females. For details, see Nishida (1992).

Reproductive Success

Given the uncontrolled conditions of nature, the relative elements of reproductive success cannot be precisely calculated. Until techniques such as DNA fingerprinting are applied consistently in the field, paternity cannot be established with certainty. Similarly until endocrine events can be monitored regularly, maternal reproductive failures such as spontaneous abortions cannot be known. For present purposes male reproductive success is measured in terms of inferred impregnations achieved. This is calculated by counting back from date of a full-term birth to the cycle of conception, to see if one male mated exclusively with a female. Female reproductive success can be counted more directly, in terms of offspring surviving to independence, i.e. past weaning.

Male reproductive success is not correlated with hunting prowess, dominance rank, or frequency of copulation. This is true across all adult males, but the alpha male is a special case. He has a much greater share of possession of meat and frequency of copulations than expected by chance.

Female reproductive success is not correlated with success as a hunter of mammals (infrequent but competitive) or as a gatherer of insects (frequent but non-competitive), nor is female reproductive success related to agonistic relations with others. (One possible exception was a mother-and-daughter pair who preyed cannibalistically on others' newborn infants. Whether this was an innovative strategy or social pathology awaits further data. For details, see Goodall 1977). Finally, female reproductive success is unrelated to frequency of copulation.

Two factors explain reproductive success: food-sharing and restrictive mating strategies. Females who receive and eat more meat have more living offspring. At Gombe, the top five female meat consumers produced on average 3.6 living offspring, while the bottom five produced on average only 1.4 (McGrew 1992). This meat was largely received from males, as were bananas and sugar cane when shared, and males favored females with whom they had practiced restrictive mating. Male involvement in nonopportunistic mating was not correlated with dominance rank (or age, or agonistic behavior directed to females), but was correlated with generosity in banana sharing and time spent grooming and in association with females. That is, females chose to conceive with generous, attentive males, or with the highest-ranking male. For details, see Tutin (1975).

Thus, ultimate reproductive success is a result of a number of interrelated proximate factors: status and fertility are a function of affinitive social relations and health; health is a function of nutrition; nutrition is a function of diet; and diet is a function of status.

Notes

Thanks to L.F. Marchant for critical comments on the manuscript, to C.E.G. Tutin and R.W. Wrangham for unpublished data, and S. Eggebrecht and F. Somerville for word processing.

References

Boesch, C. and H. Boesch. 1984. Possible causes of sex differences in the use of natural hammers by wild chimpanzees. *Journal of Human Evolution*, 13: 415-40.

Boesch, C. and H. Boesch. 1989. Hunting behavior of wild chimpanzees in the Tai National Park. *American Journal of Physical Anthropology* 78: 547-73.

Dunbar, R.I.M. 1988. *Primate Social Systems*. London: Croom Helm.

Epple, G. and V. Katz. 1984. Social influences on estrogen excretion and ovarian cyclicity in saddle back tamarins (*Saguinus fuscicollis*). *American Journal of Primatology* 6: 215-28.

Goodall, J.v.L. 1968. The behaviour of free-ranging chimpanzees in the Gombe Stream Reserve. *Animal Behaviour Monographs* 1:161-311.

Goodall, J.v.L. 1977. Infant killing and cannibalism in free-living chimpanzees. *Folia primatologica* 28: 259-82.

Goodall, J. 1986. *The Chimpanzees of Gombe*. Cambridge, Mass.: The Belkap Press of Harvard Univer. Press.

Hasegawa, T. and M. Hiraiwa-Hasegawa. 1983. Opportunistic and restrictive matings among wild chimpanzees in the Mahale mountains, Tanzania. *Journal of Ethology* 1: 75-85.

McGrew, W.C. 1975. Patterns of plant food sharing by wild chimpanzees. In *Contemporary Primatology*, ed. S. Kondo, M. Kawai and A. Ehara. Basel: Karger.

McGrew, W.C. 1979. Evolutionary implications of sex differences in chimpanzee predation and tool use. In *The Great Apes*, ed. D.A. Hamburg and E.R. McCown. Menlo Park, Calif.: Benjamin/Cummings.

McGrew, W.C. 1992. *Chimpanzee Material Culture: Implications for Human Evolution*. Cambridge: Cambridge Univer. Press.

Nishida, T. 1970. Social behavior and relationships among wild chimpanzees of the Mahali mountains. *Primates* 11: 47-87.

Nishida, T. 1983. Alpha status and agonistic alliance in wild chimpanzees (*Pan troglodytes schweinfurthii*). *Primates* 24: 318-36.

Nishida, T., ed. 1990. *The Chimpanzees of the Mahale Mountains*. Tokyo: Univer. of Tokyo.

Nishida, T. 1992. Meat-sharing as a political strategy of an alpha male chimpanzee? In *Topics in Primatology, volume 1. Human Origins,* ed. by T. Nishida, W.C. McGrew, P. Marler, M. Pickford and F.B.M. de Waal, Tokyo: Univer. of Tokyo.

Pollock. J.I. 1979. Female dominance in *Indri indri*. *Folia Primatologica* 31: 143-64.

Riss, D.C. and J. Goodall. 1977. The recent rise to the alpha-rank in a population of freeliving chimpanzees. *Folia Primatologica* 27: 134-51.

Smuts, B.B., D.L. Cheney, R.M. Seyfarth, R.W. Wrangham, and T.T. Struhsaker, eds. 1987. *Primate Societies*. Chicago: Univer. of Chicago Press.

Teleki, G. 1973. *The Predatory Behavior of Wild Chimpanzees*. Lewisburg, Pa.: Bucknell Univer. Press.

Tutin, C.E.G. 1975. Sexual behaviour and mating patterns in a community of wild chimpanzees *(Pan troglodytes schweinfurthii)*. Unpublished Ph.D. thesis, University of Edinburgh.

Tutin, C.E.G. 1979. Mating patterns and reproductive strategies in a community of wild chimpanzees *(Pan troglodytes schweinfurthii)*. *Behavioral Ecology and Sociobiology* 6: 29-38.

Uehara, S. 1986. Sex and group differences in feeding on animals by wild chimpanzees in the Mahale Mountains National Park, Tanzania. *Primates* 27: 1-13.

Wrangham, R.W. 1974. Artificial feeding of chimpanzees and baboons in their natural habitat. *Animal Behaviour* 22: 83-93.

Wrangham, R.W. 1975. Behavioural ecology of chimpanzees in Gombe National Park, Tanzania. Unpublished Ph.D. thesis, University of Cambridge.

5. FOOD SHARING AND STATUS IN UNPROVISIONED BONOBOS

Gottfried Hohmann & Barbara Fruth

Sharing of food has been reported from different primate species, including marmosets (Goldizen 1986), douc langurs (Kavanagh 1972), gibbons (Schessler and Nash 1977), chimpanzees (Lavick-Goodall 1968; Nishida 1970; McGrew this volume), bonobos (Kuroda 1984; Badrian and Malenky 1984), and in the vast literature on the topic in humans (see Kaplan 1983 for a comprehensive review). Attempts to explain the evolution and manifestation of food sharing have involved various mechanisms, including kin selection (Axelrod and Hamilton 1981), reciprocal altruism (Trivers 1971), contest over resources (Blurton Jones 1984), and selfish behavior (Moore 1984). The benefits of food sharing among close kin (e.g. mother/offspring) are obvious and do not require reciprocation. In case of food sharing among unrelated individuals, however, sharing is thought to become beneficial for the donor if the recipient reciprocates food sharing at another time and/or with another "currency" (e.g. grooming, defense, mating opportunities) or if begging for food raises the social status of the donor (de Waal 1989; Strum 1975). Sharing with distantly related individuals thus can be part of strategies to rise in status via alliance formation or food distribution, among other things. Since the status structure of bonobos groups is not yet well understood, in this chapter we will give the results of our study on food sharing, and then present a hypothesis concerning food sharing and status: that food sharing is one means of forming and maintaining alliances among females, and that it is partly through such alliances that females maintain higher status than males.

The most common mode of food sharing among primates is that observed between mother and offspring (Eibl-Eibesfeldt 1971). It involves mostly plant foods and is thought to promote independent foraging and feeding by infants (McGrew 1975; Silk 1978). By contrast, food sharing between mature individuals seems to involve predominantly animal prey (Teleki 1973; Nishida 1970) or provisioned plant foods like bananas and sugar cane (McGrew 1975; Kuroda 1984).

Reports on hunting and meat sharing are derived almost exclusively from field studies on chimpanzees (e.g. Goodall 1963; Kawabe 1966; Boesch and Boesch 1989); it is widely assumed that collective hunting and subsequent division of meat were pacemakers in human evolution (Thompson 1976; Isaak 1978). It is further understood that hunting and meat sharing are behavioral predispositions, facilitating the development and manifestation of a division of labor (McGrew 1992).

Detailed analyses of the sharing of plant foods have been made from studies of chimpanzees from Gombe (McGrew 1975) and bonobos at Wamba (Kuroda 1984). In both studies, habituated individuals were regularly provisioned with bananas (Gombe) or sugar cane (Wamba) at specific feeding sites. Although the same authors also have reported on the exchange of natural plant foods, analyses focused predominantly on data collected at the respective feeding sites. In the case of Gombe chimpanzees, sharing occurred most frequently (86 percent) between mother and offspring and only infrequently (10 percent) between male and unrelated female (McGrew 1975). This is in contrast to bonobos, where sharing between males and unrelated females exceeded the rates of all other possible dyads (Kuroda 1984; Kano 1992).

Considering the thousands of hours of observation on feeding behavior of chimpanzees collected during the last decades, it has become evident that in most populations division of natural plant foods may, indeed, be of restricted significance. One exception is the chimpanzees at Tai forest, whose sharing of natural plant food (e.g. *Coula edulis, Panda oleosa*) between mother and infant is habitual (Boesch and Boesch 1984). Compared to chimpanzees, the current knowledge on sharing of natural food among mature bonobos is still fragmentary. From studies at Wamba and Lomako it is known that bonobos share various types of natural plant food (Kano 1980; Kuroda 1984; Badrian and Badrian 1984; Badrian and Malenky 1984). Hunting for meat has also been observed at both study sites (Badrian and Malenky 1984; Ihobe 1992), but meat sharing was seen only once at Lomako (Badrian and Badrian 1984).

The grouping patterns of bonobos are more or less identical to that of common chimpanzees (McGrew this volume). Communities split into temporarily stable parties of differing size and composition. Males are philopatric, whereas females leave their natal community. In contrast to chimpanzees, bonobos more often form unisexual coalitions, male bonding is comparatively weak, and dominance relationships between sexes are biased in favor of females (White 1988; Wrangham 1986; Parish 1993; author's own data). Displacements and the outcomes of agonistic interactions suggest differences in status among different community members. However, the details of the acquisition and maintainance of social rank have not yet been studied and the same applies to the genetical relationships between community members.

This chapter reports on twenty-one cases of food sharing involving meat (two cases) and natural plant foods (nineteen cases). It presents data on (1) the type of food shared, (2) the size and composition of parties during food sharing, (3) the distribution of different roles (owner, recipients) among males and females, (4) the duration and course of food sharing episodes, and (5) the behavioral interactions related to food sharing. Data from this study are then compared with previous reports from bonobos at Lomako and Wamba as well as with data from chimpanzees where males are clearly dominant.

Methods

Data on food sharing were collected between August 1990 and July 1991 and again between February and August 1992 in Lomako (Zaire). The Lomako forest is located in the Upper-Tshuapa district of Equateur in central Zaire. Detailed descriptions of the location, climate, flora, and fauna of this area have been published by Badrian and Badrian (1984), Malenky and Stiles (1991), and White (1989, 1992). All subjects involved in this study were thought to belong to the Eyengo community (which is synonymous with the term "Rangers" used by White 1988) residing in the eastern part of the Lomako study site (Badrian and Badrian 1984). From previous studies at Lomako (e.g. Badrian and Malenky 1984; White 1988, 1992; Malenky and Stiles 1991), members of this community were accustomed to the presence of human observers. However, according to White (1992), the Eyengo community was less frequently observed and less habituated than the neighboring community ("Hedons"). Perhaps for that reason observations made during the initial part of our study were limited to times when the bonobos were engaged in arboreal activities (feeding, foraging, resting). During the course of field work, subjects became more tolerant, and later it was possible to follow parties on the ground for extended periods of time. During the first part of the study (August 1990 until July 1991), twenty-two mature community members (eight males, fourteen females) could be identified using facial features and anatomical deficiencies. This figure remained stable during the second field stay. Except for two infants born in the time between the two field periods, the exact age of the subjects was not known. Therefore, estimates on the subjects' ages were based on physical criteria such as body size, development of external genitals, physiological changes (e.g. cycling), condition of teeth, and frequency of participation in specified social interactions.

Members of the Eyengo community were observed for a total of 412 hours (corrected for simultaneous observations of two observers). Duration of constant observation (visual contact with at least one individual) varied between several minutes and eleven and a half hours. Observation distance primarily depended on whether the bonobos were in trees or on the ground, and under the latter condition varied between five and fifteen meters. Whenever possible observation started at dawn, before the bonobos left the nest site occupied during the previous night. Once contact was established, it was continued for as long as possible. The data on food sharing were collected *ad libitum*. During food sharing, interindividual distances were usually very low (less than one meter), and therefore most or all individuals involved were clearly visible to the observer. In all cases except one observations were made simultaneously by two observers from different positions. Data were recorded online and simultaneously as spoken protocols using a dictaphone (Grundig-220), an audio cassett recorder (Sony Walkman) or a SVHS camcorder (Bauer-Bosch). Data on weight and size of the fruit of *Treculia africana* were collected with a portable balance and a tape measure.

Assessments of "party size" refer to counts of clusters of bonobos and include animals of all age and sex groups, except for dependent infants. Such clusters were characterized by close spatial proximity as well as coordination of general activities like rest and locomotion. Because of the restricted visibility on the ground, scores for party size were sampled either when the subjects had occupied a feeding tree or during periods of rest and/or stationary feeding on the ground. The samples used in this analysis refer only to parties encountered during day time, but do not include counts obtained from night-nest groups.

Evaluations of the "social status" were based on the outcomes of agonostic interactions. However, use of this criterion sometimes produced conflicting results, suggesting that the individual status may be strongly affected by other factors like size and composition of parties or attendance of particular individuals.

Figures on the "adult-sex-ratio" presented in the text express the relation of mature males to mature females within a given party. In the absence of any precise data on the age of the subjects, reliable separation of adults from adolescent individuals was difficult or not possible. Therefore the assessments of sex ratios include both age groups. For calculations of adult age sex ratios, the following formula used by Kano (1982) was applied:

$$\frac{\text{adult} + \text{adolescent females}}{\text{total of adult} + \text{adol. individuals}}$$

Definition of Behavioral Categories and Terminology

Sex: In addition to heterosexual matings, female bonobos display a sexual interaction known as genito-genital rubbing, where two females make contact in a ventro-ventral position and rub their genitals laterally against each other (Kuroda 1980). A specific sound may accompany this interaction.

Begging: This behavioral category includes a number of expressive movements, gestures and vocalizations previously described by Kuroda (1984), De Waal (1988), and Kano (1992). The typical facial expression is "silent pout" (De Waal 1988), the typical gesture is extending one hand close to the mouth or hand of an animal who owns food. Vocalizations like "pout moan" (De Waal 1988) and movements like body rocking may emphasize the begging.

Agonistic behavior: Agonistic interactions involve a variety of motions, facial expressions, and vocalizations (De Waal 1988). In the field, an agonistic interaction was scored when one animal tried to displace another one, independently of whether the threatening behavior involved was lunging, an arm sway or a charging display.

When two or more individuals ate simultaneously from the same piece of food a "food sharing episode" was registered. Assessments of the duration of episodes derived from the protocols recorded during field observation. The food sharing episode started with the first food exchange and was terminated when the food was completely consumed, abandoned or when it was acquired by a new owner who did not share with the former one.

The term "food sharing party" applies to all individuals present at the time of food sharing. The term "owner" was used for an individual holding part or an entire food item close to its body and/or preventing access by other individuals. "Recipients" were individuals other than the owner who ate from the same food simultaneously.

Food was never handed out by the owner but recipients always acquired food either by active taking or begging. The third category of members of food sharing parties included individuals (1) consuming food without sharing (solo feeding) simultaneously to food sharing, (2) sitting in close proximity to those sharing but not receiving any food, (3) consuming scraps of food when the shared food was abandoned, or (4) catching bits of food dropping during food consumption by another individual.

The term "transfer" is distinct from sharing and refers to a change in ownership of food from one individual (owner-1) to another (owner-2).

Results

Analyses of food sharing presented below are based on twenty-one food-sharing episodes observed and documented in detail. The majority of food sharing occured over plant foods, but two episodes involved animal prey. Figure 5.1 presents data on (1) the type of food, (2) the number and sex of bonobos involved, (3) the duration of episodes, and (4) the occurrance of food transfers. Except for one case of *Treculia*-sharing, one individual was obviously the owner, carrying and/or holding the food item divided close to its body. The single exception was a case when three mature females and one mature male collectively consumed a *Treculia* fruit.

In the two cases of meat sharing, hunting and killing of the prey were not observed, but according to the noise that was thought to accompany the capture as well as the condition of the prey at the time of discovery by the observers the delay between capture of prey and onset of observation seemed to be very short (less than five min). The first episode involved an unidentified mammal of small size (e.g. large squirrel). The only remains found after a half hour of observation at the site of meat sharing were drops of a soft, cream-colored and strong-smelling secretion. The second case involved a medium-sized duiker *(Cephalophus sp.)* with an estimated weight of 5 to 10 kg. Sharing of the duiker lasted for 3.5 h and accounted for the longest food-sharing episode observed during this study. The remains consisted of a large piece of skin and bone fragments from the limbs and cranium. During the major part of the episode owner and recipients alternately took blood, meat, and bone from the partly opened carcass. Eighty seven minutes after onset of observation, the prey was partly dissected, the recipients had received larger pieces of meat, and sharing continued. Opening of the cranium and consumption of the brain took place approximately 180 minutes

Figure 5.1: Type of Food and Duration of Food Sharing Among Bonobos at Lomako

Food	Duration (min)	First Owner	Recipient	Second Owner	Recipient
meat	>29	F	2F (1)	–	–
meat	218	F	1M/2F (3)	F	(3)
Anonidium	>15	F	1M/1F (2)	–	–
Anonidium	90	F	(1)	–	–
Treculia	75	1M	–	1F	1M/2F (3)
"	65	1F	2F	–	–
"	82	1F	(3)	1F	–
"	81	1F	2F	1F	2F (2)
"	>92	1M	1F (1)	1F	(1)
"	>80	1F	2F (2)	–	–
"	>10	1F	1F	–	–
"	43	1F	3F (3)	–	–
"	6	1F	(1)	–	–
"	>20	1F	1F	–	–
"	90	1M	2F (3)	1F	1M/2F (3)
"	127	1F	1M/1F (2)	–	–
"	>57	1F	2F	–	–
"	61	1F	1F (2)	–	–
"	46	1M	1F	1F	–
"	53	1F	1F (1)	1F	(1)
"	>25	1F	1M/1F	–	–

F=female, M=male, figures in brackets refer to the number of immatures

after onset of observation, following transfer of the prey to another adult female. During the entire episode, all three infants present had free access to the prey and removed small pieces from the mouth or hand of adults or directly from the prey.

Time for sharing plant food varied from 6 to 130 minutes (x=62.4, SD=35.9, n=20). The episodes reported on here involved two tree species, *Treculia africana* and *Anonidium mannii,* producing fruits of extraordinary large size and weight. From *Treculia* the bonobos preferably ate the seeds, but occasionally the fibers embedding the seeds were consumed as well. Fresh *Treculia* fruits had an average weight of 7.6 kg (range: 5-30 kg, SD=6.6, n=25) and a mean diameter of 24.3 cm (range: 19-45, SD=5.7, n=25). In one fresh fruit, seeds accounted for 10.9 percent of the total weight (7 kg). Except for one episode, bonobos did not choose *Treculia* fruits still hanging on the tree but consumed fruits lying on the ground. In case of *Anonidium,* only the juicy pericarp was eaten, and bonobos were seen to eat fruits still hanging on the tree as well as fruits lying on the ground. Comparative data on size and weight for *Anonidium* are not available from Lomako, but according to the studies by Hladik and Hladik (1990) fruits may weigh up to 10 kg.

Within and between episodes variation of the mode of food sharing was high. Looking for typical features, three modes of sharing were distinguished: (1) Removing pieces of food directly from the owner's fruit, (2) taking food from the hand of the owner, (3) taking chewed food from the owner's mouth (Figure 5.2). Only in one case of food sharing (not included in the data presented here) did we observe a juvenile female passing the fruit of *Irvingia gabonensis* to an immature male.

Figure 5.2: An adult female (right) carrying a *Treculia* fruit. Another female (left) is begging for food by extending her hand toward the owner's mouth.

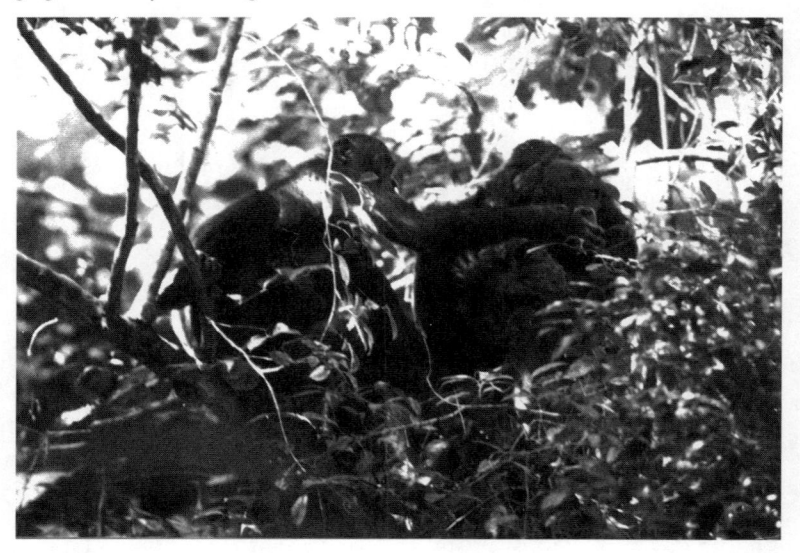

Sexual behavior occurred during eight episodes, and the total number of sexual interactions was twenty-one. The majority (fifteen cases) accounted for genito-genital rubbing among female owners and recipients. Heterosexual copulations occurred five times, three times between a male owner and a female participant and twice vice versa. Following copulation, food was transferred from males to females three times. However, in another case a male owner copulated seven times in close succession with a female vigorously begging for *Treculia* but did not share the fruit.

When sharing meat or plant foods adult recipients frequently made begging gestures, facial expressions, and related vocalizations. Begging by adults clearly resembled the behavior of infants directed to their mothers. The data currently available did not permit a quantitative analysis of the amount and intensity of begging behavior.

However, there seemed to be a correlation between intensity of begging and party size, with members of larger parties begging less often, less intensely, and for shorter periods of time compared to members of small parties.

During meat sharing, agonistic interactions were entirely absent (first episode) or mild (second episode) and restricted to displacements of potential participants by the owner (n=4) or other recipients (n=6). During sharing of plant foods agonistic interactions were also rare (n=19). However, in one episode two adult females repeatedly made joint attacks on adult males approaching a group of three females with infants and one male who were involved in food division.

Figure 5.3 includes data on party size and adult sex ratio. Mean size of food sharing parties (including owner, recipients and all individuals present but not participating) was slightly higher but still within the range of average party size (8.1 vs. 6.9).

Figure 5.3. Party Size and Sex Ratio

	Average party at day time	Food sharing party	Number of FS-individ.
n	100	10	21
party size	6.93	8.1	3.1
	(3.29)	(2.38)	(1.36)
sex ratio	0.68	0.70	0.90
	(0.23)	(0.15)	(0.15)

Mean values and standard deviation (in brackets) for party size and sex ratio. Left= day parties; middle= food-sharing parties, including owner, participants, and bystanders. The third figure (right) refers to the group consisting of owner and recipients only.

The corresponding figure in the third column shows, however, that only a small faction of a food-sharing party was actively involved in food sharing (8.1 vs. 3.1). The adult sex ratio within food sharing parties was very similar to parties not engaged in food sharing, and in both cases there was a pronounced bias in favor of females. This bias was most prominent in the factions of parties actually involved in food sharing where the number of females was more than five times higher than the number of males.

Figure 5.1 shows that in most cases (seventeen) the food that was divided was in possession of adult females, and in the four cases involving male owners food was later transferred to females. Figure 5.3 shows that on average five members of food-sharing parties were not involved in food sharing, and that the proportion of males present but not participating in food division was higher compared to females.

In order to assess both frequency and direction of food exchange within food-sharing parties, the twenty-one episodes of food-sharing were split into dyads (Figure 5.4).

Figure 5.4. Frequency and Type of Involvement in Food Sharing by Mature Males, Mature Females and Immatures of Both Sexes

Owner	Recipient			
	Male	Female	Immatures Other	Immatures Own
Female	7	31	20	13
Male	0	4	4	
Immatures	0	0	1	

The results pictured in Figure 5.4 show that female owners (n=71) shared most often with other females, frequently with immatures (own and offspring of other females), and least frequently with males. For a realistic calculation of the frequency with which males and females are involved in food sharing, it is necessary to consider the adult sex ratio within parties shown in Figure 5.3. Relating this figure to the total of forty-two dyads involving mature individuals, expected frequency of ownership would be fourteen for males and twenty-eight for females. Due to the low frequency of male participation, the observed frequencies differ significantly (Chi^2 = 10.7, p < 0.001) from the expected values.

Changes in ownership of dividable food occurred eight times. Only in one case was the transfer of food accompanied by aggressive interactions between the original and second owner. In three cases the transfer (from males to females) coincided with mating between the first (male) and second (female) owner. Figure 5.5 shows the relative time of transfer of food from one to another individual. All transfers between females occurred during the second half of the epi-

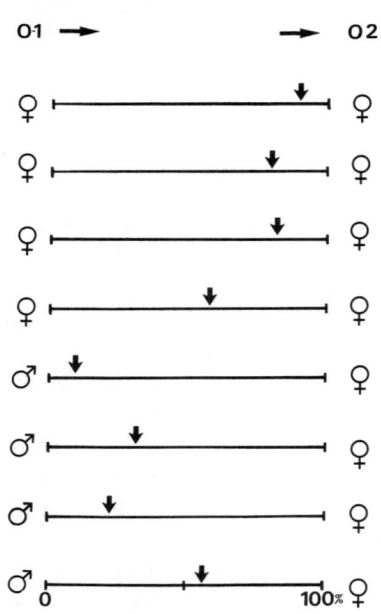

Figure 5.5: Timing of transfer of food from owner 1 (O1) to owner 2 (O2). The vertical arrows indicate the relative time of transfer in relation to the total duration of the food sharing episode (100 percent).

sode, suggesting that females tended to make small sacrifices when transferring food. Transfers from males to females occurred at earlier times. However, these differences are not significant (Mann-Whitney-U-test, U=2, n.s.).

Figure 5.6. Feeding on *Treculia Africana* Without Food Sharing

Sex of Owner	Duration (min)	Sharing (yes/no)	Begging (yes/no)
M	>60	+	−
M	>69	+	+
M	>30	+	−
M	>51	+	−
M	>58	+	−
M	>17	−	+
M	>9	−	−
M	?	+	−
M	>5	+	−
F	>10	+	−
F	>10	+	−
F	>30	+	−
F	?	−	−
F	>65	+	−
F	>43	+	−

Fifteen cases recorded for males (M) and females (F) feeding on *Treculia africana* without food sharing. In twelve cases, other individuals simultaneously share food at the same site. In two cases other individuals begged the owner for food but did not succeed in receiving it.

Figure 5.6 shows the number of single individuals feeding separately but parallel to episodes of *Treculia* sharing by other party members. The results show that males fed solitarily more often and for slightly longer times (x=37.4 min, n=9) than females (x=31.6 min, n=6).

Figure 5.7 shows the respective rates of plant food sharing between members of different age/sex classes collected at Lomako (this study) and at Wamba (Kuroda 1984). To make the data from both studies compatible, the relative frequencies of dyadic food exchanges were compared, using the figures from successful food interaction units (FIU+) presented in Table II of the paper by Kuroda (1984), and the data shown in Figure 5.4 of this chapter. Considering only natural food, the results of both study sites are similar. However, the figures for the division of artificial food collected at Wamba (Kuroda 1984; Table V) differ markedly from those for natural food. In this case, male owners share more often with both male and female recipients.

Figure 5.7: Frequencies of division of food sharing between individuals of different ages and sexes. The first two bars (black) refer to the sharing of natural plant foods observed in Lomako (this study) and Wamba (Kuroda 1984), respectively. The third bar (hatched) refers to Kuroda's data (1984) on the sharing of provisioned food among bonobos at Wamba.

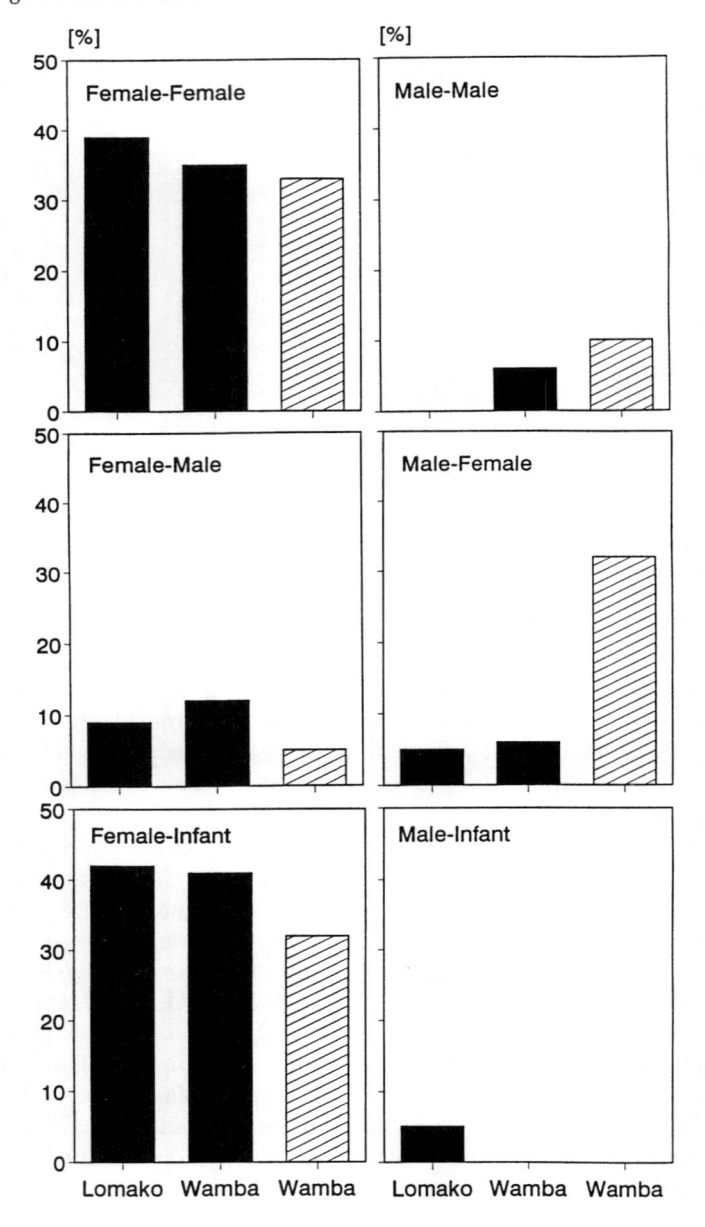

Discussion

The observations on food sharing among bonobos at Lomako described above can be summarized as follows: (1) bonobos shared both plant foods and meat, (2) with one exception (the first case of meat sharing), the food items divided were large and heavy, (3) food sharing generally involved individuals of different ages and sexes, but females were more often in possession of food and shared food more often than males, (4) female possessors most frequently shared with infants, often with mature females, and least frequently with mature males, (5) infants received/took food more often from females other than their mothers, (6) food was transferred from males to females and among females with equivalent rates, but never from females to males or among males.

Provided these results are representative features of food sharing among bonobos, the following questions arise: (1) why do females share food more frequently than males? (2) why do they share so often with infants of other females ? (3) what are the possible reasons for the observed asymmetries in direction and timing of food transfer?

Possible answers to the first question could be that males and females have different food preferences or males travel more often alone (or in male bands) than together with females, and therefore have a lower chance of participating in sharing of food obtained and divided among females. Comparison of the data on food sharing with those collected for solo feeding on *Treculia* (Figure 5.1 and 5.6) demonstrate that both sexes fed on it at rather equal rates. Moreover, the figures of Figure 5.6 indicate that, except for two cases, males fed solitarily when other individuals shared food simultaneously at the same site, and other individuals rarely begged for food from males feeding solitarily. A possible explanation of the low rate of begging for food from males could be that females possessed the better (larger/heavier) food items. The data available are not sufficient to analyze this aspect. Comparing the time of food consumption between individuals who fed solitarily and those who shared with others, the former fed significantly longer than the latter (x=51 vs. 35 min.). However, instead of being related to the size/weight of the food consumed, distinct feeding strategies seem to cause the difference in feeding time. The longer duration of consumption during sharing may be related to the reluctance of the owner to share with recipients and the modes of food distribution. Hence, there is no evidence supporting the assumption that the observed differences in food sharing express sex-related food preferences.

Did males travel more often alone (or in all-male parties) than with females? Counts of party size obtained during this study ranged between one and sixteen animals (x=5.2, SD=3.33, n=247) and the average adult sex ratio of parties was 0.51. Considering sex and total number of the individuals (except dependent infants) identified during this study, the adult sex ratio within the Eyengo community was 0.5 (eight males, fourteen females). Hence, male presence in parties corresponds well with the number of males within the community. Accordingly, males and females had equal chance to participate in food sharing.

Another possible explanation for the comparatively low rate of food sharing among males would be that the benefits gained by females exceed that of males. Division of food entails costs to the owner. According to the paradigm of sociobiology, sharing should be restricted to close kin, or else costs should be balanced by one or the other form of reciprocity (Trivers 1971). Reports from the long-term study at Wamba provide the best source of information on migration patterns available. Here, female bonobos are exogamous and males philopatric (Kano 1982). Provided the bonobos at Lomako follow the same migration patterns, kin selection does not offer a satisfying explanation, because sharing among non-kin (females) by far exceeds sharing among close kin (males). What remains is the question whether or not female community members reciprocate in food division. Unfortunately, the data necessary to analyze this aspect are not yet available. However, even in the case of a positive answer, this would not explain why males (close kin) behave so differently.

Previous studies established that in spite of the flexibility of parties, comparatively stable relationships exist among adult females, but not among males (White 1989). Although similar social ties may also be found among particular males (our observations) as well as among males and females (Kano 1982; Furuichi 1989; Kuroda 1989), data from our study are in general agreement with White's (1989) observation. It has been hypothesized that the cohesion among female bonobos may be related to defense of food resources (White 1989; Parish 1993). Observations of females collectively charging a male who owned dividable food or attempting to join a food-sharing party (see above) clearly demonstrate the ability of females to defend food resources. Parish proposed that the formation of affiliative bonds among females raises their status above those of group males (1993). Results of our study at Lomako suggest a similar tendency. However, within the group of adult females, the data collected in this study did not indicate a consistent correlation between social status and ownership of food. A group of five females who was thought to have a high social status within the community were perhaps more often in possession of food than other individuals, but within this group the role of ownership occurred with rather equal rates. It is therefore suggested that social bonding among female bonobos facilitates monopolization of food resources. Within this system, the relative status of individual females may be less important than the stability of temporary female alliances. Females who share more often with other females may reinforce existing bonds and recruit new allies. By contrast even in the few cases where parties had more than one male, males did not cooperate or share food with others.

Considering the comparatively low cost for acquisition of a *Treculia* or *Anonidium* fruit, its very large size, and the small amount of food removed by an infant, costs for an individual (Ego) sharing with an infant of another female may be almost negligible. The mother of the infant participating in eating food owned by Ego also benefits (via inclusive fitness), even if she does not receive any food. If monopolization of a food patch depends on the number of females present (White and Wrangham 1988; Wrangham 1980), Egos' ability to keep other individuals at bay may be crucial. The act of sharing with the infant of other females may be a compromise between costs (food consumed by the infant) and benefits (the presence of another female). However, the infant's mother remaining at the feeding site does not only enable her infant to consume food owned by others, but may also increase her chance to take over part of the food from the original owner. At least five cases observed during this study support this assumption. In another three cases, females attending a food-sharing party without direct participation eventually acquired small morsels by snatching it from their own infants.

Attempts to explain the few food transfers from males to females are difficult for the following reasons. First, the number of cases observed was very low (n=4), and each case involved different individuals. Second, variability in the duration of food division, the time of transfer, and the related interactions was high. In one case change of ownership occurred when two adult females charged the male owner, while in the other three cases the fruit was transferred immediately after copulation between the original (male) and second (female) owner. Considering the time spent feeding after food transfer, females acquired a large share of the food item initially owned by the male. It should be noted that in three cases, males did not participate in feeding on that food after transfer and the female owner fed solitarily (n=1) or shared with another female (n=2).

Males accepted the loss of a significant amount of food without any intervention, and this requires some explanation. The first case seems to be simple: the two females charged the male who abandoned the fruit. The two other males present did not render any support. One of them participated later in food division with the females, and the other remained close to the food-sharing party but did not receive any food. Hence, this transfer was obviously the result of cooperation among females and the lack of male alliances. In the other three cases, transfer of food was preceded by mating. Since mating increases the chance of pregnancy and paternity, males who have just copulated with a female may not compete with her over food because if copulations are a common strategy to receive food from males, the female may immediately switch to a second male and offer another copulation if the first male does not share. In this case, males who copulate but do not share may diminish an immediate chance for increasing their reproductive success. Also, a male who does not share food with a female shortly after copulation may continue to deprive the female of food later during pregnancy, when optimal nutrition will be crucial for the fetus. Consequently, the female may avoid mating with such a male in the future. Hence, the transfer of food from males to females shortly after copulation may directly and indirectly increase the reproductive success of males.

Data on food sharing among bonobos from another study site (Wamba) have been published by Kano (1980) and Kuroda (1984). Obvious differences exist with respect to meat consumption. At Wamba bonobos hunt less frequently than they do at Lomako and capture only small prey like flying squirrels (*Uromastyx sp*). Moreover, although begging for meat has been seen, bonobos at Wamba have not yet been observed to share meat (Ihobe 1992). As shown in Figure 5.7, the patterns of sharing natural plant foods are very similar at both sites. Striking differences become apparent, however, when comparing the results of the sharing of natural foods from both places with the data collected at the artificial feeding site at Wamba (Kuroda 1984). Figure 5.7 shows that when feeding on sugar cane, males at Wamba shared more often with both males and females than they did in the case of natural food. The large amount of food, its high predictability, the low costs of acquisition, and the setting of the artificial feeding site may have had severe affects on the size and composition of visiting parties. Differences in size and composition of these parties may in turn explain the observed differences in behavioral interactions, including the frequency of food sharing (White 1989).

Considering the information available from the different studies of the two *Pan* species, the sharing of food among bonobos on one hand and among chimpanzees on the other have many features in common (for bonobos see Badrian and Malenky 1984; and Kano 1992; for chimpanzees see Feistner and McGrew 1989; McGrew

1992). Striking differences seem to exist concerning the general type of food divided: while most cases of food sharing among bonobos involved plant food, it is thought that chimpanzees share predominantly meat. Asymmetries between the two species can also be found in the (1) overall frequency of food sharing, (2) participation of males and females in food sharing episodes, and (3) distribution of roles (owner, participant) among males and females.

There are different opinions about the frequencies of meat sharing and division of plant foods among chimpanzees but no supporting data. While McGrew (1975, 1992), Nishida (1970) and Silk (1978) have argued that division of plant foods is more common, Teleki (1973) and others propose that meat sharing is more prominent. Whatever the case may be, most authors agree that among chimpanzees division of plant food occurs most frequently between mother and infant and involves food items difficult to procure and/or manipulate by the infant (McGrew 1975; Silk 1978, 1979; Boesch and Boesch 1989). Hence, the patterns of food sharing among chimpanzees on one hand and bonobos on the other differ most prominently concerning the division of plant foods. The two fruits, *Treculia* and *Anonidium*, frequently shared among bonobos at Lomako are also available at the Tai National Park, and chimpanzees are known to eat and share *Treculia* (Boesch and Boesch 1984). When more data on the mode and frequency of *Treculia* sharing among Tai chimpanzees is available, the patterns of food sharing in the two *Pan* species may become even more similar. Considering the high degree of variability of food preferences, hunting activities, and modes of food acquisition reported for different communities of chimpanzees (e.g. Kawanaka 1982; Wrangham and Riss 1990), the real distinction of food-sharing between chimpanzees on one hand and bonobos on the other may be found in the composition of food sharing parties and the direction of food division rather than in the relative amount of meat or plant foods shared. Using data on meat sharing among chimpanzees, McGrew (this volume) shows the relationship between status, fertility, and health on one hand, and nutrition, diet, and status on the other. In chimpanzees, females get food mainly from adult males, and the amount of food received is correlated with higher reproductive success in females. In bonobos, it is the females who regulate the flow of food to other individuals. Considering the possible impact of the amount of food on the birthrate, food sharing could be a major device for competition among female bonobos.

The data on food sharing among bonobos presented here are based on a small sample size. More comprehensive studies are required to understand the social factors regulating food exchange and the benefits promoting this behavior. Future analyses of the nutritional value of the fruits as well as competition between bonobos and other large mammals for these particular food items may shed further light on these issues. However, even in this preliminary stage the data presented have some interesting implications. It has been proposed that food sharing among higher primates is essentially associated with hunting behavior (e.g. Etkin 1954; Tooby and DeVore 1987). However, consistent with conclusions from previous studies (Kavanagh 1972; McGrew 1975), the observations on bonobos presented above indicate that neither hunting nor meat consumption is a necessary precondition for food sharing. Moreover, contrary to previous reports from chimpanzees (e.g. McGrew 1975), division of plant food is not restricted to mother-infant dyads nor to close kin. Instead, it occurs most frequently among adult females, the faction within the community with the weakest kinship bonds.

Notes

The authors would like to thank I. Eibl-Eibesfeldt, G. Neuweiler, and D. Ploog for technical support and advice. Thanks are also due to Lombeya Bosongo Likundelio and Kambayi Bwatshia (Dept. de l'Enseignement Supérieur et Universitaire et de la Recherche Scientifique, Kinshasa) and to Zana Ndontoni and Kande Muamba (Centre de Recherche en Sciences Naturelles, Lwiro), who kindly provided permission to conduct field work. The technical and logistic support provided by the German Embassy at Kinshasa, the Gesellschaft für Technische Zusammenarbeit (Kinshasa office) and the Catholic Missions at Kinshasa, Bamanya, Boende and Befale is gratefully acknowledged. Special thanks are due to H. Dettmann, E. Ott, C. Kühn, P. Laschan, and B. Unger for their generous help and hospitality, and to R. Malenky and N. Thompson-Handler for sharing their ideas and experiences with us. We also would like to thank C. Roberts for correction of the English text and P. Wiessner, V. Sommer, and H. Hofer for critical discussions and comments. For assistance in the field we thank JP. Bontamba-Lokuli, P. Bonzenza, F. and L. Christiaans and M. Ikala-Lokuli. Financial support was provided by the Max-Planck-Society, the University of Munich, the German Science Foundation (DFG), and the German Academic Exchange Service (DAAD).

References

Axelrod, R. and W.D. Hamilton. 1981. The evolution of cooperation. *Science* 211: 1390-96.

Badrian, A. and N. Badrian. 1984. Social Organization of *Pan paniscus* in the Lomako Forest, Zaire. In *The Pygmy Chimpanzee,* ed. R.L. Sussman, 325-460. New York, London: Plenum Press.

Badrian, N. and R.K. Malenky. 1984. Feeding ecology of *Pan paniscus* in the Lomako Forest, Zaire. In *The Pygmy Chimpanzee,* ed. R.L. Sussman, 275-299. New York, London: Plenum Press.

Blurton Jones, N.G. 1984. A selfish origin for human food sharing: tolerated theft. *Ethology and Sociobiology* 5:1-3.

Boesch, C. and H. Boesch. 1984. Possible causes of sex differences in the use of natural hammers by wild chimpanzees. *Journal of Human Evolution* 13: 415-40.

Boesch, C. and H. Boesch. 1989. Hunting behavior of wild chimpanzees in the Tai National Park. *American Journal of Primatology* 78: 547-73.

De Waal, F.B.M. 1988. The communicative repertoire of captive bonobos (*Pan paniscus*), compared to that of chimpanzees. *Behaviour* 106: 183-251.

De Waal, F.B.M. 1989. Food sharing and reciprocal obligations among chimpanzees. *Journal of Human Evolution,* 18: 433-359.

Eibl-Eibesfeldt, I. 1971. *Love and Hate: The Natural History of Behavior Patterns.* New York: Holt, Rinehart and Winston.

Etkin, W. 1954. Social behavior and the evolution of man's mental faculties. *American Naturalist* 88: 129-42.

Feistner, A.T.C. and W.C. McGrew. 1989. Food-sharing in primates: a critical review. In *Perspectives in Primate Biology,* ed. P.K. Sept and S. Sept. New Delhi: Today and Tomorrow's Printers and Publishers.

Furuichi, T. 1989. Social interactions and the life history of female *Pan paniscus* in Wamba, Zaire. *International Journal of Primatology* 10: 173-97.

Ghiglieri, M.P. 1984. *The Chimpanzees of Kibale Forest.* New York: Columbia Univer. Press.

Goldizen, A.W. 1986. Tamarins and marmosets: communal care of offspring. In *Primate Societies,* ed. B.B. Smuts, D.L. Cheney, R.M. Seyfarth, R.W. Wrangham and T.T. Strusaker. Chicago: Univer. of Chicago Press.

Goodall, J. 1963. Feeding behaviour of wild chimpanzees: a preliminary report. *Symposium of the Zoological Society of London* 10: 39-47.

Hladik, C.M. and A. Hladik. 1990. Food resources of the rain forest. In *Food and Nutrition in the African Rain Forest,* ed. C.M. Hladik, S. Bahuchet and I. de Garine. Paris: UNESCO/MAB.

Ihobe, H. 1992. Observations on the meat-eating behavior of wild bonobos (*Pan paniscus*) at Wamba, Republic of Zaire. *Primates* 33: 247-50.

Isaak, G.L. 1978. The food sharing behavior of protohuman hominids. *Scientific American* 238: 90-108.

Kano, T. 1980. Social behavior of wild pygmy chimpanzees (*Pan paniscus*) of Wamba: a preliminary report. *Journal of Human Evolution* 9: 243-60.

Kano, T. 1982. The social group of pygmy chimpanzees (*Pan paniscus*) of Wamba. *Primates* 23: 171-88.

Kano, T. 1992: *The Last Ape: Pygmy Chimpanzee Behavior and Ecology.* Stanford: Stanford Univer. Press.

Kaplan, H. 1983. *The Evolution of Food Sharing Among Adult Conspecifics: Research with Ache Hunter-Gatherers of Eastern Paraguay.* Ann Arbor: University Microfilms.

Kavanagh, M. 1972. Food sharing behaviour within a group of douc monkeys (*Pygatrix nemaeus nemaeus*). *Nature* 239: 406-7.

Kawabe, M. 1966. One observed case of hunting behavior among wild chimpanzees living in Savanna Woodland of Western Tanganyika. *Primates* 7: 393-96.

Kawanaka, K. 1982. Further studies on predation by chimpanzees of the Mahale mountains. *Primates* 23: 264-384.

Kuroda, S. 1980. Social behavior of the pygmy chimpanzee. *Primates*, 21:181-97.

Kuroda, S. 1984. Interaction over food among pygmy chimpanzees. In *The Pygmy Chimpanzee,* ed. R.L. Sussman. New York and London: Plenum Press.

Kuroda, S. 1989. Developmental retardation and behavioral characteristics in the pygmy chimpanzees. In *Understanding Chimpanzees,* ed. P.G. Heltne and L. Marquard. Cambridge: Harvard Univer. Press.

Malenky, R.K. and E.W. Stiles. 1991. Distribution of terrestrial herbaceous vegetation and its consumption by *Pan paniscus* in the Lomako forest, Zaire. *American Journal of Primatology* 23: 153-69.

McGrew, W.C. 1975. Patterns of plant food sharing by wild chimpanzees. In *Contemporary Primatology,* ed. S. Kondo, M. Kawai and A. Ehara. Basel: Karger.

McGrew, W.C. 1992. *Chimpanzee Material Culture: Implications for Human Evolution.* Cambridge: Cambridge Univer. Press.

Moore, J. 1984. The evolution of reciprocal sharing. *Ethology and Sociobiology* 5: 5-14.

Nishida, T. 1970. Social behavior and relationship among wild chimpanzees of the Mahali Mountains. *Primates* 11: 47-87.

Parish, A. 1993. Bonobo females dominate males: an exception among apes. *Abstracts from the 3rd Conference of the Society for Primatology* Hamburg and Berlin: Paray.

Schessler, T. and L.T. Nash. 1977. Food sharing among captive gibbons (*Hylobates lar*). *Primates* 18: 677-89.

Silk, J.B. 1978. Patterns of food sharing among mother and infant chimpanzees at the Gombe National Park, Tanzania. *Folia Primatologica* 29: 129-41.

Silk, J.B. 1979. Feeding, foraging, and food sharing behavior of immature chimpanzees. *Folia Primatologica* 31: 123-42.

Strum, S.C. 1975. Primate predation: interim report on the development of a tradition in a troop of olive baboons. *Science* 187: 755-57.

Teleki, G. 1973. *The Predatory Behavior of Wild Chimpanzees.* Lewisburg: Bruckness Univer. Press.

Thompson, P.R. 1976. A cross-species analysis of carnivore, primate, and hominid behavior. *Journal of Human Evolution* 4: 113-24.

Tooby, J. and I. DeVore. 1987. The reconstruction of hominid behavioral evolution through strategic modelling. In *Evolution of Human Behavior,* ed. W.G. Kinzey. Albany: State Univer. of New York.

Trivers, R.L. 1971. The evolution of reciprocal altruism. *Quarterly Review of Biology* 46: 35-57.

Van Lavick-Goodall, J. 1968. The behavior of free-ranging chimpanzees in the Gombe Stream Reserve. *Animal Behaviour Monographs* 1: 161-311.

White, F.J. 1988. Party composition and dynamics in *Pan paniscus.* *International Journal of Primatolology* 9: 179-93.

White, F.J. 1989. Ecological correlates of pygmy chimpanzee social structure. In *Comparative Socioecology,* ed. V. Standen and R.A. Foley. Oxford: Blackwell.

White, F.J. 1992. Pygmy chimpanzee social organization: variation with party size and between study sites. *American Journal of Primatology* 26: 203-14.

White, F.J. and R.W. Wrangham. 1988. Feeding competition and patch size in the chimpanzee species *Pan paniscus* and *Pan troglodytes. Behaviour* 105: 148-64.

Wrangham, R.W. 1980. An ecological model of female bonded primate groups. *Behaviour* 75: 262-300.

Wrangham, R.W. 1986. Ecology and social relationships in two species of chimpanzee. In *Ecology and Social Evolution: Birds and Mammals,* ed. D.I. Rubenstein and R. W. Wrangham, Princeton, 353-78. N.J.: Princeton Univer. Press.

Wrangham, R.W. and E. Riss. 1972-1975. Rates of predation on mammals by Gombe chimpanzees. *Primates* 31: 157-70.

6. SYSTEMS OF POWER
THE FUNCTION AND EVOLUTION OF SOCIAL STATUS

Karl Grammer

Dominance, Status, and Hierarchies

Schjelderupp-Ebbe, who discovered and described pecking orders in hens (1922), laid the foundations for a vast body of research on inequality of individuals. Thirty years later, when early ethology rediscovered that behavior could be a product of natural selection, it was a small step to surmise that this principle also could apply to social structures and social sorting processes in humans.

Continuing research in this area developed quite different concepts. These concepts range from dominance and hierarchies to visual regard, status, and rank orders. Application of these concepts to observable behavior, however, can be difficult, because of some problems inherent in the definition of these concepts. Dyadic dominance, for instance, seems to be a relationship feature that can not be extended to hierarchies, because the members of groups employ a variety of strategies different from those commonly used in dyadic interactions. In contrast to dominance, therefore, social status describes power relations on a group level.

Although we can observe tactics for attaining social status reliably and repeatedly in groups, explanations for their existence are manifold. The proximate level, i.e. explanation in terms of the immediate causation and function of a behavior, and the ultimate level, i.e. explanation in terms of inclusive fitness, are best looked at separately in such an endeavor.

In this chapter I will propose that status systems have the function of promoting survival of individuals at critical life stages in which food often plays an important role. This function holds for both the powerful individual and the individual who attributes this power to another. The main points of my argument come from studies on children's peer groups and human mate selection; research in both areas is now well developed.

Among humans, control structures generated out of assertive behavior were first described by Hanfman (1935). She described a child as dominant over another child when the first child was able to control common play. The results of this work were surprising: she was not able to find a linear hierarchy. Being able to control others depends on the strategy the single child applies for controlling another child. The "little gangster" strategy, for instance, was superior to many others. A child who pursues this strategy permanently tries to demonstrate her or his power, has no interest in common play, and tries to control all the activities of the group. He or she commands other children and also takes toys despite another child's protest. Yet, a strategy can be deployed to control the little gangster. A child using this approach can be called the "destroyer". Such a child simply destroys the game, until the ganster gives up. Then he or she proposes a new game and thus gains control. Unfortunately for the destroyer, his strategy can be controlled by another strategy. The "social leader" strategy pursues the goal of playing and pays any price for doing this. He or she is able to cooperate to a high degree, announcing all of his or her own actions before carrying them out. If there is a conflict he or she complies for a certain time. Although this diplomatic behavior is susceptible to the strategy of the little gangster, the social leader is able to control the destroyer strategy. In this approach we find a high degree of circularity, which is incongruous with a hierarchical concept.

These problems were not recognized by later researchers. Esser (1968) tried to generate pecking orders out of attack and flight behavior in a group of six-to-ten-year-old boys. He found that territoriality was closely connected to the resulting hierarchy. A dominant child was able to stay in one place and hold this place against all other claims. Dominant children were constantly able to expel other children from a certain place in a room.

McGrew (1972) used a different approach. He applied the criterion of access to resources and observed it by recording acts of losing and winning object conflicts among children.

Three types of criteria are used in the different approaches. Hierarchies are the outcome (1) of control strategies, (2) of constant patterns of flight or attack behavior, and (3) of winning or losing conflicts over resources. Hierarchies defined in this way are rarely linear; circularity usually occurs. In addition, it is not clear what is really described. Is it power, status, authority or simply a leadership strategy? All we can assume is that these behavioral traits are not distributed equally in a group, and that some kind of social sorting process must have occurred among the individuals involved. What is needed is a clear definition of hierarchies, power, status, leadership, and, finally, a descriptive system that can grasp at least some of these aspects.

Dominance and the System of Explicit Power

A common outcome of aggressive encounters between two individuals is that one will flee after a certain time. Sometimes we find that one individual shows submissive behaviors after being attacked. These types of behaviors prevent the attacker from attacking further. The individual who shows the submissive signals is the "loser" in the conflict. When we see this type of episode occurring more often between two individuals, with a stable pattern over time, we are observing a dominance relationship. We then are able to predict the outcome of future aggressive encounters between the two individuals. The existence of such a relationship stems from the experience of the constant loser. The subordinate individual seems to be following the rule: "If I always lose to a particular individual, then in future contests I will show submissive behavior and do not try to fight". A dominance relationship thus is a probability estimate of the likelihood that an individual will exert power over another individual.

The resulting asymmetry in the power relations between two individuals also provides differential access to scarce resources. Ethological research has shown that dominant individuals as a rule have priority in access to food, mates, and social relationships over the subordinate individual (Bernstein 1981). Dominance in this sense describes the relative balance of power in social relationships. The proximate function is that both individuals gain advantage in such a relationship, because it creates predictability for both the dominant and the subordinate individual.

At this stage of our considerations, we have to stress again that dominance is not a personal trait, it is a relationship feature. In addition, there can be a personal tendency to strive for a dominant position in relationships. Thus we have to separate personal traits from the relationships that an individual negotiates with other individuals. If dominance describes relationships, and if we want to describe

Figure 6.1 Dominance Hierarchy

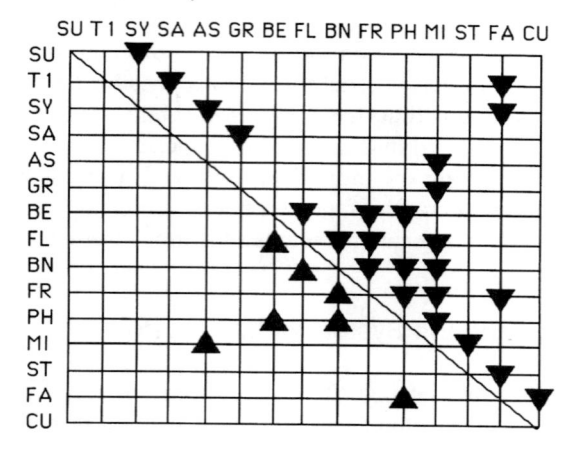

This is a dominance hierarchy generated out of winning and losing object conflicts in a group of preschool children. The children are listed vertically and vertical lines show observed dominance relations with triangles. The dominance relationships were observed by using winning and losing of object-conflicts. Downward-pointing triangles mean x dominates y, and upward-pointing triangles means y dominates x. For instance, the child BN dominates FL and is dominated by PH and FR. In an ideal rigid, transitive, and linear hierarchy, all triangles point downward. This is not the case (Schropp 1986).

relationships beyond dyads, we have to establish hierarchies. Dominance hierarchies usually are the sum of all dominance relationships in a group (Strayer and Strayer 1978). Such an approach imposes severe constraints on the construction of hierarchies. The first constraint is transitivity. This term describes the following relational mode: B is dominant over C; A is dominant over B; A, therefore, also dominates C. The second constraint is linearity. If linearity in a dominance hierarchy is high, then the percentage of relational reversals is low.

We can assume that if a given hierarchy is transitive and has a low percentage of relational reversals, the group's organization is very hierarchical. As we saw in our kindergarten studies, however, these cases are rare. As a result, the construction of hierarchies out of dominance relationships normally allows more than one solution. The one-dimensional concept of dominance, therefore, should be restricted to the description of dyadic relationships. Dominance hierachies can not emerge from a round-robin contest, because not every group member is able to repeatedly fight with every other member: a group of seven children has forty-two possible relationships! Yet we know that even in larger groups hierarchical or comparable structures exist. Thus, we need a means to describe these phenomena.

Visual Regard and the System of Implicit Power

A possible solution for the description of rank orders on the group level is to employ the concept of status. In contrast to dominance, status describes the relative position of an individual in a group of other status holders. In order to evaluate the status mechanisms, the concept of visual regard was introduced. For detailed discussion of the "attention structure" see the contribution of Barbara Hold-Cavell in this volume.

Figure 6.2 Distribution of Attention

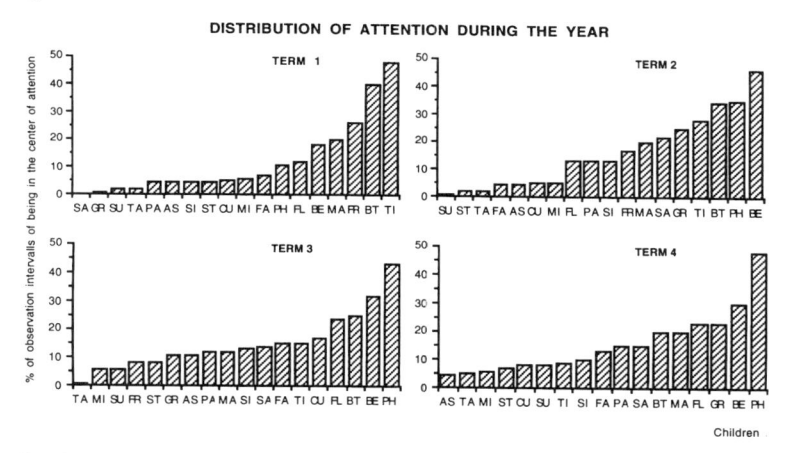

DISTRIBUTION OF ATTENTION DURING THE YEAR

This figure shows the distribution of attention in a group of preschool children. Attention is distributed hierarchically, and some children receive more attention than others. Although there is considerable stability, some children change position. Child BE has position 5 in term 1, position 1 in term 2, and position 2 for the rest of the year. Child TI, who starts at position 1 in term 1, ends up in position 11 at the end of the year. The form of the distribution shows how hierarchical the group is organized: either attention goes primarily to one or two children (term 1) or can be distributed more equally among several children (term 2), whereas in term 3 a single leader emerges and concentrates attention on himself (Grammer 1992).

Aggression, the main theme of dominance relationships, is almost negligible in attention structure. There is no direct relation between aggression and high rank, except for the fact that at the beginning of the kindergarden year, when the children enter the group, high-ranking children are much more aggressive than low-ranking children (Hold-Cavell 1985). Children use assertive behavior to establish the structure, but as soon as the structure is established this type of behavior is not necessary any more. From that stage on, high-ranking children are not more aggressive than low-ranking children, but there is an interesting physiological link. High-ranking children (regardless of sex!) have higher saliva testosterone levels. Although the total number of aggressive acts is not higher in high-ranking than in low-ranking children, high saliva testosterone levels predict the frequency of aggressive behavior and the time of the first conflict in the morning, when the children arrive at school (Schernthaner 1991). High-ranking children thus seem to concentrate their aggression to critical times of the day in the kindergarten year. Because fights or contests that are won raise testosterone level, there is a positive feedback between testosterone level, aggression, and rank. Attention structure thus does not reflect the total amount of aggressive behavior, but the likelihood that one group member will exert power over others.

The amount of attention a child receives depends on the amount of display behavior he or she performs (Hold-Cavell and Borsutzky 1986), on the child's social skills, i.e., the ability to recruit stable allies in a group (Grammer 1992), and on cooperative tendencies (Atzwanger 1991). Furthermore, unlike dominance hierarchies, which rely solely only on the assertion of power, attention structure is based on different leadership qualities. In an attention structure, an individual can be high ranking because he or she uses power, but this person can also be high ranking due to his or her social skills and cooperation. Thus, the system of explicit power is part of the system of implicit power. In this view social status is an attribution process. The function of attention structure is to provide relevant information for structuring of behavior and goals.

Dynamic Stability of Hierarchies and Rank Orders

Dominance relationships and rank in an attention structure share a feature that is necessary for understanding the concept of status and hierarchies. A dominance relationship or a rank position is stable and unstable at the same time. Both dominance relationships and attention structure show dynamic stability (Hinde and Stevenson-Hinde 1977). This seems paradoxical, because I have stated that one feature of a dominance relationship is that it creates predictability and provides a baseline for the calculation of cost-benefits in strategies. This is no longer possible if the relationship changes constantly.

In a preschool group, rank at the beginning of the year was found to correlate positively with rank at the end of the year (Grammer 1992). Thus the attention structure seems to be fairly stable. In a group of twenty-four children we found a maximum of eleven changes in rank position from one month to another. The number of changes in positions decreased during the year, and the rank order became more stable. In addition to increasing stability over the year, however, we also found disrupting events. Even a short interruption of the group life destabilizes the attention structure. It seems that the stabilizing factors need to be present constantly; there is a significant increase of aggression among high-ranking children after holidays (Hold-Cavell 1985).

As soon as stability is reached again, aggression decreases, but this decrease is followed by an increase in aggression on the part of the low-ranking children when explicit power relations ease: status struggles brew from below. We can thus conclude that the development of hierarchies causes hierarchic-specific aggression. Hierarchies or status-dependent rank orders that define status for all other group members are erected by explicit power. After they stabililize, explicit power disappears and the rank order is governed by implicit power.

Comparable conditions apply to dominance relationships. As soon as the dominance relationship is stable, the relationship itself will become invisible. This is the case because the subordinate individual will try to avoid conflicts with a dominant individual. This situation also leads to two new strategies: challenge and assertion. It is possible to explain the existence of both strategies in simple terms of cost-benefit calculations. It can be assumed that individuals try to maximize their benefits and to avoid costs (Wilson 1975) and, indeed, on a proximate level we find that children constantly try to maximize their benefits. They want to have an object 2.3 times an hour and to give away an object only 0.9 times an hour (Schropp 1986). Benefit maximation thus will automatically lead to challenging.

Challenging of an existing dominance relationship will therefore occur continually. We can assume that it will depend on the costs and the benefits that are bound to such a strategy. The subordinate child in an object conflict is confronted with high costs, because the dominant individual is very likely to fight harder (Schropp 1986). Thus the actual frequency of such challenges will be reduced. Comparable considerations apply to the assertion strategy. The dominant individual has to reestablish the relationship from time to time, so that a possible challenger will recognize the real costs of challenging. The dominant individual has to demonstrate the existing relationship by defeating the subordinate individual from time to time. This strategy has also a caveat: the dominant individual risks losing the conflict, at which point the relationship will be reversed. This cost-benefit function can be described in terms of rigidity of a dominance relationship. The index of rigidity is derived from the percentage of conflicts won by the higher-ranking individual over the lower-ranking one. Among children we found a mean rigidity of 84 percent: there is approximately a one-to-five chance of a the challenger reversing the relationship. Some of these reversals occur because an "owner rule" exists: the individual who had an object first and kept it for a longer time will also fight harder. This is true not only for children, but also for most nonhuman primates (Kummer 1978). Thus the strategies in a dominance relationship rely on a delicate balance of risk and cost-benefit considerations.

The Status Quest

Dynamic stability arises from the fact that individuals seem to strive for dominance and status. Becoming high rank or dominant is an active process. Among preschoolers, display behavior and "showing off" at the beginning of the year correlate with rank at the end of the year (Hold and Borsutzky 1986). Moreover, some children actively prevent others from showing off. Showing off and display behavior among children consists of behaviors that signal physical and psychological abilities. How else can a child actively become high ranking? In a study on support in conflicts (Grammer 1992), children show a strong tendency to support members of the group who are their friends at this given point in time. The child who is supported does not necessarily stay the friend of the supporter, so there is no bonding effect between the supporter and the supported. If we look at the status of the supporter we find that frequent involvement in supporting episodes is a trait of high rank, and being a frequent winner in supporting contests correlates with gain in rank over the year.

In addition to winning status by giving and receiving support in conflicts, we find that reciprocal supporting can reliably predict eventual rank. Reciprocity seems to be the key for high status. Atzwanger (1991) found that aggressive and cooperative behaviors are highly reciprocal, but there is no relation between aggressive behavior and rank. On the other hand, reciprocal cooperation correlates with high rank at the end of the year. This could mean that cooperation is at the heart of the status quest, and high rank in peer groups is the result of being able to recruit a group of stable and reliable allies. In other words, status must be in part agreed upon by the others.

As we move away from the level of small groups we find other pathways for the pursuit of status. In more complex societies this concept has to be extended (Congleton 1989). One possible way to measure status in complex societies is in the "quest for status goods." Accordingly, individuals strive for status goods and obtain satisfaction by acquiring them. The level of satisfaction reached does not come from the inherent properties of the goods and from the absolute level of consumption, but from the prestige value, and people tend to over-invest in high-status goods. Congleton (1989) refers to such behavior as "status-games." If somebody is pursuing status, this will generate costs for others who are doing the same. The benefit for the initiator of such strategy will be the costs that other individual incur. Status goods are redefined from time to time, because as they spread through a population they lose their value. Thus they are usually either expensive or rare goods. This situation leads to a new development in the status quest: people then tend to restrict status games to a smaller circle of people, for instance stamp collectors, beauty pageant contenders, and so on. The latter can be called micro-status in comparison to macro-status, which applies for the society as a whole.

Everyday Behavior: The Proximate Level

On a proximate level, i.e. their everyday behavior, individuals must gain satisfaction or other forms of payoff from high status or from being dominant in a relationship, otherwise they would not strive for it. Furthermore, the low-status person or the subordinate also must reap advantages, because a dominance relationship depends also on the behavior of the subordinate. In preschool classes, low-ranking children (or subdominant individuals in dyadic relationships) may indeed benefit from their position in hierarchical structures. The main advantage for the subordinate or low-status group member is, as mentioned above, predictability. Predictions are useful not only so that an individual knows how a high-ranking or dominant group member will react, but it is also possible to use this information for structuring one's own behavior and goals. A low-status individual knows that he cannot gain scarce resources easily, and thus develops alternative strategies, such as deceit. In addition, high-ranking individuals are also a source of information for a low-ranking individual, from which he or she can learn. There are also costs related to high status. High status can be challenged, and thus has to be demonstrated and reaffirmed. It seems that low-ranking children in the peer groups we studied have more free time to play than high-ranking children, who have to put a great deal of energy in stabilizing their positions, leading group activities, and so on.

The most widely recognized advantages of hierarchies is the overall reduction of aggression, but we have clearly demonstrated that

Figure 6.3 Human Life Cycles And Critical Stages

HUMAN LIFE-CYCLES AND CRITICAL STAGES: MORTALITY RATES IN GERMANY 1972/75

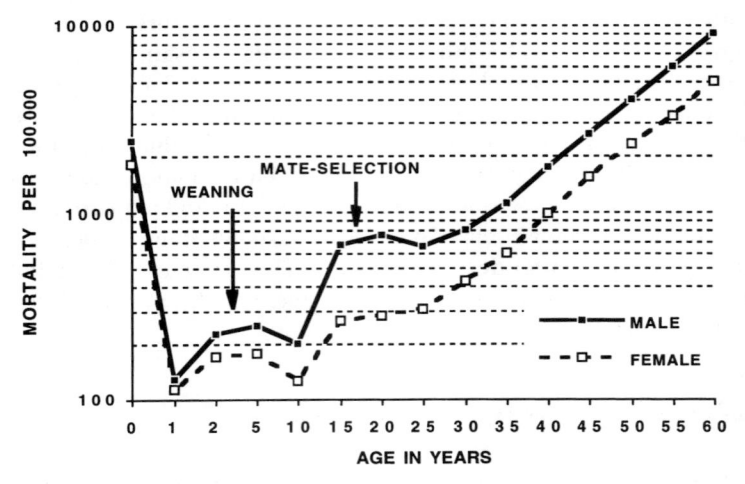

Human life cycles are marked by three stages of high mortality: birth, weaning, and first mate selection. These stages demand special adaptions. Status might be of advantage in surviving all of the three critical stages (Grammer and Atzwanger 1992).

hierarchies also produce their own patterns of aggression. The reduction of aggression thus can not be the only function of hierarchies.

Another possible proximate function is that a high-status group member has the priority of access to scarce resources. In preschool groups, high-ranking children do not get more objects than low-ranking children, but they are more likely to attack if a low-ranking child tries to get an object from them (Schropp 1986). High-ranking children are not more efficient in conflicts than low-ranking children. By contrast, we find clear advantages in the field of social relationships. High-ranking children have a higher likelihood of getting access to play partners than low-ranking children (Shibasaka 1988), and high-ranking children receive support in conflicts. For preschool children, social relations and friends seem to be the desired resources.

Dominance, Status, and the Life Cycle

Direct benefits on the proximate level must pay off in the evolutionary currency of reproductive success on an ultimate level. If this is so, a tendency for being dominant or attaining high status will become prevalent.

High status for children between the ages of three and six has an immediate effect on the quality and quantity of their social relationships. Yet it seems unclear how social status could affect the children's later reproductive success. For an explanation of the evolutionary effects of status on the reproductive success of an individual, we have to introduce the concept of life-cycle dependent strategies, for on the ultimate level behavioral and personal traits are critical for survival and reproduction.

There are different critical periods in the human life cycle that are marked by high mortality rates. These stages are critical, because they can mean the promotion or loss of the individual's genetic representation in the future gene pool of the population. The first critical stage is birth, where we find the highest mortality rates. The next critical stage is weaning, and at this stage mortality rates are rising again even in our modern society. Directly after puberty young males reach another critical stage when they begin to search for their first mates. The first two critical stages, birth and weaning, are a simple question of survival; the search for mates is a question of both survival and reproductive success (Grammer and Atzwanger 1992). If social status or dominance have any evolutionary causation, we should find positive effects for high social status on survival rates at these stages and on reproductive success. Moreover, different critical survival periods demand different adaptations. If dominance and status are critical for survival, then they will have different functions at different stages of the life cycle. With this theoretical background we can formulate a prediction: the attribution of high status to an individual at any one of the critical stages has an effect on the probability of surviving this stage and increasing the reproductive fitness.

Critical Stages and Social Networks in the Peer Group

Social status of the mother has a direct effect on the child's chances to survive the first year of life. In 1986, 8.5 children per 1,000 children born by married females in Germany did not survive their first year of life, in contrast to 13.5 per 1,000 children born to single mothers. (Schwarz 1989). Most of the single females giving birth to a child were of lower socio-economic status. Even in modern societies status can influence morbidity and mortality. This correlation will become clear when we take a look at human mate selection.

The next stage in a child's development is weaning. In traditional societies this period also marks the transition from the protective home environment to the peer group, i.e. from the relatively predictable relationships with parents and siblings to the less structured and less predictable world of peers. In this stage we can hypothesize that social status of the child in the peer group could promote survival when resources become scarce.

In a peer group, friends tend to be of similar rank, and high-ranking children have reciprocal friendships (Grammer 1992). In addition, high-ranking children are chosen more often as best friends than low-ranking children are; they are more popular. The role of the best friend is important, because best friends are more likely to share objects and best friends are more likely to accept invitations to play. If play serves learning, then even play is a critical resource. High-ranking children have a more reliable and reciprocal social network. Reliable social networks can promote survival in critical stages. It is therefore likely that children who have high status in their peer groups enjoy advantages at this critical stage for survival.

Critical Stages and Mate Choice

Asymmetric investment in offspring leads to sex specific mate-selection strategies (Trivers 1972). Females, who have an overall higher investment than males, will pursue different strategies. Internal fertilization with a limited total amount of ova present at birth and replenishable sperm leads to the potential for a higher reproductive success in individual males. Since their reproductive costs are small, their selection criteria could thus simply be the "quality" of the female. Males seem to select females according to the "good-genes" theorem. By contrast, females can reduce their reproductive costs by eliciting male investment in the offspring. In our species women select their reproductive partners accordingly. This situation leads to male-male competition over resources that are necessary for investment. Males, then, will tend to strive for high status to promote their "partner market value." A male tendency for overt status competition is the evolutionary result of female mate selection.

These differences in mate-selection criteria have been demonstrated by Buss (1989) in 36 cultures. Male status is the main selection criterion for females, whereas males value female physical attractiveness. In many societies fatness is connected to social status, and in those societies where resources are not predictable, relative fatness is the beauty standard for women (Anderson et al. 1992). Additionally, the amount of body fat correlates with free estrogen levels and a normal ovulatory cycle (Frisch 1975). Other studies have shown that fatter females have more children and fewer birth complications (Caro and Sellen 1989). Yet, this is an optimization process. Females seem to reach an optimum of fertility and have fewer health problems with a waist-to-hip ratio of 0.7. Extremes in both directions are critical for female health (Singh 1993). These facts relate food intake, social status, and critical stages directly to each other: status and, in addition, beauty of the mother (as defined above) means survival for the child. In this domain, then, food and status are causally directly connected to the passing of one's genes into the generation.

Recently Grammer and Thornhill (1993) have demonstrated that there might be a link between female beauty and parasite resistance. If this is so, female attractiveness should contribute to female reproductive status. Moreover female attractiveness also contributes to the social status of her mate. Observers contribute higher status to a male seen with an attractive female; an attractive male with an unattractive female is seen as a loser (Sigall and Landy 1973).

Figure 6.4 Mate Selection and Status

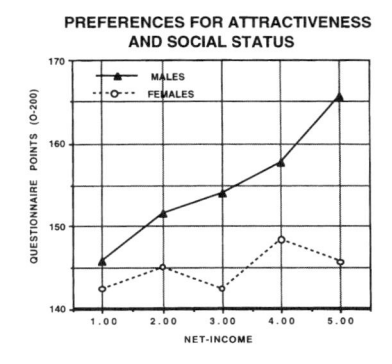

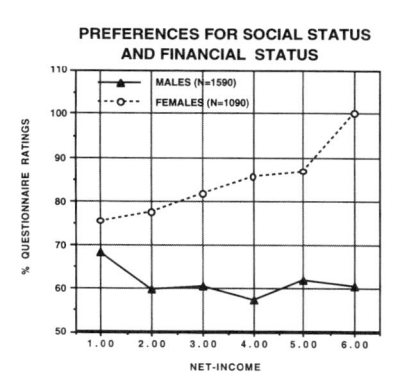

The figure on the left shows the attractiveness of a potential mate and net income. We see that males with high net income want to have very attractive partners. This is not the case for females. The figure on the right shows the status of the potential partner and net-income. Here we see that females' expectations of their partners' status varies with net income: the higher the female status, the higher the financial status of a prospective partner has to be (Grammer 1993).

Male aspirations concerning a potential female partner reflect this. The higher the male's status, the younger and the more physically attractive is the female partner (Grammer 1993). We also find the corresponding element: the more attractive the female evaluates herself, the higher she assesses her "partner market value": she seeks a potential mate in the high-status tier of society.

These facts of mate selection criteria lead us to the ultimate evolutionary function of status. Do higher-status individuals really have more offspring?

Irons (1979) showed that men in the wealthier half of a group of Persian Yomut Turkmen had significantly higher fertility than poorer men. Correlations between status (wealth) and fertility have been found also for the Venezuelan Yanomami (Chagnon 1980) and for the rural Trinidadians (Flinn 1986). Among the Paraguayan Ache, better hunters have been found to have more surviving children (Kaplan and Hill 1985). In the Kenyan Kipsigisis, there is a strong relationship between wealth (in number of cows or acres of land) and reproductive success (Borgerhoff Mulder 1988). Salaried men on the Micronesian Island Ifaluk were found to have started reproducing younger, had wives who started reproducing younger, and produced children in shorter birth intervals (Turke and Betzig 1985). Essock-Vitale (1984) showed that differential reproduction coupled to status is even true for modern societies: high status females mentioned in the Forbes magazine had a reproduction rate that was 38 percent higher than the average reproduction rate of white American females. In addition to this, the children of high-society females had a survival rate of 99 percent as compared to a mean survival rate of 97 percent. Thus we find a strong correlation between status and reproductive success.

Explicit and Implicit Systems of Power

The system of explicit power with its components of submission and dominance and the system of implicit power comprised of social skills and cooperation are a direct result of the fact that individuals constantly try to maximize their benefits in social encounters, and that other individuals attribute this ability to them. The problem with this argument is an unproved assumption: tendencies for status-seeking behavior lead to high status and thus wealth.

Explicit power can be a part of the status system of implicit power. A dominance relationship is the likelihood of winning – it represents a cost/benefit function in a relationship that can be used to predict behavior. Dominance relationships and social status also serve to assess costs and benefits for conditional strategies. Dominant and submissive behaviors are conditional strategies used whenever the benefit of acting dominant is higher than the possible costs of being submissive.

These systems, once established, are not rigid; they are systems with dynamic stability. Both systems are likely to function on an ultimate level to enhance individual survival at critical stages. Dominant behavior, status, and wealth are positively associated with a variety of mechanisms that promote reproductive success, and hence should be expected to characterize all societies to some degree. We can also expect that food will be used universally in this quest for status.

References

Anderson, J.L., C.B. Crawford, J. Nadeau, and T. Lindberg. 1992. Was the Duchess of Windsor right? A cross-cultural review of the socio-ecology of ideals of female body shape. *Ethology and Sociobiology* 13: 197-227.

Atzwanger, K. 1991. *Tit-for-tat: Strategie in der Kindergruppe? Diplomarbeit im Fachbereich Zoologie.* Wien: Universität Wien.

Bernstein, I.S. 1981. Dominance: the baby and the bathwater. *The Behavioral and Brain Sciences* 4: 419-57.

Borgerhoff Mulder, M. 1988. Reproductive success in three Kipsigis cohorts. In *Reproductive Success: Studies of Selection and Adaptation in Contrasting Breeding Systems* ed. T.H. Clutton-Brock. Chicago: Univer. of Chicago Press.

Buss, D.M. 1989. Sex differences in human mate preferences – evolutionary hypotheses tested in 37 cultures. *Behavioral and Brain Sciences* 14, no. 3: 1-49.

Caro, T.M. and D.W. Sellen. 1989. The reproductive advantages of fat in women. *Ethology and Sociobiology* 10: 51-65.

Chagnon, N.A. 1980. Kin selection theory, kinship, marriage and fitness among the Yanomamö indians. In *Natural Selection and Social Behavior: Recent Research and New Theory* ed. R.D. Alexander and D.W. Tinkle. New York: Chiron Press.

Chance, M.R.A. 1967. Attention-structure as the basis of primate rank-orders. *Man* 2: 503-18.

Congleton, R.D. 1989. Efficient status seeking: externalities, and the evolution of status games. *Journal of Economic Behavior and Organization* 11: 175-90.

Dawkins, R. 1976. *The Selfish Gene.* Oxford: Oxford Univer. Press.

Esser, A.H. 1968. Dominance hierarchy and clinical course of psychiatrically hospitalized boys. *Child Development* 39: 147-57.

Essock-Vitale, S.M. 1984. The reproductive success of wealthy Americans. *Ethology and Sociobiology* 5: 45-49.

Flinn, M.V. 1986. Correlates of reproductive success in a Caribbean village. *Human Ecology* 14: 225-43.

Frisch, R.E. 1975. Critical weights, a critical body composition, menarche and the maintenance of menstrual cycles. In *Biosocial Interrelations in Population Adaptation* ed. E.S. Watts. The Hague: Mouton.

Grammer, K. 1979. *Helfen und Unterstützen in Kindergruppen. Diplomarbeit im Fachbereich Biologie.* Hamburg: Universität München.
Grammer, K. 1992: Intervention in conflicts among children: context and consequences. In *Cooperation in Competition* ed. A. Harcourt and F. De Waal, 259-83. Oxford: Oxford Univer. Press.
Grammer, K. 1993. *Signale der Liebe.* Hamburg: Hoffmann and Campe.
Grammer, K. and K. Atzwanger. 1992. Wie du mir, so ich dir: Freundschaften, Verhaltensstrategien und soziale Reziprozität. In *Evolution, Erziehung, Schule* ed. U. Krebs and W. Adick,171-94. Erlangen, Nürnberg: Universitätsbund.
Grammer, K. and R. Thornhill. 1993. Human Facial Attractiveness and Sexual Selection: The Roles of Averageness and Symmetry. Unpublished Manuscript.
Hanfman, E. 1935. Social structure of a group of kindergarten children. *Amer. J. Orthopsychiat.* 5: 407-10.
Hinde, R.A. and J. Stevenson-Hinde. 1977. Towards understanding relationships: dynamic stability. In *Growing Points in Ethology* ed. P.P.G. Bateson and R.A. Hinde, 451-80. Cambridge: Cambridge Univer. Press.
Hold, B.C.L. 1976. Attention-structure and rankspecific behaviour in preschool children. In *The Social Structure of Attention* ed. M.R.A. Chance and R.R. Larsen. New York: Wiley.
Hold-Cavell, B.C.L. 1985. Showing-off and aggression in young children. *Aggressive Behavior* 11: 303-14.
Hold-Cavell, B.C.L. and D. Borsutzky. 1986. Strategies to obtain high regard: longitudinal study of a group of preschool children. *Ethology and Sociobiology* 7: 39-56.
Irons, W. 1979. Cultural and biological success. In *Evolutionary Biology and Human Social Behavior: An Anthropological Perspective* ed. N.A. Chagnon and W. Irons. North Scituate, Mass.: Duxbury Press.
Kaplan, H. and K. Hill. 1985. Hunting ability and reproductive success among male Ache foragers. *Current Anthropology* 26: 131-33.
Kummer, H. 1978. Analogs of morality among non-human primates. In *Morality as a Biological Phenomenon* ed. G.S. Stent. *Life Sciences Report* 9: 35-42.
McGrew, W.C. 1972. *An Ethological Study of Children's Behaviour.* London: Academic Press.
Schernthaner, U. 1991. *Hormone und Verhalten bei Vorschulkindern. Diplomarbeit im Fachbereich Zoologie.* Wien: Universität Wien.
Schjelderupp-Ebbe, T. 1922. Soziale Verhältnisse bei Vögeln. *Z. f. Psychol.* 90: 106-7.
Schropp, R. 1986. Interaction 'Objectified'. In *Ethology and Psychology* ed. J. LeCamus and J. Cosnier, 77-88. Toulouse: Univer. Paul Sabatier.
Schwarz, K. 1989. *Weniger Kinder – weniger Ehen – weniger Zukunft?* Neuwied: Strüder.
Shibasaka, H. 1988. Children's access strategies at the entrance to the classroom. *Man-Environment Systems* 17: 17-31.

Sigall, H. and D. Landy. 1973. Radiating beauty: effects of having a physical attractive partner on person perception. *Journal of Personality and Social Psychology* 28: 218-24.

Singh, D. 1993. Adaptive significance of female physical attractiveness – role of waist-to-hip ratio. *Journal of Personality and Social Psychology* 65, no. 2: 293-307.

Strayer, J. and F.F. Strayer. 1978. Social aggresssion and power relations among preschool children. *Aggressive Behavior* 4: 173-82.

Trivers, R.L. 1972. Parental investment and sexual selection. In *Sexual Selection and the Descent of Man 1871-1971* ed. B. Campbell, 136-79. Chicago: Aldine.

Turke, P.W. and L.L. Betzig. 1985. Those who can do: wealth, status, and reproductive success on Ifaluk. Ethology and Sociobiology 6: 79-87.

Wilson, E. 1975. Sociobiology: *The New Synthesis.* Cambridge, Mass.: Harvard Univ. Press.

7. FEASTS AND COMMENSAL POLITICS IN THE POLITICAL ECONOMY
FOOD, POWER AND STATUS IN PREHISTORIC EUROPE

Michael Dietler

Food is a prime political tool; it has a prominent role in social activity concerned with relations of power. There are, to be sure, many other important things that can be said about food and many other valid perspectives for understanding its significance. However, the demonstration of this political dimension and the examination of its ramifications in different contexts lie at the heart of the "food and the status quest" theme explored in this volume. In an international multidisciplinary forum of this kind, where each of us brings different conceptual orientations, research goals, and methodological approaches, it is advisable to begin with a few remarks about the nature of a potential archaeological contribution to understanding food as a political tool, about the relevance to archaeology of investigating ancient societies from the perspective of the political dimension of food, and about my choice of subject and approach.

As a representative of the archaeological contingent among the contributors to this volume, I must acknowledge straight away that the data with which we grapple present us with several limitations peculiar to our field. We cannot observe people's behavior directly, we cannot ask them questions, and we are, in fact, left with only partially preserved remnants of material culture, food refuse, and human bodies themselves to interpret the actions of people living in ancient societies. This means that we must rely heavily upon information from ethnographic and historical studies in order to derive insights into the operation of social systems. These studies can help us both to make sound inferences about the people who made and used the archaeological material we are studying and to evaluate the plausibility of different competing interpretations. This means also that our perspective on ancient societies generally lacks the fine resolution available in ethnographic studies. In the question of food and status, for example, we have for some time been relatively adept at using faunal, pollen, seed, and plant remains to reconstruct a general picture of diet. However, subtleties in the daily manipulation of dietary and culinary variations, the kind of activity that Appadurai (1981) has identified as household "gastro-politics", remain largely invisible to our analytical lens. On the other hand, this often frustrating deficiency is offset to some extent by the possibility of observing processes of change in societies from a long-term diachronic perspective unavailable to other intellectual disciplines. This time depth, in fact, constitutes the major potential contribution and the raison d'être of archaeology. As archaeologists, we may be able to answer questions about the origins and development of various kinds of social relations and processes that are important for understanding contemporary societies and that cannot be addressed by other means.

Although this has yet to be adequately explored, the political dimension of food is, fortunately, one such phenomenon about which archaeology has some potential to furnish a long-term perspective, provided that analysis is focused upon the aspects of this issue that are amenable to archaeological investigation. Moreover, I would assert that archaeologists themselves stand to benefit greatly from addressing this issue, because a focus on the political dimension of food may provide them with fresh and productive insights into larger questions of social relations in the specific societies they are investigating (Dentzer 1982; Gras 1983; Bender 1985; Bats 1988; Dietler 1990a; Hayden 1990; Murray 1990). It is possible to move beyond the traditional focus on generalized diet (or "what they ate") in the archaeological analysis of food by seeing food as a pervasive and critical element in the articulation and manipulation of social relations. For this reason I have chosen to focus on the role of feasts and what I call "commensal politics" in the political economy and, through this perspective, to explore what can be discerned of the relationship between food, power, and status in prehistoric European societies.

Feasts and Commensal Politics

There are several reasons why it is productive to focus on feasts, by which I mean communal food consumption events that differ in some way from everyday practice. Feasts are, in fact, ritualized social events in which food and drink constitute the medium of expression in the performance of what Cohen (1974) has called "politico-symbolic drama." As public ritual events, in contrast to daily activity, feasts provide an arena for the highly condensed symbolic representation of social relations. Like all rituals, they express idealized concepts, that is the way people believe relations exist or should exist rather than how they are necessarily manifested in daily activity. However, in addition to this idealized representation of the social order, they also offer the potential for manipulation by individuals or groups attempting to alter or make statements about their relative position within that social order as it is perceived and presented. As such, feasts are subject to manipulation for both ideological and more immediately personal goals.

Feasts are a particularly powerful form of ritual activity that also have the pragmatic virtue of being potentially visible in the archaeological record. Because of their inherent emotive and symbolic power, feasts are very often intimately embedded in rites of passage or life-crisis ceremonies, such as funerals; it is this feature that often renders them archaeologically detectable as distinct events. Moreover, the culinary nature of feasts generally necessitates the use of containers for both preparation and consumption. Very frequently, as in the last 8,000 years of European prehistory and history, these containers tend to be made of ceramic or metal that remain preserved extremely well in the archaeological record even when they are broken. Although we often have difficulty measuring the structural "complexity" of food patterns, as that term is defined by Douglas (1984), we do at least have the potential to learn a good deal about the complexity of presentation of food for consumption by examining the range of containers in use in different contexts.[1]

The potency of feasts as a form of ritual activity derives from the fact that food and drink serve as the medium of expression, and that commensal hospitality constitutes the syntax in a ritual of consumption, a preeminently political activity (Douglas and Isherwood 1979; Bourdieu 1984; Appadurai 1986). Food and drink are highly charged symbolic media because they are a basic and continual human physiological need. They are also a form of "highly condensed social fact" (Appadurai 1981: 494) embodying relations of production and exchange and linking the domestic and political economies. I would insist, incidentally, that drink must be included in any consideration of food and status. Alcoholic beverages are, after all, simply food with certain psychoactive properties (resulting from an alternative means of preparation) that tend to amplify their importance in the ritual contexts in which power relations are negotiated and formalized (Mandelbaum 1965; Heath 1976; Dietler 1990a).

Both food and drink are also a highly perishable form of good; their full politico-symbolic potential is realized in the drama of consumption events that constitute a prime arena for the reciprocal conversion of what Bourdieu (1977) calls "economic and symbolic capital." Public distribution and consumption of a basic need derives added symbolic salience from its demonstration of confidence and managerial skill in the realm of production. More important, however, consumption is played out in the extremely powerful idiom of commensal hospitality. I believe this feature is critical to understanding the political dimensions of feasts, and it is for this reason that I have chosen to focus on what may be called "commensal politics."[2]

Commensal hospitality may be viewed as a specialized form of gift exchange that establishes the same relations of reciprocal obligation between host and guest as between donor and receiver in the exchange of other more durable types of objects (Mauss 1966). The major difference is that food is destroyed in the act of commensal consumption at a feast. Unlike durable valuables it cannot be recirculated (or "reinvested") in other gift exchange relationships, and it must be produced anew through agricultural and culinary labor in order to fulfill reciprocal obligations.

A clarification should be raised here, however, because food can also be used for nondestructive exchange in the same fashion as durable valuables, as, for example, in the *moka* exchanges of the Melpa (Strathern 1971), the *gimaiye* exchanges of the Siani (Salisbury 1962), or the *abutu* exchanges of Goodenough Island (Young 1971). In contrast to the prepared food consumed at feasts, this food may be either raw (e.g. yams, sacks of flour), processed (e.g. cooked or smoked meat), or even live potential food (e.g. pigs or cattle). In the case of live animals, in particular, the potential for long-term reinvestment is obvious; but even the more perishable forms may be quickly redeployed to a certain extent in other local exchange networks or in subsequent commensal hospitality (e.g. see Hogbin 1970; Feil 1984). The exchange of food in this manner may take place completely outside of a commensal consumption context that one would properly call a feast, as with the *moka* (Strathern 1971); or a feast may serve as the arena for such exchanges. In the latter case, different kinds of foods may be used for the feast and the exchange transaction, as in the Abelam yam exchange, where long yams are exchanged and short yams are eaten with soup and greens (Kaberry 1941-2). Although both of the two political uses of food described above (commensal consumption and nondestructive gift exchange) may take place at feasts, it is important for the purposes of this discussion that the distinction between them is not obscured by subsuming them both under the general term "feasting." Commensal consumption (which is taken here to be the definitive attribute of a feast) places obvious limitations on the possibilities of the guest/receiver to reemploy the food she has received in the fulfillment of reciprocal obligations of other exchange relationships; it removes goods permanently and immediately from circulation. It is thus a less fluid (and perhaps more subtle) use of food in manipulating social relations than is the nondestructive exchange pattern that may or may not accompany a feast.[3]

In addition to the commensal politics involved in food and drink consumption and possible simultaneous exchanges of food, feasts also frequently serve as a public venue for the concurrent prestation or exchange of various kinds of durable valuables, as with the Kwakiutl "potlatch" (Codere 1950; Suttles 1991) or the *kelo* feasts of Choiseul Island (Scheffler 1965). This latter feature is one of the important functions feasts often serve in the larger regional political economy: they act as the nodal contexts that articulate regional exchange systems. Commensal hospitality establishes relationships between exchange partners, affines, or political leaders and provides the social ambiance for the exchange of valuables, bridewealth, and other goods that circulate through a region. Feasts also serve to provide links to the gods or ancestors, which can be used to define the structure of relations between social groups or categories within a region or community (Friedman 1984). They also provide an important mechanism for the process of labor mobilization that underlies the political economy. While serving all these broader functions, feasts simultaneously offer myriad possibilities for individual manipulation of commensal politics.

The critical point is that commensal hospitality centering around food and drink distribution and consumption is a practice that, like the exchange of gifts, serves to establish and maintain social relations. This is why feasts are often viewed as mechanisms of social solidarity that serve to establish a sense of community. However, as Mauss (1966) pointed out, these are relations of reciprocal obligation, which translate into a relationship of social superiority and inferiority unless and until the equivalent can be returned. In this feature, the potential of hospitality to be manipulated as a tool in defining social relations, lies the crux of commensal politics. Hospitality is, of course, only one of many potential fields of political action (Bourdieu 1977; Modjeska 1982; Lemonnier 1990); but its special attribute is that, because of the intimate nature of the practice of sharing food, of all forms of gift presentation it is perhaps the most effective at subtly euphemizing the self-interested nature of the process.

Feast Patterns

Three different patterns may be distinguished in a schematic fashion in the ways feasts are used and in the functions they serve within the political economy. I am not really proposing here a typology of kinds of feasts, but rather a dissection of the political dimension of feasting as an institution. The first of these feast patterns is directed toward the acquisition of social power, and the latter two are directed toward the maintenance of existing inequalities in power relations. The first two operate primarily through an emphasis on quantity, and the last operates through an emphasis on style. The first two work through the idiom of donor/receiver, superiority/subordination relations within an inclusive binding exchange dyad, whereas the latter works through the idiom of diacritical exclusion in an insider/outsider relationship.

Entrepreneurial Feasts

The first of these feast patterns, which I will call the "entrepreneurial feast," involves the competitive manipulation of commensal hospitality toward the acquisition of what Bourdieu (1977) calls "symbolic capital" which translates into informal political power and economic advantage.[4] By informal political power I mean what is often called "prestige," or what Salisbury (1962) called "free-floating power." That is, an ability to influence group decisions or actions which derives not from the authority vested in a particular formalized status or role, but rather from the relations created and reproduced in the process of personal interaction. In this case, those are multiple relations of reciprocal obligation and sentiments of social superiority/subordination between host and guests, created through generous displays of hospitality. The power derived from this sort of commensal politics may range from a subtle and temporary affirmation of elevated status (such as attitudes of superiority and deference) to demands for certain rights and leading managerial roles in group decisions. In societies without formal specialized political roles, hosting feasts is very often a major means of acquiring and maintaining the prestige necessary to exert leadership. In societies where institutionalized political roles or formal status distinctions exist, but without fixed hereditary rules for determining who may fill them, competitive feasting is often the means by which individuals assume and hold these roles and statuses. In all cases, this kind of power is continually being renegotiated and contested through competitive commensal politics.

This type of feasting has been described by various anthropologists in many contexts ranging from Melanesia to Central America to Asia to Africa (e.g. Hocart 1916; Powdermaker 1932; Cancian 1965; Scheffler 1965; Young 1971; Tosh 1978; Kennedy 1978; Friedman 1984; Volkman 1985; Rehfisch 1987; Hayden and Gargett 1990). In societies with an egalitarian political ethos, the self-interested manipulative nature of the process may be concealed or euphemized by the fact that it is carried out through the socially valued and integrated institution of generous hospitality, and it may even be perceived by the participants as a leveling device. However, this apparent leveling is merely the conversion of economic capital into "symbolic capital" (Bourdieu 1977: 171-83). Feasts may be used as a form of what Firth (1983) has called "indebtedness engineering" every bit as much as the prestation of valuables. This is quite clear in the cases where feasting is recognized by the participants to be openly aggressive (Scheffler 1965; Rehfisch 1987), but it is equally operative in cases where competitive manipulation is more subtly euphemized.

Commensal hospitality may be manipulated in the entrepreneurial feast pattern for economic advantage as well as for political power, especially through the institution of the work-party feast; this was particularly true of societies in the past. The work-party feast is a labor mobilization device with a worldwide distribution in which a group of people are called together to work on a specific project for a day and are then treated to a meal and/or drink, after which the host owns the proceeds of the day's labor. Before the development and spread of the monetary economy, this was virtually the only means (excluding slavery) by which a group larger than the family could be mobilized for a project requiring a larger communal effort. This is particularly true of societies without centralized political authority, but even obligatory forms of *corvée* labor organized by chiefs normally operate within this idiom by providing refreshments for workers. There is actually a range of work-party types running between what Erasmus (1956) called "exchange" and "festive" forms of labor. In the former, the quantity of food and drink offered is relatively small but the obligation to reciprocate labor services at the work parties of others is strong. These are not normally effective in mobilizing very large groups. In the "festive" type, much larger work groups can be organized, and these are also more effective at recruiting labor without reference to kinship and neighborhood affiliation. Moreover, the obligation to provide reciprocal labor services is minimal or nonexistent, but the quantities of food and drink required are much greater. Work-party feasts on this end of the spectrum are viewed by the participants more as finite exchange transactions. These should not be regarded as mutually exclusive binary types but rather as poles of a continuum in which examples tending toward both extremes may be employed in the same society for different purposes (Erasmus 1956; Dietler 1989).

Work-party feasts are important in the political economy for two reasons. In the first place, as with all other types of feast, they provide an opportunity to make public statements about prestige (Kennedy 1978: 118). In the second place, they act as a mechanism of indirect conversion in multicentric economies, which provides a potential catalyst for increasing inequality in social relations. This latter aspect may be illustrated by reference to an ethnohistorical study on precolonial iron production conducted among the Samia people in western Kenya (Dietler 1989).

The Samia are an agricultural people with a traditionally acephalous form of political organization. Until the influx of European industrially produced iron in the 1920s, all of the iron used over an area of several thousand square kilometers, encompassing both Samia and the neighboring Luo territory, was derived from a single ore source in the Samia hills. This fact is reflected in the Luo name for the principal object produced from this ore, a large iron hoe blade called *Kwer Nyagot*, or "Hoe, Daughter of the Hills." The production of these hoes was based upon a system fueled by large feasts. A wealthy man with a large number of wives capable of preparing a substantial quantity of beer and food would call together all the willing men of the area on a given day to mine ore from the Samia hills. There was no obligation to participate, but men were drawn to do so by the reputation of the host for generous hospitality. After gathering the ore, these men were treated to a lavish feast, and the host was left with a large supply of iron ore. No further compensation was required. A smelter and a smith were then called to convert the ore into hoes, and they were compensated by being given some of these hoes. The hoes, some of which still survive as heirlooms, were extremely valuable. Although used for subsistence agriculture, they formed part of the prestige sphere of exchange: their acquisition required the giving of livestock and they were even used along with cattle as bridewealth in marriage transactions (Dietler 1989).

While this method of engaging in iron production was in principle open to all Samia men, in practical terms its effective manipulation was limited to those wealthy enough to provide sufficiently large feasts to mobilize a large work-party. Moreover, there is an obvious link between subsistence production, marriage, and iron production, which would insure that an initial position of advantage in access to this process would tend to have a spiraling effect in augmenting wealth and prestige. That is, wealth in cattle was necessary to obtain many wives, whose labor could produce a large feast. But once this was achieved, the hoes gained through the institution of the work-party feast could be used to obtain more wives (through conversion to stock used as bridewealth or used directly in marriage transactions); and the increased productive capacity represented by these women could be used to amass the supplies for a large feast more effectively and frequently, and to engage again in iron production. Men without the initial "capital" to produce a large feast were effectively excluded from the cycle.

This example serves to illustrate how feasts may act as a means of conversion among spheres of exchange in a multicentric economy. While grain is so low on the scale of value that no one would be willing to accept even a huge quantity of it in direct exchange for prestige goods, its conversion into beer and food in the context of a feast is a prime means of acquiring prestige and mobilizing the labor by which prestige exchange objects ultimately can be obtained. It also demonstrates the way in which entrepreneurial feasts serve as a conduit for reciprocal conversions of economic and symbolic capital (Bourdieu 1977). People are drawn to participate in such "festive" work parties by the reputation of the host for generous hospitality. This reputation is an aspect of symbolic capital acquired through the expenditure of economic capital in previous feasts. But through the institution of the work-party feast, this symbolic capital is used to harness the labor of others for the acquisition of further economic capital. Finally, this example also illustrates how the manipulation of this practice can lead to increasing social and economic inequality. When one segment of a community becomes adept at managing this entrepreneurial device and begins to act consistently as hosts of large work-party feasts while others find themselves continually serving as guests/workers, then one has the beginnings of a pattern of labor exploitation by which some individuals or groups are able to dominate the system and extract wealth and prestige from the labor of others (Barth 1967; Dietler 1989).

The entrepreneurial feast pattern operates on a variety of scales and in numerous contexts within a given society. It may extend from the private hosting of a pot of beer among a small group of friends to the hosting of trade partners from another community to the sponsorship of major community life crisis ceremonies and religious festivals. Guests may include members of the local community or people from other communities. The extent of the symbolic capital derived from these activities varies according to the context, lavishness, and range of guests convened. The host may be either an individual household, a kinship unit, or an entire community. In the latter cases there are usually certain individuals who act as managers and derive prestige from their role in successfully organizing and executing feasts that represent the group to outsiders; hence prestige accrues to both the hosting group as a whole and to certain influential individuals who can mobilize group activities.

While most households will engage in some form of this kind of feasting behavior, hosting large-scale feasts requires considerable planning, time, and labor (for both agricultural production and culinary preparation), as well as large surplus stocks of food and/or drink. The kinds of food and drink available in prehistoric societies would generally have had very limited storability, especially once prepared for consumption. This would necessitate, in most cases, a large labor force for final preparation and serving just prior to the feast as well as command of a large ready supply of agricultural produce. The institutional arrangements for mobilizing these large supplies of labor and food vary a great deal from society to society, but in all cases the organization and execution of a large feast requires the host to be a good manager. It is usually advantageous for a household sponsoring a feast to be able to provide a large portion, if not the bulk, of the labor and raw materials from its own reserves, and a high incidence of polygyny among Big-men and other types of informal leaders is often cited in this connection (Geschire 1982; Friedman 1984; Lemonnier 1990). As noted above, in some cases work-party feasts may also be employed to harness the labor of others in differentially increasing the productive base of certain households. In most cases of very large feasts, however, the host must mobilize additional food and labor contributions through personal networks of social obligation. These networks of support are established by adept building up of symbolic capital over the years through various arenas of prestige competition and various deployments of economic capital. Hence a large, lavish feast is not just an isolated event. It is a moment of public drama in a continuous process of political manipulation that serves as an advertisement of the scale of the support base that a social manager has been able to construct through various transactions at the same time that it produces further social credit and symbolic capital.

Patron-Role Feast

Returning to our discussion of the major political roles of feasts, the second feast pattern that may be distinguished, and that I will call the "patron-role feast," is the formalized use of commensal hospitality to symbolically reiterate and legitimize institutionalized relations of unequal social power. This corresponds to a form of what has traditionally been called "redistribution" in the literature of economic anthropology (Polanyi 1957; Sahlins 1972), or what Pryor (1977), paying closer attention to the actual flows of material goods, has called "centric transfers." The operative principle behind this form of commensal politics is the same as for the previous type: the relationship of reciprocal obligation engendered through hospitality. In this case, however, the expectation of equal reciprocation is no longer maintained. Rather, the acceptance of a continually unequal pattern of hospitality symbolically expresses the formalization of unequal relations of status and power, and this acceptance ideologically naturalizes the formalization through repetition of an event that induces sentiments of social debt. On the one hand, those who are continually in the role of guests are symbolically acknowledging their acceptance of "minister" status (Mauss 1966: 72) vis-à-vis the continual host. On the other hand, the role of continual and generous host for the community at large comes to be seen as a duty incumbent upon the person who occupies a particular elevated status position or formal political role. Institutionalization of authority depends on this binding commensal link between unequal partners in a patron/client relationship.

This is the principle that lies behind the regular lavish hospitality expected of chiefs in many societies. This sense of obligation for generosity in a commensal context is nicely encapsulated in the Baganda definition of the essential qualities of a good chief: "beer, meat and politeness" (Mair 1934: 183). One might also cite Casati's (1891:248) observation about such duties among the Azande: "A chief must know how to drink; he must get drunk often and thoroughly" (Washburne 1961: 10). This is not, as has sometimes been posited, a functionally adaptive means of providing balanced food security for a population. Rather, it is a politico-symbolic device for legitimizing status differences (Friedman 1984; Hayden and Gargett 1990).

Chiefs raise food supplies for this lavish public hospitality in a variety of ways (Schapera 1938; Richards 1939; Hunter 1961: 384-89). Tribute in food and drink often furnishes a certain part, with individuals obligated to provide the chief with a portion of their own production. The work-party feast (especially in the more obligatory *corvée* form), directed toward the extensive fields of the chief, is another very common mechanism of mobilizing food stocks for such purposes. Moreover, chiefs are very often ostentatiously polygynous in comparison to their people, providing a large pool of household labor and they sometimes have attached forms of dependent labor, such as slaves.

Diacritical Feasts

The third major feast pattern, which I call the "diacritical feast," involves the use of differentiated cuisine and styles of consumption as a diacritical symbolic device to naturalize and reify concepts of ranked differences in social status (Elias 1978; Goody 1982; Bourdieu 1984). Although it serves a somewhat similar function to the previous pattern (i.e. the naturalization and objectification of inequality in social relations), it differs from it in several important respects. In the first place, the basis of symbolic force shifts from quantity to style. Moreover, the emphasis shifts from a commensal bond between unequal partners to a statement of exclusive and unequal commensal circles: obligations of reciprocal hospitality are no longer the basis of status claims and power. This is the distinction made by Goody (1982) when he differentiated between "hieratic" and "hierarchical" systems of stratification in his discussion of the origins and significance of cuisine. This practice transforms elite feasts into what Appadurai (1986: 21) has called "tournaments of value" that serve both to define elite status membership and to channel social competition within clearly defined boundaries.

Diacritical stylistic distinctions may be based upon the use of rare or expensive foods or food service vessels and implements. Or they may be based upon differences in the complexity of the pattern of preparation and consumption of food and the specialized knowledge (or "cultural capital": Bourdieu 1984) this entails. Because this type of feasting relies upon style for its symbolic force, it is subject to emulation by those aspiring to higher status. This can result in the gradual spread through a society of food practices by what Appadurai (1986) has described as a "turnstile effect," as happened in ancient Greece with the expansion of the *symposion* (wine-drinking party) from its aristocratic origins throughout urban society (Dentzer 1982; Murray 1990). Such emulation can be thwarted only by the imposition of sumptuary laws or by the use of exotic foods and consumption paraphernalia, access to which can be controlled through elevated expense or limited networks of acquisition. In the absence of effective monopolization, the symbolic force of elite food practices can eventually become "devalued" and this may provoke continual shifts in elite style as it reacts to the process of emulation.

In looking for evidence of diacritical feasting practices in the archaeological record, care must be taken not to confuse these with the kinds of practices that may be used to differentiate feasts in general, as public ritual events, from everyday informal consumption.[5] In many cases, this distinction is marked simply by differences in the sheer quantity of food and drink proffered and consumed, or by a change in the location and timing of consumption. However, the same classes of devices used as symbolic diacritica in marking social distinctions may be employed to distinguish ritual from quotidian practice by serving as "framing devices" that act as cues establishing the ritual significance of events (Miller 1985: 181-3). Feasts may be marked by special foods (e.g. ones which are expensive, rare, especially rich, particularly sweet, etc.). Alternatively, special service vessels may be employed for this purpose. Finally, atypical complexity in recipes or in the structure of service and consumption may be used to invoke such distinctions. The archaeologist must rely upon a critical evaluation of the context and association of the evidence in order to distinguish between diacritical feasts marking social classes or categories and the diacritical use of cuisine to mark feasts as special events. For example, types of ceramic fine tableware that are found only in funerary contexts, but in all funerary contexts, are more likely representative of feasts as special events, whereas large bronze drinking vessels found in a limited number of wealthy burials most likely indicate feasts marking social classes.

While there is an obvious correlation with increasing social stratification and complexity of structures of political power, these three feast patterns should not be interpreted as strict evolutionary stages. Rather, they constitute a progressively inclusive repertoire of forms of commensal politics. That is, although there are and have been societies in which only entrepreneurial feasts operate, societies in which diacritical feasts are found are also likely to have each of the two other types. Where cuisine is used as a diacritical symbolic device between classes, competitive commensal politics still will be used by individuals or groups jockeying for relative status within those classes, and unequal commensal hospitality will be simultaneously used to legitimize institutionalized political authority roles. Likewise, both entrepreneurial and patron-role feasts are likely to be operative where the latter type is found: the use of redistributive hospitality by chiefs or other "patrons" to maintain their authority does not preclude the use of competitive hospitality by others to define their relative statuses below that of the chief (or indeed its use by clients to curry favor with patrons [Barlett 1980]), or its use by chiefs of different areas to negotiate and define their relative statuses vis-à-vis each other.

Prehistoric Europe

How can this perspective on feasts and commensal politics help us to understand the development of social relations in prehistoric European societies, and what can we say about long-term developments in the matter of food and politics? I will address this question in two ways. First, I will offer a very brief and schematic sketch of what can be discerned in this domain during the course of European prehistory, and then I will employ a more detailed examination of the period most familiar to me, the Early Iron Age, to illustrate how an examination of food, power, and status can provide a window of entry for new understanding of particular ancient societies.

Very little can be ascertained about commensal politics during the Paleolithic, the period of prehistory contemporary with the Ice Ages, which ended about 10,000 years ago. From preserved faunal and floral evidence archaeologists have been able to piece together a partial and tentative picture of the diet of peoples living in different regions at different times (Dennell 1983; Mellars 1985; Gamble 1986). These studies indicate a great deal of regional and temporal variation within a general pattern of reliance on variable proportions of wild animal foods, particularly large game animals such as mammoth, reindeer, deer, bovids, and horse. During most periods a fairly wide range of animals was utilized, but during some periods and in certain areas a more specialized focus on specific species (e.g. reindeer or mammoth) appears to have been practised. Fish may have developed into a food resource of some importance in a few areas late in the Paleolithic (Jochim 1983; Hayden et al. 1987). Very little evidence exists of the wild plant contribution to the diet, but it has been suggested that peoples of at least the Upper Paleolithic (i.e. the last phase, from about 35,000 to 10,000 years ago) relied upon a "hunter/collector" subsistence strategy in which, in contrast to the alternative "forager/gatherer" strategy now practised in several modern tropical contexts, plant foods formed a much less important contribution to the diet than did meat (Binford 1980, 1982; Gamble 1986).

This would mean that periodic events of meat sharing by successful hunters or leaders of hunting groups may have provided a basis for acquiring prestige and informal leadership roles within the rather small and flexible social groups that lived together. Interpretative caution is suggested by Wiessner's (this volume) analytical survey of data from modern forager societies (or what Hayden calls "simple hunter-gatherers"), which indicates that most such societies have well-developed social mechanisms that serve to dissipate the political potential of the use of food in this way. However, as she further points out, some of the limitations on the manipulative use of food in modern forager societies may be a feature of their integration into the larger regional and world political economy, which has tended to diminish the role of local leadership. Hunter-gatherers of at least late Paleolithic Europe may well have had much more developed institutions allowing the acquisition of informal leadership and social power than modern hunter-gatherers (Mellars 1985). Interestingly, Wiessner's data (this volume) also suggest that modern hunters have the greatest prestige in societies that rely most on meat in their diet (i.e. those closest to the hunter/collector pattern proposed for Upper Paleolithic Europe).

In any case, it is not clear when this pattern might have developed. Anatomically fully modern humans (*Homo sapiens sapiens*) appeared in Europe only at the beginning of the Upper Paleolithic, and we do not really have any firm basis for analogical inferences for hominid behavior during the several hundred thousand years before that period, when archaic Homo sapiens and Neanderthals were present in Europe. If De Waal's (1986, 1989) interpretations of chimpanzee behavior are considered, there may be some justification for extending food-sharing behavior and its potential manipulation for social and political purposes back to some early common ancestral species (see Isaac 1978a, 1978b); although this remains a hotly contested issue in the archaeological literature (cf. Binford 1981; Marshall 1993).

Feasts as distinct events are, to say the least, very difficult to detect in the Paleolithic archaeological evidence. Butchery patterns in the faunal remains certainly demonstrate that cooking operations (e.g. boiling, marrow extraction, roasting) were sufficiently developed by the Upper Paleolithic to offer possibilities for some minor complexity of culinary elaboration (Le Tensorer 1985). Moreover, some of the large concentrations of animal bones that often have been interpreted as mass kill sites, such as at La Solutré, certainly would have provided extraordinary quantities of food that might have served feasting events (Mohen 1986). However, this interpretation requires that these sites can be demonstrated, in the light of modern taphonomic understanding of site formation processes, to represent single-episode deposits of human origin; and the realization of this goal remains difficult. It may be surmised that the large seasonal concentrations of population proposed for several areas in late Paleolithic Europe quite probably would have included feasting among the ritual activities serving to establish and maintain social relations (Jochim 1983; Mellars 1985), and that these would have served equally as a venue for commensal politics. However, the physical evidence for such feasts is lacking and, for the most part, in the Paleolithic one can advance little beyond plausible surmises.

The succeeding Mesolithic period witnessed the adaptation of a diet based on hunted and gathered foods to a progressively more forested and temperate post-glacial environment beginning about

10,000 years ago (Tringham 1971; Dennell 1983). Variety seems to have been a common characteristic of the food repertoire. A range of somewhat smaller woodland animal species was hunted, including especially red deer, but also various other types of deer, pig, ovicaprids, and aurochs. Birds and small mammals also formed part of the diet; fish and shellfish were eaten in significant quantities in some areas, leading to possibilities for sedentary occupation (Rowley-Conwy 1983; Price 1985). Evidence of plant foods is still very meager and ambiguous, but a rich variety was available for exploitation (Clarke 1976; Jochim 1976), and bone chemistry studies may eventually provide a more reliable picture of the vegetal component of the diet than have scarce floral and seed remains (Price 1989). Some evidence also exists for the exploitation of honey (Dennell 1983: 126), and it is of interest in the context of this discussion that this would have presented improved possibilities for early production of alcoholic beverages (Brothwell 1969: 165).

We are, again, in a rather poor position to understand commensal politics during this period. Presumably meat sharing was still a potentially common means of establishing prestige. Indeed, the shift toward smaller, less gregarious animals and the use of the bow and arrow may have more readily allowed greater individual manipulation of this means of acquiring prestige, as the strategy of hunting may have relied less on group effort and more on individual skill. However, the broader resource base, particularly the foraging exploitation of stationary, predictable resources (such as shellfish) might well have mitigated the relative nutritional importance of hunting. It is unclear in what ways this might have affected its symbolic importance in particular cases (as modern ethnographic studies show, there is no necessary direct correlation) or to what extent commensal political strategies, insofar as they were developed, may have shifted toward the control of foraging and culinary labor. In the case of culinary labor, one might expect manipulations leading eventually to gender-based patterns of labor exploitation within "household" units. Several scholars have entertained the possibility that "complex hunter-gatherer" societies may have developed during this period in several areas of Europe (e.g. Price 1985), and that this might be associated with a circumvention of the structural barriers to the political use of food described by Wiessner (this volume) for "forager" societies. Unfortunately, however, our ability to detect feasts in the archaeological record remains little better than during the preceding period.

With the spread of agriculture and animal domestication through Europe, we begin to perceive the operation of feasts in society more directly. These new techniques of food production appeared first in

Greece and the Balkans during the seventh millennium B.C. (largely as an extension of practices developed earlier in the Middle East). They then spread, in a complicated pattern and through a variety of social processes, westward along the Mediterranean coastal zones; and somewhat later (during the sixth millennium B.C.), these techniques of food production were carried through the heart of central and western Europe with a complex known as the "Bandkeramik" culture. After several millennia of adoption of agriculture by indigenous hunter-gatherer societies and the gradual territorial expansion of agricultural societies, by the fourth millennium B.C. subsistence over virtually the whole of Europe had come to rely on these techniques (Tringham 1971; Dennell 1983; Whittle 1985; Barker 1985). Eventually, the dominant crops everywhere were wheat and barley, and the dominant food animals were cattle, pigs, sheep, and goats. These, of course, varied a great deal locally in relative importance, and they were combined with other complexes of cereals, legumes, vegetables, fruits, and animals in the elaboration of local culinary traditions. For example, grapes for the production of wine and olives became a crucial feature of the Aegean diet during the third millennium B.C. (Renfrew 1972: 304-7), and this eventually became a general Mediterranean pattern. Because of the sedentary nature of settlements and the prevalence of storage and techniques such as parching grain, the evidence for reconstructing specific local diets is generally much better during the Neolithic than for preceding periods. In a few cases of extraordinary preservation, such as the numerous Alpine lake dwellings of France, Switzerland, and Germany, it has even been possible to suggest reconstructed recipes (Jacomet and Schibler 1985).

Bender (1978, 1985) has suggested that the initial spread of agriculture may be related to demands generated by competitive political relations on productivity and production in some hunter-gatherer societies. This political activity would have evolved in the context of regional exchange networks for valuables and marriage partners. Hayden (1990) has further developed this idea in suggesting specifically that the competitive manipulation of food for the acquisition of power by "accumulators" among "complex hunter-gatherers" was the catalyst responsible for the origins and spread of agriculture. While these arguments were only marginally directed at Europe, they may well provide an explanation for the spread of agriculture into many regions where it is clear that the change involved a transfer or transformation of techniques rather than a movement of people (Voytek and Tringham 1989).

What is clear in the European evidence is that, from early in the Neolithic, food containers and sometimes food remains began to appear in funerary contexts over a very wide area (Tringham 1971: 87, 124, 154, 190; Whittle 1985: 89-91, 160, 197-99), indicating that the ritual consumption of food played an important role in the "politico-symbolic drama" of funerary ritual. In fact, from the Neolithic on, pottery became by far the most common and consistent item of funerary furniture throughout Europe.[6] This is not necessarily an indication of the first appearance of this funerary role for feasts, since it may simply be due to the vastly superior preservation qualities of the containers of durable ceramic material that were first manufactured by early agricultural societies. It does, however, give us our first solid evidence of this connection.

Broad generalization about pan-European burial patterns is extremely difficult (indeed foolhardy) due to the great amount of regional and temporal variation. For example, in the earliest Neolithic societies of southeastern Europe burials were often in pits within settlements, whereas many Bandkeramik burials are clustered in independent cemeteries of single graves. In some regions (particularly in western and northern Europe), burials were at first collectively grouped in large "megalithic" tombs. Nevertheless, with the caveat that meaningful analysis must really be based upon regionally specific patterns, it is possible to offer a few tentative general observations relevant to the central theme of this paper. In the earlier phases of the Neolithic, the food consumption containers found in graves are generally of the same type as those found on settlements. This may be interpreted as indicating that ritual distinction of consumption was most likely to have been marked by quantity rather than by the style of presentation. Later, pots of a different shape or style from those representative of domestic contexts are characteristic of burials or ceremonial sites in some regions (e.g the "grooved ware" found on English henge monuments), and greater quantitative differences in vessels included in graves are sometimes notable. These features most probably indicate an elaboration of complexity in feasting ritual through both relative quantity and stylistic means, although there seems little convincing evidence of the development of diacritical feasting practices until perhaps the Beaker burials of the final Neolithic, or Chalcolithic, period (Sherratt 1986).[7]

The growing importance of feasts in the political economy during the Neolithic may also be detected indirectly in several features, including the construction of large monuments (particularly in western Europe) and the expansion of exchange networks. Massive earthen burial mounds, megalithic tombs, earthwork enclosures, and standing stone arrangements (such as Stonehenge or the alignments of Carnac) are all evidence of large communal labor projects that almost certainly relied upon work-party feasts for their mobilization. These would have been sponsored by individuals or groups that would have gained prestige in addition to labor in the process; the visibility of the monument would have been, in addition to its other cultural significance, a conspicuous advertisement of the scale of the labor capable of being mobilized. Whether these may have been *corvée* projects organized by chiefs or "festive labor" projects executed through entrepreneurial feasts is difficult to determine. Renfrew (1973) has suggested that the size of some of the latest projects necessarily implies centralized political authority, but this seems questionable. Many of the monuments show evidence of having been built in sections, and it is quite conceivable that they were constructed by smaller work parties over time or, for example, by neighborhood or lineage-based labor groups (each mobilized by separate feasts) working in competition with each other (Startin and Bradley 1981; Bradley 1984). A similar process has been convincingly suggested to explain the construction of early ceremonial monuments in Peru (Burger 1992). Given the possibilities for labor mobilization through feasts (Dietler 1989), it seems prudent to critically question claims for the necessity of institutionalized central political authority behind large-scale monuments and labor projects.

Neolithic England has produced a series of curious large earthwork structures called "causewayed enclosures" that offer further evidence for feasting. These are far from homogeneous in their structure and associated materials, and caution should be used in treating them as a uniform phenomenon (Burgess et al. 1988). However, aside from the labor mobilization involved in their construction, several of these have yielded evidence of meat consumption on a large scale and other features that suggest that they may have been communal centers for feasting and exchange (Smith 1965; Bradley 1984). One may surmise – albeit on the basis of an association established by ethnographic analogy rather than a great deal of archaeological evidence that feasting also played a prominent role in the growth of the exchange networks through which objects such as flint and various kinds of stone axes were circulating over large areas by the later Neolithic (Clough and Cummins 1979; Bradley and Edmonds 1993). Feasts would have been important in this context both in production and exchange, that is, in mobilizing mining parties for stone quarrying and in exchange transactions between trade partners.

Given the nature of the archaeological record and the difficulty of distinguishing between entrepreneurial and patron-role feasts on purely material grounds, it is difficult to say precisely at what point the latter may have developed during the Neolithic. This must be judged on the basis of other evidence from settlements and burials that indicates the emergence of institutionalized political roles and hierarchical status differences, a process that was quite variable in different areas of Europe (Bradley 1984; Whittle 1985; Shennan 1993).

During the succeeding Bronze Age, which began in some areas during the late third millennium B.C., an increasing emphasis on eating and particularly on drinking equipment placed in burials is evident; it is possible to fairly clearly detect status differentiation associated with such culinary material in many areas (Coles and Harding 1979). In certain cases this is represented by markedly different quantities of essentially similar ceramic tableware, pointing toward quantity as the primary indicator of status. However, in other cases the clear beginnings of differentiated cuisine and the diacritical feast pattern may be detected in the use of rare and precious materials for exclusively elite feasting equipment (such as gold cups and bowls: Taylour 1983: 118-24, 144, 146), or the similar use of items that require considerable specialist expertise in their manufacture (such as sheet bronze cauldrons and buckets: Hawkes and Smith 1957). This diacritical drinking and culinary pattern is particularly marked in some extremely elaborate and opulent graves of the Mycenaean state in the Mediterranean region. However, it can also be detected in various areas of temperate Europe, particularly in some extravagant tumulus graves constructed during the latest (or "Urnfield") period of the Bronze Age, such as those of Saint-Romain-de-Jalionas in France (Verger and Guillaumet 1988), Hart an der Alz in Bavaria (Müller-Karpe 1959: 156), or Ockov in Slovakia (Paulik 1962), with their collections of impressive sheet-bronze feasting gear. This incorporation of bronze vessels in feasting ritual is not accidental; feasts quite probably played a major role in the articulation of the extensive exchange networks that were responsible for the circulation of metal resources across Europe, and commensal politics was critical for the operation of the prestige goods economies that relied upon bronze objects.

During the Iron Age (roughly the last eight centuries of the first millennium B.C.), the evidence for studying feasting becomes even more extensive and detailed. As will be shown in the following section, it has the potential to be exploited to great benefit in specific cases. To a certain extent this increased visibility of evidence is due to the equipment used in the elaboration of diacritical feasting practices. The Early Iron Age cemetery of the Austrian salt-mining community of Hallstatt, for example, is richly endowed with sheet bronze feasting vessels (Merhart 1969). The chiefly tumulus burials of the West Hallstatt domain contain yet more spectacular sets of bronze, gold, and ceramic feasting gear (imported from the Mediterranean states and produced locally), and similar kinds of objects continued to be used during the Late (or La Tène) Iron Age (Ruoff 1985; Kaenel 1985). This evidence is supplemented by traces of a trade in wine between the Mediterranean states and the societies of western Europe that began during the seventh century B.C. (Dietler 1990a, 1992). In the last century before the Roman conquest of Gaul this trade resulted in the importation of perhaps forty million amphoras of Roman wine into the region (Tchernia 1983). For this latter period, our knowledge of feasting in this area is further enhanced by contemporary descriptions of feasting practices provided by Greek and Roman authors (e.g. Athenaeus IV, 152c-d). Moreover, as early as the sixth century B.C., decoration on bronze *situlae* from northern Italy (themselves used in feasting) provide us with detailed pictorial renderings of feasts in progress (Bonfante 1981; Ruoff 1985). Although it falls outside the scope of this paper, the evidence pertaining to feasting in the literate Mediterranean state societies (Greek, Etruscan, and Roman) is, of course, even more abundant. It includes literary descriptions and visual depictions on ceramics, metalwork, and murals; this has given rise to numerous analyses that provide significant insights into social relations and processes (Dentzer 1982; Gras 1983; Murray 1990).

Early Iron Age Western Europe

Having painted with a rather broad brush this hasty portrait of what can be discerned of the evolving role of feasts during European prehistory, I will examine the Early Iron Age situation in western Europe in somewhat greater detail. This analysis is offered because I believe it demonstrates that an approach to the interpretation of these ancient societies based upon the perspective of commensal politics has the potential to be very useful in explaining several features that previously have been poorly understood. Specifically, I believe that an understanding of the relationship between food, power, and status is essential to understanding the process of colonial interaction that had a major influence on the development of the indigenous societies of Iron Age western Europe. As will be shown, this colonial encounter was largely articulated through the institution of feasting.

The earliest contacts between the Mediterranean states and the native societies of this region (see Figure 7.1) occurred in the latter half of the seventh century B.C. and were in the form of a ship-based trade conducted by Etruscan merchants along the littoral zone of southern France (Bouloumié 1980; Morel 1981; Py 1985, 1990;

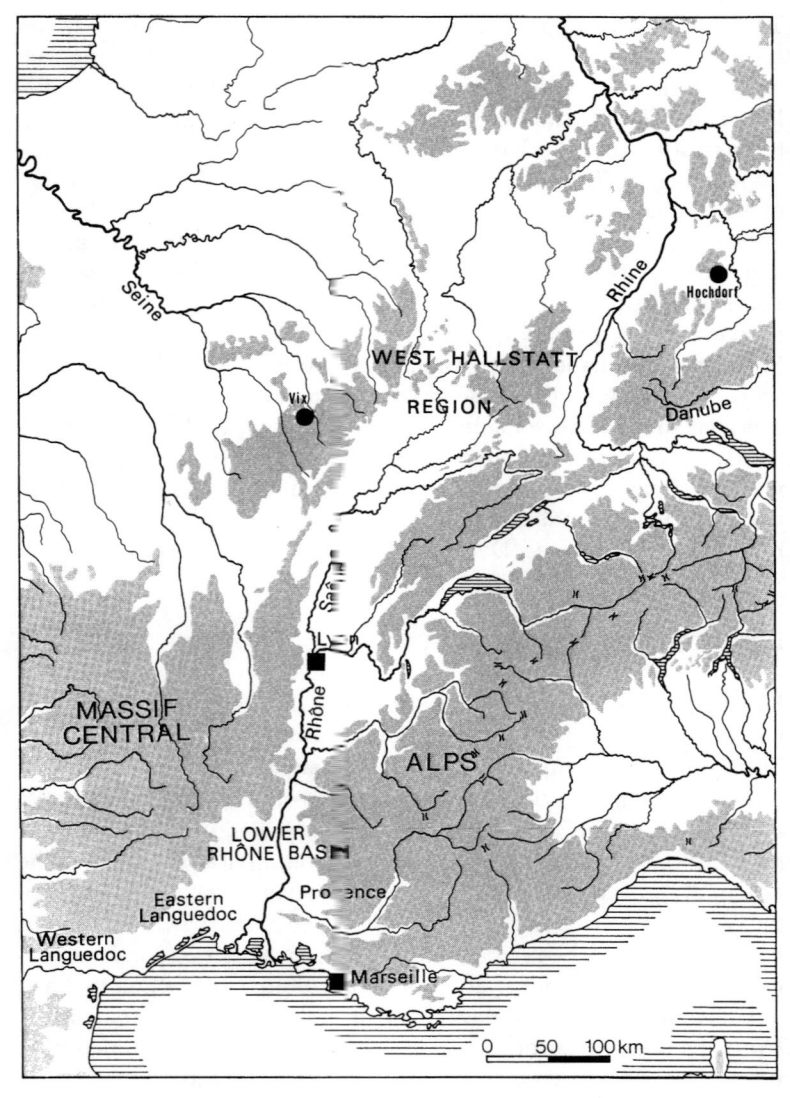

Map of regions and sites mentioned in discussion of Early Iron Age.

Dietler 1990b). The abundant evidence of imports from settlement excavations, shipwrecks and surface survey is overwhelmingly dominated by one class of objects: those related to drinking wine. This material consists of over 90 percent Etruscan wine transport amphoras, with a scattering of Etruscan *bucchero nero* pottery and East Greek pottery (in both cases, with forms almost exclusively restricted to wine-drinking cups and flagons). This pattern is in marked contrast to that of contemporary trade in other areas, such as at Carthage and on Sardinia, where the range of imports is much greater (Morel 1981) or in eastern Spain, where wine amphoras are notably absent (Rouillard 1991). This feature is significant in terms of the nature of indigenous demand that it demonstrates.

At approximately 600 B.C., Greeks from Asia Minor founded the colonial city of Massalia at the site of modern Marseille on the coast of southern France (Gantes 1990; Morel 1990, 1992). Over the course of the sixth century, Massalia gradually eclipsed the Etruscans as the main agents of trade with the indigenous peoples of the area. Significantly, the pattern of trade remained the same, with wine again being the main component, but in this case it was predominantly wine produced at Massalia and transported in a distinctive form of amphora with a characteristic heavily micaceous fabric (Bats 1990; Bertucchi 1992). Along with its own wine, Massalia also traded to the natives pottery imported from Athens (again, almost exclusively wine-drinking items) and began producing its own tableware in imitation of models from its Ionian homeland. The two major series of these wares are called "Pseudo-Ionian" and "Grey-Monochrome" (Lagrand 1963; Py 1979-80; Arcelin-Pradelle 1984). A good deal of this pottery was also imported by the natives, and again the pattern is striking. Among all the forms in evidence at Marseille (Villard 1960: 59-61), wine-drinking cups and pitchers were the only Greek forms imported in any significant quantity into native contexts. The only other popular forms that they imported were derivatives of native tableware produced by the Greeks especially for consumption by the natives. Parallel production of these wares soon began in indigenous territory as well, showing for the first time in western Europe a technique borrowed from the Greeks: throwing on a potter's wheel. Again, wine-drinking cups and pitchers were the only Greek forms reproduced in significant quantity, and the rest consisted of native-derived tableware forms (Lagrand 1963; Py 1979-80; Arcelin-Pradelle 1984; Dietler 1990b: 229-94).

From the mid-sixth century on, Greek and Etruscan objects began to appear in an area called the Western Hallstatt Culture, several hundred kilometers north of southern France up the Rhône valley, in Burgundy, southern Germany, and Switzerland (Frankenstein and Rowlands 1978; Wells 1980; Kimmig 1983). Again, it is striking that the objects imported are connected almost entirely with drinking. However, there are some significant differences with southern France in the nature of these objects and the contexts in which they are found. In the first place the objects in the Hallstatt area are far less numerous than in the south, but they are often far more spectacular. Wine amphoras are relatively few; in fact, there are single sites in the south with more amphoras than have been found in the entire Hallstatt region combined (Dietler 1990a, 1995). Fine Attic drinking ceramics are relatively better represented on some sites in the Hallstatt area than they are in the south. Whereas in the south they consist almost entirely of drinking cups, in the Hallstatt region both cups and kraters are well represented (the latter were used in the Greek world for mixing wine and water before drinking it) (Villard 1988). Finally, there are a number of truly spectacular bronze wine-mixing vessels of a type that have never been found in southern France. Objects such as the 1.6-meter tall krater from a tumulus burial at Vix in Burgundy (Joffroy 1979), the *lebes* with griffin heads from the nearby La Garenne tumulus (Joffroy 1979), and the 500-liter *dinos* from the Hochdorf tumulus near Stuttgart (Biel 1985) were exceptional even within the Greek world where they were made (Fischer 1973; Rolley 1982).

The contexts in which these objects were found are also quite different for the two regions (Dietler 1990a, 1990b, 1995). In the Hallstatt zone, the objects are confined almost entirely to a small number of elaborate tumulus burials and to a few defended hilltop settlements (the so-called *Fürstensitze*) around which these tumuli are clustered (Pare 1991). The few amphoras and Attic drinking ceramics appear on the settlements, and the bronze vessels and other rare luxury goods appear in the burials, where they are regularly associated with the most opulently furnished graves in a central wooden chamber with a four-wheeled wagon and a lavish array of indigenous prestige items (such as gold neck rings and other jewelry, and native feasting equipment). In the south, Mediterranean imports are relatively rare in graves and when they occur they are neither of a spectacular nature nor associated in any characteristic way with wealthier or more elaborate burials (Dietler 1995). Most of the Mediterranean imports appear as domestic debris in settlement deposits. Moreover, they are not confined to any particular type or size of settlement, but are spread over many different varieties. In fact, by the late sixth century B.C. they are found on virtually every settlement in the lower Rhône basin (Dietler 1990b).

The traditional explanation for this pattern of contact and cultural borrowing has been a concept called "Hellenization" (Jacobsthal and Neuffer 1933; Benoit 1965; Bouloumié 1981; Kimmig 1983). This is, in brief, the assumption that "barbarians" would automatically wish to emulate the "higher culture" of the Mediterranean civilizations whenever they had the benefit of coming into contact with it, and that the gradual absorption of Mediterranean goods, practices, and beliefs is a natural and ineluctable, if somewhat clumsy, process. It should be immediately apparent that this is a highly unsatisfactory explanation. In the first place, it is not an explanation at all, but, at best, merely a description of a process. Moreover, it is not even an accurate description. A close look at the evidence shows, first, that the pattern of cultural borrowing in both regions was not one of general emulation, but rather was highly limited, specific, and coherent. The natives of both southern France and the Hallstatt region were interested in wine and feasting paraphernalia, and very little else. Secondly, such a crude blanket concept can do little to explain the significant differences in the contexts in which these objects are found. Moreover, an anthropological perspective on consumption makes it clear that demand is never a simple response to the availability of goods: it follows a social logic that is determined by power relations within a society (Douglas and Isherwood 1979; Bourdieu 1984; Appadurai 1986).

I believe that an approach to this problem of colonial contact from the perspective of commensal politics goes a long way toward shedding new light on this issue and helping us to understand larger social processes at work here. In the first place, it must be recognized that one is dealing in these two regions, the lower Rhône basin and the Hallstatt zone, with societies organized very differently (Dietler 1995). Scholars in general agree that the settlement and funerary data indicate that in the Hallstatt case we are dealing with a society showing marked social stratification and centralized, hierarchical political control (Frankenstein and Rowlands 1978; Wells 1980; van der Velde 1985), which included a regionally shared iconography of elite status representation. On the other hand, the lower Rhône basin was occupied by societies with a low level of institutionalized social ranking and without any regionally extensive political centralization (Dietler 1990b, 1995).

In the case of Hallstatt importations of Mediterranean goods, it appears that there was never a significant influx of Mediterranean wine. Rather, rare, exotic, and spectacular drinking vessels were imported for use by the elite in the context of feasting activities. These vessels were not prestige goods destined for redistribution, but were goods reserved exclusively for use and burial within the highest stratum of the social scale. Their adoption does not constitute an attempt to imitate the Greek symposium, as has sometimes been claimed (Bouloumié 1988); this can be readily seen by their admixture in tombs with native drinking horns, buckets, and plates. Rather, it represents the incorporation of exotic items into an established repertoire of feasting equipment in a pattern of diacritical social symbolism that was already well established. These items are preeminent "luxury goods" in the sense defined by Appadurai (1986: 38), that is, "rhetorical" signs within the domain of political representation and action. Their value in this context derives from their exotic origin and their perception as spectacular and "costly", in the sense of being unattainable except by a very few. They may be recognized as a further ideologically "naturalizing" extension of the emphasis on diacritical symbolism in feasting gear already noted in this region during the Bronze Age.

This process may be seen in the same vein as what Goody (1982) described as the development of differentiated cuisine as a diacritical symbolic device in hierarchical societies, where commensal circles and marriage networks come to be restricted along class divisions. In this case, transport and communication impediments precluded the incorporation of exotic Mediterranean food ingredients (such as wine) in the elite cuisine on a regular basis, but the vessels in which food and drink were served offered a more durable and visible means of differentiating elite consumption at feasts. Another feature that offers support for the interpretation presented here is that for virtually the first time in the European archaeological record women also were buried with elaborate sets of feasting gear, including Mediterranean imports. The Vix tumulus, for example, was a female burial. This indicates that men and women were united as a class in the symbolic use of feasts as a statement of social differentiation. It may also indicate a possible shift in the role of wives within the elite class from food preparers and servers to commensal partners, a shift linked to the development of specialist food preparers, which Goody (1982) views as associated with the distinction between "hierarchical" and "hieratic" societies.

In the lower Rhône basin the situation is quite different. There, I would contend that the notable influx of Mediterranean wine had an effect similar to the colonial introduction of steel axes and shell valuables in New Guinea (Salisbury 1962; Strathern 1971; 1982, Young 1971) and money and wage labor in many small-scale acephalous societies (Dalton 1978; Robbins 1973). Specifically, it initiated an escalation of social competition centered around the institution of feasting.

In small-scale societies without specialized or institutionalized political roles the competitive manipulation of commensal hospitality provides a major avenue for the acquisition of informal political power and economic advantage by virtue of the role of entrepreneurial feasts as a conduit for the reciprocal conversion of economic and symbolic capital. However, while in principle operation in this domain is open to all households and everyone has access to the basic means of producing feasts, in practice there are constraints that often result in some individuals developing privileged access to the benefits of the system. Successful manipulation on a large scale requires large ready surplus stocks of agricultural resources for conversion into food and drink, control of a large pool of labor for culinary processing, and the establishment and management of a network of social resources to provide additional support. These do not materialize out of nothing; large feasts are, after all, merely the final event in a long and complex process of management of resources and relationships (Scheffler 1965: 216). Constructing the support base necessary to become a major successful operator in this domain normally requires years of skillful "investment" in symbolic capital and social credit (building a reputation for generous hospitality, organizing and sponsoring community festivals, representing the community to outsiders in exchange feasts, helping others in their feasting efforts, etc.) as well as the gradual harnassing of labor resources (e.g. the acquisition of multiple wives, the cyclical expansion and exploitation of work-party feasts). Within different societies there are established paths by which adept managers are able to "build their careers" in the arena of commensal politics; these paths require time, work, and skill, and they involve managers in complex networks of obligations and alliances.

The sudden availability of an alien source of drink (i.e. in this case Mediterranean wine) in such a system might initially have been viewed by those individuals or groups who already had an established advantage in the sphere of commensal politics as a way to augment their existing prestige and power. These "Big-men," "leaders" (Lemonnier 1990), "managers" (Scheffler 1965), lineage elders, or other culturally appropriate types of successful accumulators of political influence would most likely be the first to orchestrate contact with external agents (Salisbury 1962; Strathern 1971). Wine would have been viewed simply as an added element in the scale of their hospitality; it would be desirable because of its superior storage and transport qualities over native grain beers and because it would not require direct production (and perhaps also for its enhanced psychoactive effects due to higher alcohol content). This would explain the initial enthusiastic acceptance of wine as a trade item despite the apparent lack of demand for other aspects of Etruscan and Greek culture.

However, in the absence of an effective monopoly on access to the sources of wine, it could soon have become a threat to the base of the social power of these informal leaders. It would allow those who had previously been relatively disadvantaged in their ability to engage in commensal politics on a significant scale (e.g. young men, minor managers) to quickly obtain the means to do so and to mobilize large work parties. Access to effectively operating in this arena of social competition would no longer be limited by the traditional system of slowly building up the requisite support base. Rather, drink could be obtained by furnishing goods sought by Mediterranean traders or by providing labor services for them in exchange for amphoras of wine, thus circumventing the traditional route to engaging as a significant player in this theater of political competition. This broadening of the recruitment base for leadership contestants would most likely have resulted in an escalation of competition carried out through the institution of feasting, with increasing demand for both Mediterranean wine and native drinks and food. Competition would have continued to be particularly focused in the arena of feasting because this was the domain through which the colonial encounter was first articulated and in which challenges to status claims were first made.

Further support for this scenario may be derived from a consideration of the two new styles of pottery that began to be produced during the sixth century BC: Pseudo-Ionian and Grey-Monochrome. These are hybrid wares, combining imported production techniques (the wheel and controlled-draught kilns), imported decorative concepts, and some imported forms with native forms and motifs. This phenomenon of borrowing, once again, has most often been explained simply as a case of imitation through "Hellenisation" (Benoit 1965). However, things are not quite that simple. While it might be somewhat plausible to explain the imitation of Greek drinking forms in this way, the same is not true for the adoption of the potter's wheel. In fact, a suggestion that this stems from a desire to imitate the Greeks misses the point entirely. The adoption of this technique was not as simple a matter as importing Greek objects or copying Greek forms or decoration; it involved significant material costs. These included both permanent workshop equipment (such as the wheel, closed kilns, clay purification tanks, and storage facilities) as well as new specialized knowledge, and completely new motor skills. In brief, it involved a change in the basic organization of part of the ceramic industry from what, in the terminology of Peacock (1982) and van der Leeuw (1984) is called a "household industry" to a "workshop industry." I emphasize that this is a change only in part of the industry, because domestic cooking and storage pots continued to be made by the same methods as before. Such a development implies by its very nature a significant increase in demand for the range of ceramics produced by the new workshops, because an increased volume of production is the only advantage that the use of the wheel confers. An increase in demand can result from the development of new means of transport that allow the expansion of the demand catchment zone, or it can result from an increase in the consumption of such ceramics within the same local area. Since there is no evidence for the former, the latter is the more likely explanation. Considering that the range of forms produced in the new wares is almost entirely confined to Greek-style drinking cups and pitchers and native-derived tableware, it seems highly probable that this increase in demand is tied in with an inflation in the scale of feasting activities, which is also indicated by the evidence of the amphoras.

In summary, it seems that the nature of colonial interaction in the Hallstatt area can be explained primarily by reference to developments in the diacritical feast pattern of the classification of the political dimensions of feasting set up earlier; whereas colonial interaction in the south was manifest through the entrepreneurial feast pattern. Undoubtedly, commensal hospitality was also being manipulated in both the entrepreneurial and patron-role feast patterns in the Hallstatt area by various social groups and persons jockeying for position within the system of social stratification. However, Mediterranean objects were incorporated only into the diacritical feast sphere of activity. In the south, the latter pattern was not yet developed. Hence, it becomes easier to understand why no spectacular bronze vessels have been found in that region despite the fact that they probably all entered western Europe through the port of Massalia. The Pseudo-Ionian and Grey-Monochrome productions were not items destined for exclusive elite consumption. As with the imported amphoras, they are found on a wide variety of settlements of all types and sizes, and they are found in most domestic structures on those sites. Such a diacritical use of cuisine would have been inappropriate in the south French context, where power and status competition was pervasively carried out through the binding idiom of commensal hospitality.

Conclusion

In conclusion, I hope that this rather rapid and schematic dash through European prehistory has served at least to suggest two things of some utility within the multidisciplinary discussion of the issue of "food and the status quest" to which this volume is directed. First, archaeology does have the potential to contribute to an understanding of the long-term historical development of the ways in which food is employed in the quest for power and status. Secondly, an approach to archaeological data through the perspective of "commensal politics" has the potential to reveal significant new insights into social processes and relations in ancient societies. These are both avenues of research that have yet to be developed and exploited to any significant extent in archaeology; but given further conceptual and methodological refinements, they hold considerable promise of advancing understanding beyond current frontiers.

Notes

My hearty thanks to Polly Wiessner and Wulf Schiefenhövel for the invitation to participate in this most enjoyable encounter and for the lavish hospitality and transport provided by the Max Planck Gesellschaft. Thanks also to Polly for helpful editorial suggestions and the generous extension of her home and table. I am also most grateful to all my commensal companions for stimulating and enlightening discussion that took place in both the formal symposium and the numerous informal symposia (in the original sense) during our stay at the Ringberg castle.

1. The techniques being developed for the physico-chemical analysis of the organic contents of ancient vessels (Biers and McGovern 1990) hold considerable promise for improving our knowledge of culinary complexity, but this field is still in the preliminary experimental stages.
2. Given the diverse disciplinary backgrounds of participants in this volume, it is perhaps advisable to emphasize that I use the term "commensal" in its more literal, original sense (from Latin *com mensalis*) having to do with sharing a table, or eating together, rather than in its more specialized usage in biology. Needless to say, the table is simply a handy Eurocentric metaphor; people in many societies around the world eat together without this device.
3. Brian Hayden (this volume) employs a more inclusive range of activities under the rubric of feasting and develops a somewhat different typology of patterns. These differences do not necessarily indicate disagreement, but rather simply reflect our contrasting focuses of analysis on "commensal politics" versus the competitive use of food as a more generalized phenomenon.
4. The term "entrepreneurial feast" should not be misunderstood as some sort of crude formalist economic concept, nor as an attempt to distinguish a type of specialized feast involving openly aggressive contests (as distinct from, for example, a

"harmonious egalitarian" community celebration). I use the term metaphorically to refer to an effective political role of feast events of various kinds rather than necessarily to refer to the conscious intention of the hosts. While this role is sometimes fully, or at least partially, recognized by the participants, much of the effectiveness of this political mechanism derives from the fact that it often entails a kind of collective misrecognition or euphemization of the self-interested nature of the practice. Likewise, in using the term "competitive" I am not referring only to activities that involve an overt aggressive challenge. Prestige and free-floating power are always competitive in that they describe conditions of relative dominance and subordination between people. Hence, commensal politics is always competitive in its effects, even though the process may be thoroughly euphemized. I would maintain, for example, that celebratory feasts of community identity and unity are simultaneously arenas for entrepreneurial manipulation (see the earlier discussion of the nature of public ritual).

5. Of course, quotidian meals are also "ritualized" events. They are highly structured sequences of action that serve to shape the "habitus" of individuals, inculcating dispositions guiding practice and naturalizing the social order (Mauss 1936; Bourdieu 1977). They differ from more formal ritual events mainly in being less consciously public performances.
6. A more detailed and nuanced analysis of this pattern is, of course, necessary. At a minimum one ought to differentiate between service or table wares that would be associated with food and drink consumption and cooking pots that might, for example, simply indicate gender roles.
7. It is important to point out that a general increase in the complexity or elaborateness of the decoration of tablewares in comparison to cooking wares (or of ceramics in general in comparison to a previous period) is not necessarily an indication of the use of style in the development of diacritical feasts. This may simply be related to an increasing "complexity" of food consumption patterns (Douglas 1984) through symbolic emphasis on distinctions such as that between ritual and quotidian dining practice. The diacritical feast pattern rests on an exclusive sumptuary use of style in food consumption rituals by certain social groups or classes whatever the relative complexity of food patterns.

References

Appadurai, A. 1981. Gastropolitics in Hindu South Asia. *American Ethnologist* 8: 494-511.

Appadurai, A. 1986. Introduction: commodities and the politics of value. In *The Social Life of Things: Commodities in Cultural Perspective*. ed. A. Appadurai, 3-63. Cambridge: Cambridge Univer. Press.

Arcelin-Pradelle, C. 1984. *La céramique grise monochrome en Provence*. Supplement 10 of the Révue Archéologique de Narbonnaise. Paris: Boccard.

Athenaeus. *The Deipnosophists*, vol. II, trans. C. B. Gulick, 1928. London: Heinemann.

Barker, G. 1985. *Prehistoric Farming in Europe*. Cambridge: Cambridge Univer. Press.

Barlett, P. F. 1980. Reciprocity and the San Juan fiesta. *Journal of Anthropological Research* 36: 6-30.

Barth, F. 1967. On the study of social change. *American Anthropologist* 69: 661-70.

Bats, M. 1988. *Vaisselle et alimentation à Olbia de Provence, v. 350 – v. 50 av. J. C. : modèles culturels et catégories céramiques*. Supplement 18 of the Revue Archéologique de Narbonnaise. Paris: CNRS.

Bats, M., ed. 1990. *Les amphores de Marseille grecque*. Etudes Massaliètes 2. Lattes: A. D. A. M.

Bender, B. 1978. Gatherer-hunter to farmer: a social perspective. *World Archaeology* 10: 204-22.

Bender, B. 1985. Prehistoric developments in the American midcontinent and in Brittany, northwest France. In *Prehistoric Hunter-Gatherers: The Emergence of Cultural Complexity*, ed. T. D. Price and J. A. Brown, 21-57. New York: Academic Press.

Benoit, F. 1965. *Recherches sur l'hellénisation du Midi de la Gaule*. Aix-en-Provence: Annales de la Faculté des Lettres, no. 43.

Bertucchi, G. 1992. *Les amphores et le vin de Marseille, VIe s. avant J.-C. – IIe s. après J.-C.* Révue Archéologique de Narbonnaise, Supplément 25. Paris: CNRS.

Biel, J. 1985. Die Ausstattung des Toten. In *Der Keltenfürst von Hochdorf: Methoden und Ergebnisse der Landesarchäologie*, ed. D. Planck, J. Biel, G. Süsskind and A. Wais, 78-105. Stuttgart: Konrad Theiss.

Biers, W. B. and P. E. McGovern, eds. 1990. *Organic Contents of Ancient Vessels: Materials Analysis and Archaeological Investigation*. Philadelphia: MASCA Research Papers in Science and Archaeology, vol. 7.

Binford, L. R. 1980. Willow smoke and dogs' tails: hunter-gatherer settlement systems and archaeological site formation. *American Antiquity* 45: 4-20.

Binford, L. R. 1981. *Bones: Ancient Men and Modern Myths*. New York: Academic Press.

Binford, L. R. 1982. The archaeology of place. *Journal of Anthropological Archaeology* 1: 5-31.

Bonfante, L. 1981. *Out of Etruria: Etruscan Influence North and South*. Oxford: BAR International Series, no. 103.

Bouloumié, B. 1980. Recherches sur les importations étrusques en Gaule du VIIIième au IVième siècle avant J. C. Doctorat d'état dissertation, University of Paris.

Bouloumié, B. 1981. Le vin étrusque et la première hellénisation du Midi de la Gaule. *Revue Archéologique de l'Est et du Centre-Est* 32: 75-81.

Bouloumié, B. 1988. Le symposion gréco-étrusque et l'aristocratie celtique. In *Les princes celtes et la Méditerranée*, 343-83. Paris: La Documentation Française.

Bourdieu, P. 1977. *Outline of a Theory of Practice*. Cambridge: Cambridge Univer. Press.

Bourdieu, P. 1984. *Distinction: A Social Critique of the Judgment of Taste*. Cambridge, Mass.: Harvard Univer. Press.

Bradley, R. 1984. *The Social Foundations of Prehistoric Britain.* London: Longman.
Bradley, R. and M. Edmonds. 1993. *Interpreting the Axe Trade: Production and Exchange in Neolithic Britain.* Cambridge: Cambridge Univer. Press.
Brothwell, D. and P. Brothwell. 1969. *Food in Antiquity: A Survey of the Diet of Early Peoples.* New York: Praeger.
Burger, R. 1992. *Chavin and the Origins of Andean Civilization.* London: Thames and Hudson.
Burgess, C., P. Topping, C. Mordant and M. Maddison, eds. 1988. *Enclosures and Defences in the Neolithic of Western Europe.* Oxford: BAR International Series, no. 403.
Cancian, F. 1965. *Economics and Prestige in a Maya Community.* Stanford: Stanford Univer. Press.
Casati, 1891. *Ten Years in Equatoria and Return with Emin Pasha,* vol. 1. London: Frederick Warne and Co.
Clarke, D. L. 1976. Mesolithic Europe: the economic basis. In *Problems in Economic and Social Archaeology,* ed. G. Sieveking, I. H. Longworth, and K. E. Wilson, 449-81. London: Duckworth.
Clough, T. H. M. and W. A. Cummins, eds. 1979. *Stone Axe Studies.* London: Council for British Archaeology.
Codere, H. 1950. *Fighting with Property: A Study of Kwakiutl Potlatching and Warfare, 1792-1930.* Seattle: Univer. of Washington Press.
Cohen, A. 1974. *Two-Dimensional Man: An Essay on the Anthropology of Power and Symbolism in Complex Society.* Berkeley: Univ. of California Press.
Coles, J. M. and A. F. Harding. 1979. *The Bronze Age in Europe.* London: Methuen.
Dalton, G. 1978. The impact of colonization on aboriginal economies in stateless societies. *Research in Economic Anthropology* 1:131-84.
Dennell, R. 1983. *European Economic Prehistory: A New Approach.* New York: Academic Press.
Dentzer, J.-M. 1982. *Le motif du banquet couché dans le Proche-Orient et dans le monde grec du VIIe au IVe siècle avant J.-C.* Bibliothèque des Ecoles Françaises d'Athènes et de Rome, no. 246. Paris: Boccard.
De Waal, F. 1986. The integration of dominance and social bonding in primates. *The Quarterly Review of Biology* 61: 459-79.
De Waal, F. 1989. Food sharing and reciprocal obligations among chimpanzees. *Journal of Human Evolution* 18: 433-59.
Dietler, M. 1989. The work-party feast as a mechanism of labor mobilization and exploitation: the case of Samia iron production. Paper presented at the 88th Annual Meeting of the American Anthropological Association, Washington, D. C.
Dietler, M. 1990a. Driven by drink: the role of drinking in the political economy and the case of Early Iron Age France. *Journal of Anthropological Archaeology* 9: 352-406.
Dietler, M. 1990b. Exchange, Consumption, and Colonial Interaction in the Rhône Basin of France: A Study of Early Iron Age Political

Economy. Ph.D. Dissertation, Univer. of California, Berkeley.
Dietler, M. 1992. Commerce du vin et contacts culturels en Gaule au Premier Age du Fer. In *Marseille grecque et la Gaule*, (Etudes Massaliètes 3), ed. M. Bats, G. Bertucchi, G. Congès, and H. Tréziny, 401-10. Lattes: A. D. A. M Editions.
Dietler, M. 1995. Early "Celtic" socio-political relations: ideological representation and social competition in dynamic comparative perspective. In *Celtic Chiefdom, Celtic State*, ed. B. Arnold and D. B. Gibson, 64-71. Cambridge: Cambridge Univ. Press.
Douglas, M. 1984. Standard social uses of food: introduction. In *Food in the Social Order*, ed. M. Douglas, 1-39. New York: Russell Sage.
Douglas, M. and C. Isherwood. 1979. *The World of Goods: Towards an Anthropology of Consumption.* New York: Norton.
Elias, N. 1978. *The History of Manners.* (Original German language edition, 1939). New York: Pantheon.
Erasmus, C. J. 1956. Culture structure and culture process: the occurrence and disappearance of reciprocal farm labor. *Southwestern Journal of Anthropology* 12: 444-69.
Feil, D. K. 1984. *Ways of Exchange. The Enga Tee of Papua New Guinea.* St. Lucia: Univer. of Queensland Press.
Firth, R. 1983. Magnitudes and values in Kula exchange. In *The Kula: New Perspectives on Massim Exchange*, ed. J. W. Leach and E. Leach, 89-102. Cambridge: Cambridge Univer. Press.
Fischer, F. 1973. KEIMHΛIA. Bemerkungen zur kulturgeschichtlichen Interpretation des sogenannten Südimports in der späten Hallstatt- und frühen Latène-Kultur des westlichen Mitteleuropa. *Germania* 51: 436-59.
Frankenstein, S. and M. J. Rowlands. 1978. The internal structure and regional context of Early Iron Age society in southwestern Germany. *Bulletin of the Institute of Archaeology, London* 15: 73-112.
Friedman, J. 1984. Tribes, states, and transformations. In *Marxist Analyses and Social Anthropology*, ed. M. Bloch, 161-202. London: Tavistock.
Gamble, C. 1986. *The Paleolithic Settlement of Europe.* Cambridge: Cambridge Univer. Press.
Gantes, L.-F. 1990. Massalia retrouvée. *Les Dossiers d'Archéologie* 154: 14-21.
Geschire, P. 1982. *Village Communities and the State: Changing Relations Among the Maka of South-Eastern Cameroon Since the Colonial Conquest*, trans. J. Ravell. London: Kegan Paul.
Goody, J. 1982. *Cooking, Cuisine and Class: A Study in Comparative Sociology.* Cambridge: Cambridge Univer. Press.
Gras, M. 1983. Vin et société à Rome et dans le Latium à l'Epoque archaïque. In *Modes de contacts et processus de transformations dans les sociétés anciennes*, 1067-75. Rome: Collection de l'Ecole Française de Rome, no. 67.
Hawkes, C. F. C. and M. A. Smith. 1957. On some buckets and cauldrons of the Bronze and Early Iron Ages. *The Antiquaries Journal* 37: 131-98.

Hayden, B. 1990. Nimrods, piscators, pluckers, and planters: the emergence of food production. *Journal of Anthropological Archaeology* 9: 31-69.

Hayden, B. and R. Gargett. 1990. Big man, big heart? A Mesoamerican view of the emergence of complex society. *Ancient Mesoamerica* 1: 3-20.

Hayden, B. , B. Chisolm and H. P. Schwarcz. 1987. Fishing and foraging: marine resources in the Upper Paleolithic of France. In *The Pleistocene Old World: Regional Perspectives*, ed. O. Soffer, 279-92. New York: Plenum.

Heath, D. B. 1976. Anthropological perspectives on alcohol: an historical review. In *Cross-cultural Approaches to the Study of Alcohol: An Interdisciplinary Perspective*, ed. M. Everett, J. Waddell, and D. Heath, 41-101. The Hague: Mouton.

Hocart, A. M. 1916. The common sense of myth. *American Anthropologist* 1916: 307-18.

Hogbin, I. 1970. Food festivals and politics in Wogeo. *Oceania* 40: 304-28.

Hunter, M. 1961. *Reaction to Conquest: Effects of Contact with Europeans on the Pondo of Southern Africa*. London: Oxford Univer. Press.

Isaac, G. 1978a. The food sharing behavior of protohuman hominids. *Scientific American* 238: 90-106.

Isaac, G. 1978b. Food sharing and human evolution: archaeological evidence from the Plio-Pleistocene of East Africa. *Journal of Anthropological Research* 34: 311-25.

Jacobsthal, P. and E. Neuffer. 1933. Gallia Graeca: recherches sur l'hellénisation de la Provence. *Préhistoire* 2: 1-64.

Jacomet, S. and J. Schibler. 1985. Die Nahrungsversorgung eines jungsteinzeitlichen Pfynerdorfes am unteren Zürichsee. *Archäologie der Schweiz* 8: 125-41.

Jochim, M. 1976. *Hunter-gatherer Subsistence and Settlement: A Predictive Model*. New York: Academic Press.

Jochim, M. 1983. Paleolithic cave art in ecological perspective. In *Hunter-Gatherer Economy in Prehistory*, ed. G. N. Bailey, 212-19. Cambridge: Cambridge Univer. Press.

Joffroy, R. 1979. *Vix et ses trésors*. Paris: Librairie Jules Tallandier.

Kaberry, P. M. 1941-2. Law and political organization of the Abelam tribe, New Guinea. *Oceania* 12: 79-95, 209-25, 331-63.

Kaenel, G. 1985. Boire et manger à la fin de La Tène en Suisse occidentale. *Archäologie der Schweiz* 8: 150-59.

Kennedy, J. G. 1978. *The Tarahumara of the Sierra Madre: Beer, Ecology, and Social Organization*. Arlington Heights, Il. : AHM.

Kimmig, W. 1983. Die griechische Kolonisation im westlichen Mittelmeergebiet und ihre Wirkung auf die Landschaften des Westlichen Mitteleuropa. *Jahrbuch des Römisch-Germanischen Zentralmuseums Mainz* 30: 5-78.

Lagrand, C. 1963. La céramique "pseudo-ionienne" dans la vallée du Rhône. *Cahiers Rhodaniens* 10: 37-82.

Lemonnier, P. 1990. *Guerres et festins: paix, échanges et compétition dans les Highlands de Nouvelle-Guinée.* Paris: CID – Editions de la Maison des Sciences de l'Homme.

Le Tensorer, J.-M. 1985. L'alimentation à l'"Age de la Pierre Taillée", Paléolithique-Mésolithique. *Archäologie der Schweiz* 8: 118-24.

Mair, L. P. 1934. *An African People in the Twentieth Century.* New York: Russell and Russell.

Mandelbaum, D. 1965. Alcohol and culture. *Current Anthropology* 6: 281-93.

Marshall, F. 1993. Food sharing and the faunal record. In *From Bones to Behavior: Ethnoarchaeological and Experimental Contributions to the Interpretation of Faunal Remains*, ed. J. Hudson, 228-46. Carbondale: Southern Illinois Univer.

Mauss, M. 1936. Les techniques du corps. *Journal de Psychologie* 22: 363-86.

Mauss, M. 1966. *The Gift: Forms and Functions of Exchange in Archaic Societies*, trans. I. Cunnison (original 1925). London: Routledge and Kegan Paul.

Mellars, P. 1985. The ecological basis of social complexity in the Upper Paleolithic of southwestern France. In *Prehistoric Hunter-gatherers: The Emergence of Cultural Complexity*, ed. T. D. Price and J. A. Brown, 271-97. New York: Academic Press.

Merhart, G. von. 1969. *Hallstatt und Italien.* Mainz: Habelt Verlag.

Miller, D. 1985. *Artefacts as Categories: A Study of Ceramic Variability in Central India.* Cambridge: Cambridge Univer. Press.

Modjeska, N. 1982. Production and inequality: perspectives from central New Guinea. In *Inequality in New Guinea Societies*, ed. A. Strathern, 50-108. Cambridge: Cambridge Univer. Press.

Mohen, J.-P. 1986. Les festins préhistoriques. In *La table et le partage*, 131-144. Paris: La Documentation Française.

Morel, J.-P. 1981. Le commerce étrusque en France, en Espagne et en Afrique. In *L'Etruria mineraria: Atti del XII Covegno di Studi Etruschi e Italici, Firenze 1979*, 463-508. Florence: Leo Olschki.

Morel, J. -P. 1990. Marseille dans le mouvement colonial grec. *Les Dossiers d'Archéologie* 154: 4-13.

Morel, J. -P. 1992. Marseille dans la colonisation phocéenne. In *Marseille grecque et la Gaule*, Etudes Massaliètes 3, ed. M. Bats, G. Bertucchi, G. Congès, and H. Tréziny, 15-26. Lattes: A. D. A. M. Editions.

Müller-Karpe, H. 1959. *Beiträge zur Chronologie der Urnfelderzeit nördlich und südlich der Alpen.* Berlin: de Gruyter.

Murray, O. 1990. Sympotic history. In *Sympotica: A Symposium on the Symposion*, ed. O. Murray, 3-13. Oxford: Clarendon.

Pare, C. 1991. *Fürstensitze* Celts and the Mediterranean world: developments in the West Hallstatt Culture in the 6th and 5th centuries B.C. *Proceedings of the Prehistoric Society* 57: 183-202.

Paulik, J. 1962. Das Velatice-Baierdorfer Hügelgrab in Ockov. *Slovenská Archeológia* 10: 6-96.

Peacock, D. P. S. 1982. *Pottery in the Roman World: An Ethnoarchaeological Approach.* London: Longmans.

Polanyi, K. 1957. The economy as instituted process. In *Trade and Markets in the Early Empires*, ed. K. Polanyi, C. Arensberg, and H. Pearson, 243-69. New York: The Free Press.

Powdermaker, H. 1932. Feasts in New Ireland: the social function of eating. *American Anthropologist* 34: 236-47.

Price, T. D. 1985. Affluent foragers of Mesolithic Southern Scandinavia. In *Prehistoric Hunter-Gatherers: The Emergence of Cultural Complexity*, ed. T. D. Price and J. A. Brown, 341-63. New York: Academic Press.

Price, T. D. 1989. The reconstruction of Mesolithic diets. In *The Mesolithic in Europe*, ed. C. Bonsall, 48-59. Edinburgh: John Donald.

Pryor, F. 1977. *The Origins of the Economy: A Comparative Study of Distribution in Primitive and Peasant Economies.* New York: Academic Press.

Py, M. 1979-80. Ensayo de clasificación de un estilo de cerámica de Occidente: los vasos pseudojonios pintados. *Ampurias* 41-42: 155-202.

Py, M. 1985. Les amphores étrusques de Gaule méridionale. In *Il commercio etrusco arcaico*, ed. M. Cristofani, P. Moscati, G. Nardi, and M. Pandolfini, 73-94. Rome: Consiglio Nazionale delle Ricerche.

Py, M. 1990. *Culture, économie et société protohistoriques dans la region nîmoise*, 2 vols. Rome: Ecole Française de Rome.

Rehfisch, F. 1987. Competitive beer drinking among the Mambila. In *Constructive Drinking: Perspectives on Drink from Anthropology*, ed. M. Douglas, 135-45. Cambridge: Cambridge Univer. Press.

Renfrew, C. 1972. *The Emergence of Civilisation: The Cyclades and the Aegean in the Third Millennium B. C.* London: Methuen.

Renfrew, C. 1973. Monuments, mobilization and social organization in Neolithic Wessex. In *The Explanation of Culture Change: Models in Prehistory*, ed. C. Renfrew, 539-58. London: Duckworth.

Richards, A. 1939. *Land, Labour and Diet in Northern Rhodesia.* London: Oxford Univer. Press.

Robbins, R. H. 1973. Alcohol and the identity struggle: some effects of economic change on interpersonal relations. *American Anthropologist* 75: 99-122.

Rolley, C. 1982. *Les vases de bronze de l'archaïsme récent en Grande Grèce.* Naples: Centre Jean Bérard.

Rouillard, P. 1991. *Les Grecs et la péninsule ibérique du VIIIe au IVe siècle avant Jésus-Christ.* Publications du Centre Pierre Paris, 21. Paris: Diffusion de Boccard.

Rowley-Conwy, P. 1983. Sedentary hunters: the Ertebølle example. In *Hunter-Gatherer Economy in Prehistory*, ed. G. N. Bailey, 111-26. Cambridge: Cambridge Univer. Press.

Ruoff, U. 1985. Wegzehrung ins Jenseits? *Archäologie der Schweiz* 8: 142-49.

Sahlins, M. 1972. *Stone Age Economics.* London: Tavistock.

Salisbury, R. 1962. *From Steel to Stone: Economic Consequences of a Technological Change in New Guinea.* Melbourne: Melbourne Univer. Press.

Schapera, I. 1938. A *Handbook of Tswana Law and Custom.* London: Oxford Univer. Press.

Scheffler, H. W. 1965. *Choiseul Island Social Structure*. Berkeley: Univer. of California Press.

Shennan, S. J. 1993. Settlement and social change in Central Europe, 3500-1500 B.C. *Journal of World Prehistory* 7: 121-61.

Sherratt, A. 1986. Cups that cheered. In *Bell Beakers of the Western Mediterranean*, vol. 1, ed. W. H. Waldren and R. C. Kennard, 81-106. Oxford: BAR International Series, no. 331.

Smith, I. F. 1965. *Windmill Hill and Avebury*. Oxford: Oxford Univ. Press.

Startin, W. and R. Bradley. 1981. Some notes on work organization and society in prehistoric Wessex. In *Astronomy and Society During the Period 4000-1500 B.C.*, ed. C. Ruggles and A. Whittle, 289-96. Oxford: BAR.

Strathern, A. 1971. *The Rope of Moka: Big-men and Ceremonial Exchange in Mount Hagen, New Guinea*. Cambridge: Cambridge Univer. Press.

Strathern, A. 1982. Two waves of African models in the New Guinea Highlands. In *Inequality in New Guinea Societies*, ed. A. Strathern, 35-49. Cambridge: Cambridge Univer. Press.

Suttles, W. 1991. Streams of property, armor of wealth: the traditional Kwakiutl potlatch. In *Chiefly Feasts: The Enduring Kwakiutl Potlatch*, ed. A. Jonaitis, 71-133. Seattle: Univer. of Washington Press.

Taylour, W. 1983. *The Mycenaeans*. London: Thames and Hudson.

Tchernia, A. 1983. Italian wine in Gaul at the end of the Republic. In *Trade in the Ancient Economy*, ed. P. Garnsey and C. R. Whittaker, 87-104. London: Chatto and Windus.

Tosh, J. 1978. *Clan Leaders and Colonial Chiefs in Lango: The Political History of an East African Stateless Society c. 1800-1939*. Oxford: Clarendon.

Tringham, R. 1971. *Hunters, Fishers and Farmers of Eastern Europe, 6000 – 3000 B.C.* London: Hutchinson.

Van de Velde, P. 1985. Early state formation in Iron Age Central Europe. In *Development and Decline: The Evolution of Sociopolitical Organization*, ed. H. Claessen, P. van de Velde, and M. Smith, 170-82. South Hadley, Mass.: Bergin and Garvey.

Van der Leeuw, S. 1984. Dust to dust: a transformational view of the ceramic cycle. In *The Many Dimensions of Pottery*, ed. S. E. van der Leeuw and A. C. Pritchard, 707-92. Amsterdam: Univer. of Amsterdam.

Verger, S. and J.-P. Guillaumet. 1988. Les tumulus de Saint-Romain-de-Jalionas (Isère). Premières observations. In *Les princes celtes et la Méditerranée*, 231-40. Paris: La Documentation Française.

Villard, F. 1960. *La céramique grecque de Marseille (VIe-IVe siècle), essai d'histoire économique*. Bibliothèque des Ecoles Françaises d'Athènes et de Rome, no. 195. Paris: Bocard.

Villard, F. 1988. Des vases grecs chez les Celtes. In *Les princes celtes et la Méditerranée*, 333-41. Paris: La Documentation Française.

Volkman, T. A. 1985. *Feasts of Honor: Ritual and Change in the Toraja Highlands*. Urbana: Univer. of Illinois Press.

Voytek, B. and R. Tringham. 1989. Rethinking the Mesolithic: the case of south-east Europe. In *The Mesolithic in Europe*, ed. C. Bonsall, 492-99. Edinburgh: John Donald Publishers.

Washburne, C. 1961. *Primitive Drinking: A Study of the Uses and Functions of Alcohol in Preliterate Societies.* New York: College and Univer. Press.

Wells, P. 1980. *Culture Contact and Culture Change: Early Iron Age Central Europe and the Mediterranean.* Cambridge: Cambridge Univer. Press.

Whittle, A. 1985. *Neolithic Europe: A Survey.* Cambridge: Cambridge Univer. Press.

Young, M. 1971. *Fighting with Food: Leadership, Values and Social Control in a Massim Society.* Cambridge: Cambridge Univer. Press.

8. FEASTING IN PREHISTORIC AND TRADITIONAL SOCIETIES

Brian Hayden

Although feasting has featured prominently in a number of anthropological monographs (Codere 1950; Strathern 1971; Young 1971), it has not been an important focus of comparative or general theoretical interest either in anthropology or archaeology. Nor has feasting ever been accorded a particularly prominent role in evolutionary schemes. Yet, on the basis of work that I have conducted over the past ten years, I would like to explore the possibility that feasting, and particularly competitive feasting, may have played a pivotal role in cultural evolution. I suggest that competitive feasting was a critical mechanism in some societies whereby food surpluses were used to create debts, hierarchical and centralized political control, and increased production.

This system may have originated in favored locations during the Upper Paleolithic period; however, it appears to have become widespread only during the Mesolithic and subsequent food-producing periods. In fact, the competitive-feasting complex may have been the principal reason for the domestication of the first animals and plants. I suggest that economically-based competitive feasting occurred only under certain resource conditions, notably where resources were abundant and invulnerable to overexploitation. Individuals were induced to participate in competitive feasts on the basis of self-interest, i.e. the possibility of increasing their wealth, influence, or chances for survival.

In this paper, I will define competitive feasting, discuss the mechanics of feasting systems, identify the ways that such feasting systems can be recognized archaeologically, briefly note some prehistoric occurrences, and discuss implications for the emergence of competition, domestication and warfare.

Definition

While most, if not all, societies have feasts, not all feasts are competitive in nature. Among generalized hunter/gatherers (characterized by limited, fluctuating resources vulnerable to overexploitation), sharing and egalitarian ethics prevail. Obligatory sharing of food, a lack of private ownership in most spheres, and a proscription on ego-centered, self-aggrandisive behavior are typical of generalized hunter/gatherers, and are probably highly adaptive given the resource conditions of these groups. I have explored these relationships elsewhere (Hayden 1981, 1990a), and others before me have emphasized their importance (Lee 1972; Harris 1971; Winterhalder 1986). Feasts in these societies are exclusively celebratory or serve functions related to rituals and the creation of social bonds. There is no obvious, and usually not even implicit, competitive aspect to these feasts, and there is certainly no involvement of economic or subsistence elements in any competition. Competition that may exist at these feasts among egalitarian hunter/gatherers usually revolves around ritual knowledge and the ability to acquire mates. These characteristics provide the contrast necessary for viewing the competitive feasts as a distinctive phenomenon.

The competitive feast can be situated along a broad range of types of feasting, including the celebratory feast and others discussed by Michael Dietler in this volume. I use a slightly different feast classification from Dietler since competition and practical benefits are my main interest. At the broad level of general feasts, we can distinguish at least three major categories (see Figure 8.1). First are the "celebratory feasts" described above, held primarily in order to reinforce social bonding between individuals of approximately equal social standing. Often these are ritual in nature. Second are "reciprocal aid" or exchange work-party feasts. These generally involve meals after mutual aid in clearing land, sowing or harvesting crops, or in other types of work, such as barn raising. Third are the commensal (table) feasts. Within this group, the following types can be distinguished:

1. Economic feasts, which in turn can be broken down into competitive-productive feasts involving loans and interest in relation to food production, and "festive work-party feasts," where organizers try to attract people (labor) to work for them on a

one-time basis to accomplish a specific task that will benefit the organizers, such as gathering iron ore or smelting it.
2. Redistribution feasts, which seek to bond (or control) labor (people) to organizers on a more permanent basis than the festive work-party feast. In both cases material distributions are used to achieve the respective goals, although the quantities, value, and types of materials used are often quite different. Where control of labor is the key to wealth or military success, redistributive feasts become highly competitive.
3. Diacritical feasts are used to create exclusive elite circles that exclude lower classes, display status and belonging of the participants, and engage in rank competition within the group.

In reality pure forms of some of these feasts may be rare; in many cases feasts may exhibit several or all of the characteristics of the subtypes, differing only in relative emphasis on economic gain, control over labor, and diacritical displays. Competition for economic gain and control over labor very frequently occur together as feasting goals. For the remainder of the discussion I will treat them both as characteristics of what I shall refer to as "competitive feasts."

As I use the term, the competitive feast has four basic characteristics:

1. Economic: Competition in competitive feasts always has an economic basis. The group that can produce and marshal the greatest amount of food, the best-quality food, and the most skilled labor for producing or acquiring specialized exchange items is recognized as "winning" a competition. Other ways of competing often also occur in the competitive feast (e.g. ritual knowledge, oratory, gambling), but these other competitive domains do not play as fundamental a role as the economic ability to produce and use goods for competitive feasts.
2. Self-aggrandizement: Self-aggrandizing speeches and behavior are prominent either on the part of organizing individuals or host groups. Typically, speeches boast of the accomplishments of Big men, chiefs, clans, or communities. Prominent individuals attempt to demonstrate their superior strength by endurance tests involving smoking, drinking, pain, eating (e.g. consumption of oil), physical strength, or other similar displays. Frequently, dances and ritual displays involving elaborate costumes and orchestrated dancing also play an important part in the competitive displays.
3. Food competition: While many possible techniques can be employed to aggrandize one's self or one's group, food always

features prominently in competitive displays. Here, I employ a broad definition of food that includes drink and intoxicants. Food plays such a central role partly due to the definition of a feast; other competitive behaviors, such as competitive exchanges between individuals, can take place without the use of food. However, I would like to suggest that both the use of feasting foods and the larger group context inherent in feasts are recurrent, common elements because they serve the underlying purposes of the organizers and participants well. The appeal of delicacies and drink is used to draw individuals into participating in competitive feasts, while the emotional bonds created through the giving and accepting of valued foods serves to reinforce loyalties between supporters and organizers. These emotions may well have their roots in our primate heritage, where the giving and accepting of food is a sign of hierarchical relationships or mutual support. Moreover, if it is true that economic production is the underlying basis of competition in competitive feasts, it would be natural to compete directly using food as well as the products that abundant surpluses could provide in the form of specialist craft products and trade items.

4. Practical self-interest motivations: The ultimate purpose of organizing competitive feasts and participating in them is to provide practical benefits. Although reasons for participating in these feasts are often couched in terms that appeal to higher and more noble values, practical benefits for participants and especially organizers are always relatively apparent. By practical benefits, I refer to (1 direct material gains in the form of "gifts" or returns on investments, (2) indirect benefits such as increases in power or control within communities, and (3) less obvious benefits of attracting highly skilled or industrious labor to the labor pool of participating families, kin groups, or communities on the understanding that they will make contributions to the group in exchange for benefits that the group can provide. I distinguish all of these practical benefits from the frequently mentioned aim in ethnographic works of increasing one's status (equated with renown or prestige, e.g., Young 1971: 211), which by itself seems to have only a psychologically soothing benefit rather than any benefit of practical nature.

Thus, critical characteristics of the competitive feasts are the economic basis of competition, self-aggrandizing behavior, the prominent role of food, and expectations of practical benefits. How precisely does the competitive feast translate into practical benefits? In order to deal with this question, a more detailed examination of the mechanics of competitive feasting is required.

Mechanics of Feasting

In order to understand the function of the competitive feast, several important factors must be taken into consideration. First, the competitive feast is predicated upon the availability of, or potential for, food surpluses. Second, given such conditions, there will always be a few individuals who will recognize that a vast untapped source of wealth and power exists because of those surpluses. From an ecological point of view, we can expect some individuals to attempt to exploit any new or untapped source of energy. The primary problem that ambitious individuals would have faced when starting out in egalitarian communities would have been, first, how to get people to produce surpluses, i.e. to do more work than necessary for their own subsistence needs; and, secondly, how to concentrate the benefits of those surpluses in the hands of the ambitious. I have called such ambitious individuals "accumulators" (Hayden and Gargett 1990), while others have called them "aggrandizers" (Gould 1982; Clark and Blake 1991), or "acquisators" (Benedict 1934). To accommodate all these terms, one might refer to these people as individuals with "Triple A" personalities. Whatever one chooses to call them, aggressively ambitious personalities regularly arise in small numbers in all societies. In the truly egalitarian societies exemplified by generalized hunter/gatherers, their competitive activities are severely curtailed. It is only under conditions of nearly guaranteed subsistence and surpluses that Triple A personality types are allowed to unfold their ambitious socioeconomic games.

While there may be alternate solutions to the problems of how to induce surplus production and how to control some of that surplus, I would like to argue that the competitive feast provided one of the most obvious and effective vehicles that Triple A individuals could devise to achieve this and other goals. As a result, in favorable economic conditions throughout the world, competitive feasting emerged, to benefit organizers and participants alike.

Starting from an egalitarian basis as represented by generalized hunter/gatherers, there are few means by which single individuals or even groups of individuals can establish control over anyone else's labor or surplus. Control cannot be established by means of force, kinship, or supernatural threats. Individuals targeted for control will simply either walk away or band together and get rid of those trying to impose control. In contrast, a highly effective means of concentrating control in one's own hands is the establishment of contractual debts freely entered into under individual volition. Effective contractual arrangements involving material goods depend to a large degree on the recognition of individual ownership of goods, especially resources.

While contractual relationships could provide the basis for Triple A individuals to concentrate power in their own hands, they would also have needed a means to lure individuals into these contractual relationships and a means to achieve some advantage over others in these contractual arrangements. I suggest that typical contracts consisted of loans or "gifts" of highly valued foods or other goods that the partner in the contract agreed to pay back, together with a supplement for the privilege of using the materials loaned. Many anthropologists and popular writers have emphasized the "gift" aspect of competitive feasts such as in the potlatch and Maya cargo feasts, making competitive feasts seem like irrational, economically self-destructive behavior for which the only reward was an increase in social status with no practical benefits. However, Mauss (1954: 1) long ago pointed out that these prestations are only voluntary and altruistic in some emic idealistic views. In reality, the return of the loaned materials is obligatory, while the entire contractual arrangement is based on economic self-interest.

It is precisely economic self-interest that Triple A individuals (ambitious, aggressive accumulators/aggrandizers/acquirers) use as the main lure to engage others in contractual relationships. Not only does the reciprocal competitive feast establish a network of debts that skillful manipulators can control to various extents, but it also motivates – even requires – individuals to produce surpluses well beyond what they require for their own subsistence needs.

These contractual agreements can provide very enticing economic benefits. According to the terms of the agreement, there is always supposed to be a supplement when loans are repaid. This, in effect, provides the person making the loan with something for nothing – an automatic increase in their net wealth. In addition, it allows industrious individuals to produce and invest large amounts of wealth that they do not have to worry about storing, caring for, or preventing from spoiling. This, in turn, frees those making the loans to produce even more surpluses, thereby steadily increasing their own net wealth.

From the borrower's point of view, the benefits of entering into a contract involve the ability to use someone else's capital to obtain objectives, such as marriage, or to make loans and to try to derive a benefit from those investments above what eventually will be owed.

For instance, I may borrow five pigs with a promise to return seven pigs in one year, and then use the five pigs as loans to other people to try to obtain eight pigs within the year, yielding a net increase of one pig for myself for a minimal amount of work. Contemporary banks use this same strategy in charging differential interest rates on borrowings and loans, keeping the difference for themselves. Another reason for borrowers to enter into these agreements is that after they pay back the person who originally loaned them five pigs, the roles generally become reversed, and it is the partner who now receives seven pigs and must return these, plus another supplement of several additional pigs or something else of equivalent value.

Obviously, if this cycle were to continue, the world would soon be overrun with pigs, and people would be incapable of supporting them. Thus, equivalencies are established in terms of rare or labor-intensive nonconsumable items that are generally referred to as "primitive valuables" or "prestige items" or other similar terms. These prestige items can be substituted for value foods whenever this is desired. From time to time, valuable foods are also consumed in special contexts.

Getting something for nothing and getting other people to do one's producing for oneself have always been effective lures for getting people to enter into contractual agreements. For many people they are still irresistible, as modern-day advertisers and con artists who offer free gifts to their targets are well aware. These same lures operate in traditional societies, as is more than apparent in Strathern's (1971) description of the *moka* system in New Guinea, and Boas's (1897, 1921) and Codere's (1950) descriptions of the potlatch among the Kwakiutl of British Columbia. All of these authors use modern economic terms such as "credit", "investment", and "interest" to describe these systems. They make explicit comparisons between these traditional "gift-giving" systems and modern economic practices of "high finance".

Typically, the supplement or "interest", expected on a loan is quite high, ranging from 50 percent to 100 percent, or even much higher for risky loans. Given the inherently inflationary nature of these systems, families are frequently pushed to their maximum willingness to produce surpluses in order to avoid defaulting on debts. Defaulting can result in the rupture of relationships between families, clans, and communities, which carry important economic, political, marital, and defense consequences. These can be in the form of outright retaliation or simply lack of support for important undertakings; few people would risk involvement with families that were obvious failures. However, as ethnographers clearly illustrate, actual interest gained from loans was frequently far below what was expected, and total defaulting on loans was not unknown, resulting in bitter disputes. In the event of losing one's investment due to defaulting or bad luck, it would simply be necessary to begin working again to replace the lost investment. If one wanted to retain a position in the competitive feasting system and maintain a good credit reputation, it would be necessary to work doubly hard to ensure that full contractual expectations were honored, and to produce the surplus necessary for starting up the loan cycle again. Thus, Triple A personalities often might end up working much harder than other individuals in the community if things did not turn out favorably for them; however, they might also reap great benefits if luck, climate, and the gods were favorable. Everyone involved clearly must have recognized the risks involved, just as modern investors in stock markets recognize the risks they take when buying stocks. However, the lure of potential large increases in wealth was, and remains, irresistible for many people.

Contractual agreements can and do occur on an individual-to-individual basis without involving competitive feasting. However, as far as I know, the competitive feast occurs in all tribal societies where contractual agreements occur, and therefore we should suspect that competitive feasts have important advantages. The advantages I perceive are that competitive feasts enable Triple A individuals to lure a much wider range of people into contractual or semi-contractual agreements by adding the lure of free delicacies, spectacular entertainment rituals, socially exciting dances, and the possibilities of receiving unusual items for adornment or other purposes as gifts. Triple A individuals seem to use all the psychological means at their disposal to create an appealing event, and then try to extract promises of contributions from supporters and participants to produce the event. Ambitious organizers use appealing feasts as "hooks" to engage others in contractual agreements. The great volumes of materials amassed for loaning and consumption at these events also enable organizers to retain considerable amounts for themselves when the feasts are successful and, just as important, to enable them to develop a much more widespread degree of control in community affairs due to the large numbers of debts that are generated and the central role of organizers in the debt structure.

In all such events, a certain amount of the profit from investments or recruited labor is used for consumption or as giveaways. This provides a "lure" for people to attend feasts, and a taste of even greater advantages if they become more active supporters and contribute more energetically to contractual arrangements and future feasts. This is why, even today, aggressive cults and fund-raising groups try to recruit people or their labor by initially offering them "free" meals.

The organizers then use acceptance of their meal as an indication of an implicit agreement to render a service or donation to the group.

Gosden (1989) has argued that in subsistence economies, labor is often the major constraint to the production of wealth. Clearly, committed labor in the form of contractual partners and supporters for competitive feasts frequently appears to be the key to success. The more important labor is, the higher the interest rates should be in contractual relations, and the more lavish should be the gifts that are bestowed on supporters and participants in order to entice producers into contributing to the events and to lure them from other communities or groups also seeking to attract productive individuals. Ability to give goods or benefits is probably a major criterion in a group's ability to attract and keep productive wives, while the deaths of important group figures are used as prime opportunities to display group wealth and initiate additional contracts. The ability to give is constantly cited by ethnographers as an important characteristic of Big Men and chiefs.

I suspect that labor is most critical for corporate groups such as those in the American Northwest Interior and Coast, and that societies organized into corporate groups therefore tend to give away much more without an immediate expectation of return. However, once individuals commit themselves to joining either corporate groups or feasting support groups, they are expected to make substantial contributions, and to organize others in their kin groups to contribute in order to receive benefits themselves. In this manner, although a great deal can be consumed or given away at feasts, even more is expected to be produced as a result of luring productive labor to one's group and establishing contractual commitments to produce certain amounts of surplus goods.

In order to legitimize competitive activities involving surpluses of initially egalitarian communities, Triple A individuals need to make them seem attractive to large segments of their community (hence the lure of attractive potential benefits) and to couch the events in respectable contexts. Since celebratory religious feasts are common among most egalitarian societies, these probably provided the respectable initial context for developing competitive feasts. Such ritual feasts also provided a means of attracting participants and displaying the success, wealth, or power of host groups via rich costumes, orchestrated dances, and dramatic rituals. The strengthening of social bonds among participants in celebratory feasts could also be manipulated to serve the goals of Triple A organizers. The advantages of organizing the feasts in terms of loans and debts, and the advantages of being able to use supernatural authority to encourage support of competitive feasts are most likely the reasons behind the recurrent pattern of 'Triple A personalities' also assuming the most important ritual roles in their communities, whether they are house chiefs on the Northwest Coast of Noth America or Big Men in New Guinea. Ritual and religion were essentially used as pretexts. Such individuals could conceivably even turn defaulted loans to their advantage by offering debt cancellations in return for rights to the owned resources or important services of the defaulters.

There are many other implications of the model of competitive feasts, but they would be difficult to explore given the constraints of this chapter. Some of them include recourse to open conflict in the face of major defaulting, thus engendering endemic conflict and competition over surpluses even within communities or between allied communities; the progressive disenfranchisement of members of the community who do not participate in competitive feasts or presentations, resulting in the emergence of proto-elites vs. a poor, denigrated segment of communities; the development of craft specialization and prestige display art; record-keeping and numeration systems ranging into the hundreds or thousands; the attempt to use successful ancestors as links to supernatural and hence temporal authority and power; polygyny among successful competitors; the emergence of fragile or easily offended egos; pressure to increase the local labor and productive forces, i.e. strong motivations for the first time in history to have large numbers of children and to engage in public projects that would increase yields such as irrigation, terracing, and drainage projects.

The preceding discussion presents in brief outline form the mechanics of the competitive feast. It is ultimately a means of generating surpluses and turning them into material and political advantages for those that are most skillful in manipulating the economic and social factors central to its operation. It is based on a system of loan investments and/or recruitment of the labor into corporate groups or support groups that make such investments as a group. In its most common form, the system is predicated on reciprocal exchanges and the return of "gifts" plus supplements. To default on such contracts is to declare hostilities and to become "rubbish" unworthy of support in any other endeavors. If every participant honors all of their contractual agreements, everyone should benefit economically, and this is the lure of the system.

Archaeological Recognition of Competitive Feasts

Given these characteristics, how can the development of the competitive feast be traced in terms of cultural evolution? Reciprocal contractual agreements with supplements paid on loans are impossible to directly document in the archaeological record, yet these are the central features of the competitive feast. Thus, in order to trace the development of the competitive feast it is necessary to employ more indirect indicators, such as those associated with the actual production, exchange, and consumption of items used in the feasts. It is fortunate for archaeologists that food and prestige items provide the ultimate base for making the competitive feast function, because these are precisely the kinds of remains that archaeologists deal with. Six different categories of archaeological remains can be used to indicate the presence of competitive feasts: (1) abundant resource bases capable of providing surpluses, (2) special foods used for feasting, (3) special vessels used for serving feasting food, (4) the use of prestige items that food surpluses could be converted into, (5) the occurrence of special grounds or structures where feasting events could be held, and (6) the occurrence of Triple A individuals having more wealth and influence than others in the community. I will briefly discuss these six lines of evidence.

Resource Characteristics

On the basis of empirical ethnographic generalizations and theoretical considerations, competitive feasting should occur only where the resource base is abundant and invulnerable to overexploitation. Competitive feasting is found only among complex rather than generalized hunter/gatherers; complex hunter/gatherers are characterized by abundant and invulnerable resources. Examples include the Northwest Coast cultures, the Calusa of Florida, and the Jomon of Japan. Most tribal horticulturalists rely on even richer invulnerable resources. Resources can be evaluated either directly by estimating their abundance for given environments, or they can be estimated indirectly by estimating human population (and dependent livestock) densities and degrees of sedentism for specific localities.

Special Foods

In order to lure people into participating in feasts, and in order to create the greatest debts possible, surplus foods used both for consumption and for investment at feasts emphasize foods that are the rarest, most difficult to procure, or most labor-intensive to produce. Highly labor-intensive preparations also are frequently involved. These foods are the delicacies, and generally the richest, largest, sweetest, and most succulent foods that can be obtained by specific groups. I have argued elsewhere (Hayden 1990a) that the domesticated pigs of New Guinea are valued much more highly than wild pigs because they are specially fattened by yams. These pigs therefore represent a considerable labor investment, and because of their higher fat content which is highly desired by all hunter/gatherers (Speth and Spielman 1983) and may well be part of an evolutionary "taste" for rich food, I conclude that they are much more desirable. The same argument can be made about domesticated cattle, about the specially grown clover and cinquefoil roots for feasts on the Northwest Coast, and about most other important foods in competitive feasting. In the competitive feasts among the Highland Maya of Mexico that I have studied, maize is not only a valued food, but for feasting purposes it is ground to an exceedingly fine paste requiring many more hours of grinding than normal. The paste is then strained through a specialized fine ceramic sieve, and then made into a special ritual food called *atole*, which is sometimes mixed with other special foods such as ground cacao or honey. Specialized foods can often be recognized archaeologically on the basis of their occurrence outside normal habitat ranges, of genetic transformations resulting from breeding or rearing, of unusual size, and of unusual preparations.

Feasting foods as well as actual feasts themselves can often be recognized by copious food leftovers and much greater wastage than usual (Mercer 1985: 100); this is often observed even in the context of contemporary feasting (Wilson 1989). For example, animal bones often are not completely broken up for marrow, and may not even be completely disarticulated, and feasting refuse tends to occur in considerable quantities in single deposits.

Special Vessels and Features

Special vessels, implements, and facilities are frequently required for producing feasting types of foods in feasting quantities. I have already mentioned one example involving the special strainers of the Maya used to make atole, which is also cooked in special, large-sized cooking vessels. Dietler (1990) provides other examples of specialized vessels used for brewing large quantities of beer for feasts and work groups. Large earth ovens for cooking pork during New Guinea feasts are examples of special facilities.

Although these examples can sometimes be difficult to identify archaeologically, special serving vessels are very common in competitive feasts and are easy to identify where they are made of materials that preserve well. Large-size, elaborately decorated, and/or difficult-to-obtain materials are frequently used for serving vessels and utensils in order to impress participants and guest/competitors with the importance of the events and to impress them with the success, wealth, or high quality of labor of the host group. At a slightly more advanced level of cultural development, Clark and Parry (1990) and Underhill (1991) have shown that competitive aspiring chiefs sponsor the manufacture of elaborate serving vessels because these items are so prominent in feasts and displays of wealth and status. Such items can even be used as part of the competitive gift exchange. Examples include the elaborate wood and horn bowls used to hold grease on the Northwest Coast as well as large food serving and eating vessels of this area, and special large gourds on ritually woven supports for serving atole among the Maya as well as carefully carved or painted versions of these gourds. In fact, the remarkable Peten polychrome vessels of the Classic Maya period appear to be direct analogs of contemporary painted and carved gourd vessels used in ritual contractual relationships and competitive feasting. Recently, Clark and Blake (1990) have argued that the earliest ceramics that occur in Mexico were used as status items for serving foods by high-status individuals at important events, such as feasts. These early ceramics are very finely made, requiring considerable skilled labor, and they include dish forms as well as tecomate forms that imitate the shape of gourds that are used to serve atole today. Similar arguments can be advanced for early ceramic assemblages in many parts of the world as well as in our own contemporary culture, where fine china is still used for important feasting occasions. The finely carved wood bowls of Melanesia, and intricate, labor-intensive baskets of the American Southwest and West Coast provide further examples of prestige containers. Unfortunately, wooden and gourd vessels do not preserve very well although it is sometimes possible to determine that these materials were being used because of the appearance of domesticated (unusually large) gourds or the use of lacquer, as among the Jomon assemblages in Japan.

Prestige Items

Limits on how much surplus food can be produced, stored, or consumed; the inherent inflation of competitive feasting; and the desire of Triple A individuals to increase debts and profits mandate that food value be convertible into some other form of value, generally a nonperishable material. This is a very significant development that sets human cultures apart from those of other primates. In virtually all competitive feasting contexts, "primitive valuables" or prestige items play extremely important roles. Shells, especially the difficult-to-obtain dentalium shells, often are featured prominently. However, other items generally include elaborately carved stone, ivory, bone, horn, or antler; objects fashioned of native copper; special ceramics; and labor-intensive ceremonial tools such as jade axes and decorated maces. In order to obtain rare materials, regional exchange networks become established. These are among the most visible components of most competitive feasting systems for archaeologists, even though if they were considered in isolation, it would be difficult to distinguish competitive feasting origins of these exchange patterns from simple direct exchange for practical purposes (Pires-Ferreira and Flannery 1976; Rappaport 1968). When considered with other indicators, however, the competitive feasting origin of certain regional exchange networks and prestige items should be more apparent.

Feasting Facilities

One clear expectation of the competitive feasting model is that some feasting facility ought to be present. These may simply be open-air feasting grounds for large feasts such as in Mexico, Amazonia, Turkey, and New Guinea; however, special structures at least for the highest-ranking competitors can be expected to be found in many communities. These specialized feasting structures may occur only where the common residence pattern is of independent nuclear or small extended families. Where residential corporate groups dominate the community, as on the Northwest Coast and among the Iroquois, it is generally the corporate residence that is used as a feasting structure, with the most successful and wealthy corporate groups having the largest and most spacious structures.

Where residential corporate groups are not large or strong, the special feasting structures used by organizers may consist of temporary shelters; men's houses or special sacrificial houses, as in New Guinea; unusually large Big-men's or chief's residences; and specialized "ritual" structures whose primary function I believe was for competitive feasting, e.g., Neolithic enclosures. Unfortunately, archaeological excavations have rarely occurred on a scale sufficient to identify or even detect feasting structures or open-air grounds. Even worse, the material description of these facilities by ethnographers has generally been totally inadequate for archaeologists to be able to create material models of such structures or to make any estimates as to where within communities these facilities should occur and what their relationship to cooking or refuse facilities for feasts might be.

Triple-A-Personality Expression

Finally, in situations where competitive feasting and contractual loans are important, archaeologists expect to find material evidence of strong Triple A personalities together with the accumulations of wealth and power that they strive to obtain. Burial evidence of acquired status involving lavish burial goods and unusual burial treatment are the most common indicators of the existence of such individuals. However, the existence of unusually large structures of successful feasters, some craft specialization, and the emergence of some form of site hierarchy can also be used as indicators.

Prehistoric Competitive Feasts

While none of the above indicators might be used alone to convincingly argue for the existence of competitive feasting systems in the past, the occurrence of a number of these indicators together provides much more compelling grounds for arguing that such systems did exist. Due to the vagaries of preservation, excavation sampling, and cultural choices in these areas, we cannot always expect all indicators to be present before identifying a prehistoric competitive feasting system. However, this is standard procedure for all polythetic typologies, which is probably the type of classification most frequently used archaeologically and ethnographically.

Certainly, one of the best candidates for a prehistoric competitive feasting system is the European Neolithic. In this case, (1) an abundant invulnerable resource base can be identified (developed domestic plants and animals that had become cost-competitive in relation to wild foods), (2) special hunted or grown foods can be identified (e.g., the most labor-intensive domesticated animals and plants such as cattle and wheat), (3) ceramic vessels may have been used primarily for feasting, (4) regional exchange networks clearly existed, involving celts, maceheads, jet, and amber, (5) feasting sites have been identified within causewayed enclosures and in front of and inside megalithic tombs with copious feasting refuse, and (6) Triple A individuals are buried in the megalithic tombs, in some instances accompanied by high-status items such as ceremonial axes. In some areas, it is also possible to argue for settlement hierarchies, while the massive size of some of the enclosures, such as Avebury, indicate a remarkable degree of competition and a staggering degree of control over large amounts of surplus labor. The conflict and emphasis on ancestors that also tends to accompany developed competitive feasting systems is also evident in the European Neolithic.

On the basis of analogies with the American Northwest Coast cultures, I think it is highly probable that competitive feasting systems also were operating in the rich coastal and riverine environments of Mesolithic Europe, where fish, deer, sea mammals, and shellfish provided an abundant, invulnerable resource base. The archaeological evidence is much more sparse than for the Neolithic due to preservational factors, however, regional exchange networks are clearly in evidence, as is an appropriate resource base revealed by high site densities. In many Mesolithic-type cultures elsewhere in the world, such as the Jomon of Japan and the Natufian of the Levant, there are other indicators of competitive feasting types of systems. In the Jomon, the larger settlements are characterized by "ritual" plazas suitable for feasting events, and at these sites some individuals are given special treatment in slab-lined tombs. Foods include many delicacies and condiments that people took special efforts to produce; and lacquered vessels also are present. Regional exchange was strong, and there are numerous ritual or prestige items, including phallic scepters and prestige ceramics (Hayden 1990a).

Before the Mesolithic, the evidence becomes less clear. However, I would like to at least suggest that a few of the Upper Paleolithic communities living in the richest environments, harvesting seemingly inexhaustible herds of caribou and other animals, probably also developed competitive feasting systems similar to those of the Northwest Coast, although they were more mobile. The elaborately carved prestige items of the Upper Paleolithic imply private ownership, socioeconomic inequality, competition, craft specialization, and the acquisition of great wealth by some individuals or groups. The sharp increase in site densities and component thickness during the late Upper Paleolithic reflect an abundant resource base. Elsewhere, (Hayden 1990b, 1993) I have suggested that the major form of wealth may have been the labor-intensive production of dried storable meat together with buckskin, which is also labor-intensive to produce.

Implications

On the basis of ethnographic comparisons, it seems clear that private ownership of procured resources and ownership of resource procurement locations and personal items is not characteristic of generalized hunter/gatherers. It is only among complex hunter/gatherers using abundant and invulnerable resources that private ownership and competitive feasts seem to occur. Perhaps storage of seasonal surpluses facilitates these developments, but, storage does not appear to be the critical element, as indicated by the Calusa, who did not store food on a significant scale (Widmer 1988). There is no indication that complex hunter/gatherers, private ownership, storage, economically based competition, or competitive feasting occurred anywhere prior to the Upper Paleolithic; in the Upper Paleolithic these occurrences must have been restricted to only a few favored localities. In the Mesolithic, with a new suite of technological inventions that expanded resources, especially involving fish and grains, complex hunter/gatherers became much more common in many different environments.

It is at this point, I suggest, that competitive feasting became relatively common. And it is at this point that the first domesticates begin to appear in the archaeological record, a development that is probably far from coincidental. In fact, due to the labor-intensive nature of initial domesticates, the motivation in competitive feasts to produce bigger, richer, more succulent foods, and the ability of the system to motivate people to produce foods requiring extra labor investment, initial domestication can be viewed as a direct outcome of competitive feasting in environments favorable to the raising of animals and growing of plants (Hayden 1990a). In all the ethnographic descriptions of competitive feasts that I have examined, emphasis is always on the labor-intensive aspect of the foods used in the feast. Anyone who has gardened without the benefit of modern fertilizers and tools will readily appreciate what is involved in producing unusually large varieties of food or varieties with other desirable characteristics.

While the production of larger and richer foods was initially far too labor-intensive for such foods to be used for daily domestic consumption, genetic selection over time and the development of farming and animal raising techniques probably eventually made some of these labor-intensive feasting foods cost-competitive in relation to naturally occurring wild foods. It would have been at this point that the use of domesticated food would have intensified and spread much more widely, as in the European Neolithic expansion. At this point, too, Triple A individuals would have had to find or develop other kinds of labor-intensive or rare foods to use as lures in their competitive feasts. This same process is followed throughout the world even today. Elites are constantly developing desirable, labor-intensive or rare materials, including foods, to distinguish themselves from others and to provide motivation for participating in competitive organizations. Elites know that many people will compete to obtain the "best" that is available. Because these items are widely desired, other entrepreneurs are constantly seeking ways to make them available to more and more people, eventually developing technologies that substantially reduce costs. Thus, aluminium, plastics, and complex industrial goods like automobiles all began as labor-intensive elite consumable items and became commonplace items as the technologies were refined. Similar developments can be seen with elite exotic food fads in contemporary society, and this undoubtedly occurred in prehistoric times, although at a much slower pace.

Competitive feasts are thus primarily mechanisms for converting surpluses in subsistence economies into wealth and power. As such, I would argue that they probably continued to function at the level of the general populace, in one form or another, right up until the establishment of military power, taxes, and the absolute authority associated with the emergence of state types of organization. With increasing complexity and size of political organisation, competitive feasts probably have become increasingly concentrated and restricted to the elites and their administrators. In the Maya area, for instance, there were two levels of feasting. The highest-ranking members of the political system held feasts among themselves, and they required prospective candidates trying to advance in the political hierarchy to hold more public feasts. The success of the candidates in procuring and organizing supporters, including financial support, was used as an important criterion for determining who would obtain higher political positions. Similar arrangements probably characterized many chiefdoms. Even in contemporary Industrial society, promotion may depend in part on the display of competence and achievement through the holding of business or political dinner feasts with appropriate displays of prestige items and socially accepted self-aggrandizement. To the extent that such dinners or parties are used as criteria for promotion to desirable or powerful positions, they constitute competitive battlegrounds for Triple A personalities, and they can be considered as a special industrial type of competitive feast. On the other hand, the introduction into traditional communities of wage labor and individually run businesses such as village shops has generally been the death knell of the subsistence-based community competitive feasting in the Maya Highlands and elsewhere.

References

Benedict, R. 1934. *Patterns of culture*. Boston: Houghton Mifflin.
Boas, F. 1897. The social organization and the secret societies of the Kwakiutl Indians. *Report of the U.S. National Museum for 1895*. Washington, D.C.
Boas, F. 1921. Ethnology of the Kwakiutl, parts I and II. *Bureau of American Ethnology* 35.
Clarke, J. and M. Blake. 1990. The development of early formative ceramics in the Soconusco, Chiapas, Mexico. Paper presented at the

55th annual meeting of the Society for American Archaeology, Las Vegas.

Clarke, J. and M. Blake. 1991. The power of prestige: competitive generosity and the emergence of rank societies in lowland Mesoamerica. In *Factional Competition and Political Development in the New World*, ed. E. Brumfiel and J. Fox. Cambridge: Cambridge Univer. Press (forthcoming).

Clark, J. and W. Parry. 1990. Craft specialization and cultural complexity. *Research in Economic Anthropology* 12: 289-346.

Codere, H. 1950. *Fighting with Property*. Seattle: Univer. of Washington Press.

Dietler, M. 1990. Driven by drink: the role of drinking in the political economy and the case of early Iron Age France. *Journal of Anthropological Archaeology* 9: 352-406.

Gosden, Ch. 1989. Debt, production, and prehistory. *Journal of Anthropological Archaeology* 8: 355-87.

Gould, R. 1982. To have and have not: The ecology of sharing among hunter-gatherers. In *Resource Managers: North American and Australian Hunter-Gatherers*, , ed. N. Williams & E. Hunn, 69-92. Australian Institute of Aboriginal Studies: Canberra.

Harris, M. 1971. *Culture, Man and Nature*. New York: Crowell.

Hayden, B. 1981. Research and development in the stone age: technological transitions among hunter/gatherers. *Current Anthropology* 22: 519-48.

Hayden, B. 1990a. Nimrods, piscators, pluckers, and planters: the emergence of food production. *Journal of Anthropological Archaeology* , 9: 31-69.

Hayden, B. 1990b. The right rub: hide working in high ranking households. In *The Interpretative Possibilities of Microwear Studies* 14, ed. B. Graslund, 89-102. Uppsala: Societas Archaeologica Upsaliensis.

Hayden, B. 1993. The cultural capacities of Neanderthals. *Journal of Human Evoluition* 24:113-46.

Hayden, B. and R. Gargett. 1990. Big man, big heart? A Mesoamerican view of the emergence of complex society. *Ancient Mesoamerica* 1: 3-20.

Lee, R. 1972. Work effort, group structure and land use in contemporary hunter-gatherers. In *Man, Settlement and Urbanism*, ed. P. Ucko, R. Tringham, and G. W. Dimbleby, 177-85. London: Gerald Duckworth and Co., Ltd.

Mauss, M. 1954 (originally 1924). *The Gift*. trans. I. Cunnison. New York: Free Press.

Mercer, R.J. 1985. A Neolithic fortress and funeral center. *Scientific American* 252, no. 3: 94-101.

Pires-Ferreira, J. and K. Flannery. 1976. Ethnographic models for formative exchange. In *The Early Mesoamerican Village*, ed. K. Flannery, 286-91. New York: Academic Press.

Rappaport, R. 1968. *Pigs for the Ancestors*. New Haven: Yale Univer. Press.

Speth, J. and Spielmann. K. 1983. Energy source, protein metabolism, and hunter-gatherer subsistence strategies. *Journal of Anthropological Archaeology* 2: 1-31.

Strathern, A. 1971. *The Rope of Moka*. Cambridge: Cambridge Univer. Press.

Underhill, A.P. 1991. Pottery production in chiefdoms: The Longshan period in northern China. *World Archaeology* 23: 12-27.

Widmer, R. 1988. *The Evolution of the Calusa: A Nonagricultural Chiefdom on the Southwest Florida Coast.* Tuscaloosa: Univer. of Alabama Press.

Wilson, D. 1990. Discard distributions and the measurement of human behavior. Paper presented at the 55th annual meeting of the Society for American Archaeology, Las Vegas.

Winterhalder, B. 1986. Diet choice, risk, and food sharing in a stochastic environment. *Journal of Anthropological Archaeology* 5: 369-92.

Young, M. 1971. *Fighting with Food.* Cambridge: Cambridge Univer. Press.

Figure 8.1 Major Catagories of Feasts

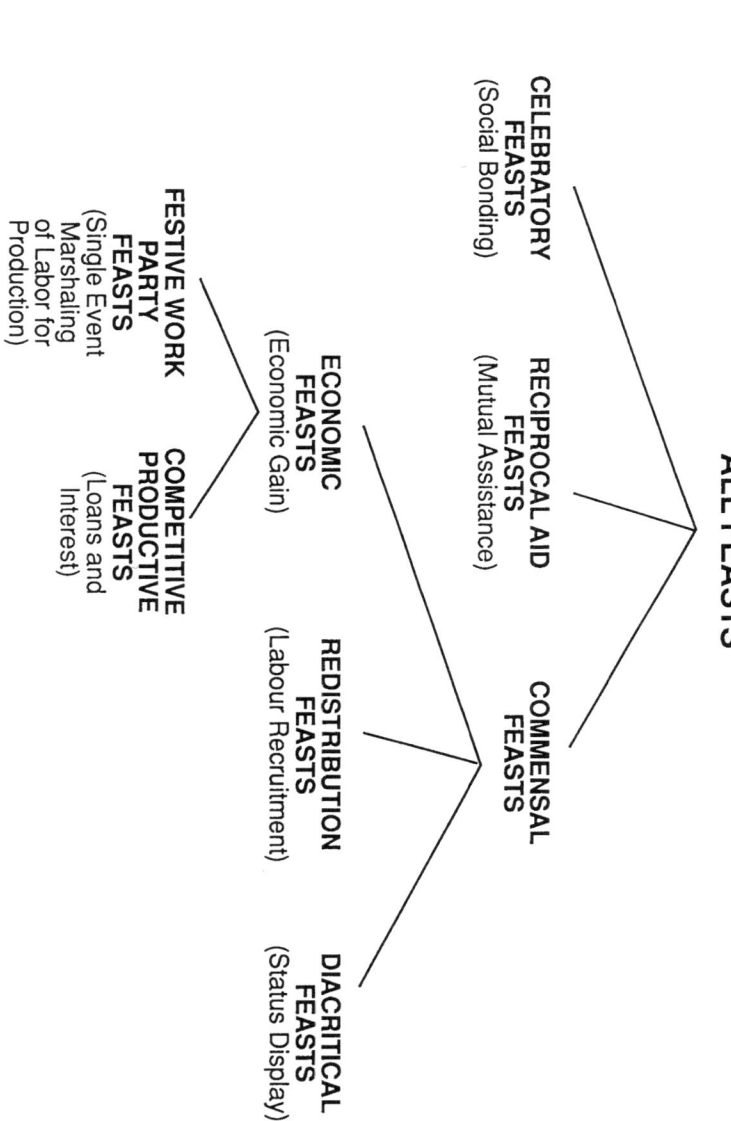

- **ALL FEASTS**
  - **CELEBRATORY FEASTS** (Social Bonding)
  - **COMMENSAL FEASTS**
    - **RECIPROCAL AID FEASTS** (Mutual Assistance)
    - **ECONOMIC FEASTS** (Economic Gain)
      - **FESTIVE WORK PARTY FEASTS** (Single Event Marshaling of Labor for Production)
      - **COMPETITIVE PRODUCTIVE FEASTS** (Loans and Interest)
    - **REDISTRIBUTION FEASTS** (Labour Recruitment)
    - **DIACRITICAL FEASTS** (Status Display)

9. FOOD PRODUCTION AND SOCIAL STATUS AS DOCUMENTED IN PROTO-CUNEIFORM TEXTS

Peter Damerow

In this chapter I shall present findings on a transitional stage of human development that seems crucial for the emergence of civilization. These findings, on the ancient Uruk civilization, indicate that food rations were deliberately scaled to rank, and that rationing had economic and power dimensions. The stage of cultural development to be discussed is the historical transition from life in rural communities to an urban civilization. There is an obvious gap in our knowledge about this stage of development of human culture. We know much about the so-called primitive peoples of today because these people and their culture can still be studied directly. We also know something about early civilizations because an abundance of written sources and archeological remains is available to us in sites as diverse as Mesoamerica, China, Egypt, and – of interest here – Mesopotamia, or, more generally the Near East. But the transition from band and village societies to urbanism is poorly understood.

Sociocultural mechanisms of food production and distribution differ profoundly among cultures such as, for example, Australian aborigines on the one hand and the Old Kingdom of Egypt on the other. The same is true for social status. Egalitarian hunter-gatherer communities seem a world apart from a society where the social strata extended from slaves to pharaoh. How did the tremendous bureaucracies controlling food production and distribution in early civilizations, constituting vast status differences, emerge from food production and the status quo in rural communities? Despite the existence of historical sources documenting parts of this process I am unable to provide a full answer. All I can offer is a survey of what has been learned up to today about this process from certain documents written at the dawn of literacy. Together with the archaeologist Hans Nissen and the Assyriologist Robert Englund I have been working for some years on deciphering archaic texts of ancient Mesopotamia and its neighbors. Our knowledge of these texts is still poor. Although they provide a fascinating insight into food production and distribution in the transition period from a rural to a centralized, redistributive economy, it is still too early to draw general conclusions. I shall therefore concentrate on examples.

I shall begin with a survey of the text material and then describe and interpret some archaic texts germane to the relationship between food production and social status. I shall close with some remarks on what I think we can learn from these about the development of early civilization.

Archaic Writing Systems

It is well known that Mesopotamia was the center of a writing system known as cuneiform, which was used for about 3,000 years. Tablets of clay served as writing material. Script was produced by impressing a stylus into the smooth surface of wet clay, leaving the wedge-shaped markings that inspired the modern name of this writing system. This script was used to record many languages over a long period of time, most of which are well understood since the cuneiform script was deciphered in the middle of the nineteenth century. The oldest clay tablets displaying the developed system of cuneiform writing were written about the middle of the third millenium B.C. However, at the end of the nineteenth century A.D., a substantial collection of texts was excavated in Susa, the urban center of a region east of southern Babylonia known in cuneiform documents of the third millenium as "Elam". These texts seemed to date from a much earlier period. Drawings of more than 200 of these texts were published in 1905 (Scheil 1905). They depict a pictographic writing system called "proto-elamite" that has many similarities to later cuneiform writings (Damerow and Englund 1989). In particular it displays the same kind of number notation impressed vertically or obliquely into the clay by means of a round stylus. Only a short time later, however, it turned out that proto-elamite writing was not the direct precursor of cuneiform. Beginning with some texts unearthed before 1915, more and more clay tablets were excavated in the center of southern Mesopotamia (Falkenstein 1936; Langdon 1928) indicating another system of pictographic writing (Damerow, Englund, and Nissen 1988a, 1988b).

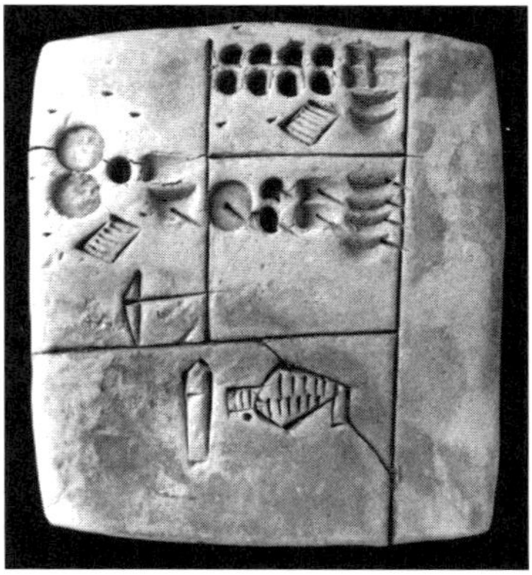

It was immediately obvious that this system was the true precursor of cuneiform, and it was therefore designated proto-cuneiform writing. Proto-cuneiform and proto-elamite texts are together known as "archaic texts." Archaic writing in this sense covers the period from about 3100 to 2800 B.C. So far, about 5,500 proto-cuneiform and 1,500 proto-elamite texts or text fragments have been excavated at several sites in southern Mesopotamia and the highland area of Persia. The creation of these archaic writing systems was closely linked to the early urbanization process in the Near East during the so-called Late Uruk Period (Adams and Nissen 1972; Algaze 1989). The oldest texts are proto-cuneiform from the area of the ancient city of Uruk itself, the main site of proto-cuneiform text findings in general. It seems to be well established now that the proto-elamite writing system was created under the influence of this proto-cuneiform script. Proto-elamite was used for only a short time.

Figure 9.1
Archaic account (approx. 3000 B.C.) of barley groats and malt (see figure 5)

The great majority of the archaic texts are administrative documents (Nissen, Damerow, and Englund 1993). Nearly all concern the allocation of human labor and the distribution of human products, particularly basic means of nutrition and subsistence. Many of these texts contain information about food production and distribution. They are probably the most important sources for any investigation of production processes in the early period of urban civilization. Moreover, these texts bear direct witness to the stratification of the society in this period. The archaic writing system was essentially an instrument used by elites controlling major parts of or even the entire production of the society.

It may be useful to elaborate a little more the special character of the proto-cuneiform and proto-elamite writing systems before I turn to examples of those texts. According to our modern understanding, writing codifies language. In most writing systems a few signs with phonetic values enable us to map spoken sentences. And in principle this is true for the cuneiform writing system, although it is more accurate to describe it as "logo-syllabic," since the signs can be used either for whole words or the sounds of syllables. The archaic texts, however, seem to have been written before the invention of this phonetic idea. We have been unable up to now to identify with certainty any phonetic codification of spoken language in these texts. This may be the result of our still very limited understanding of sign combination.

However, even if we discovered such phonetic writings in the texts, this would not really change the situation, since most signs recorded economic and administrative transactions. I doubt that an archaic scribe would have been able to write down ideas or facts in prose, even if his training and position had allowed that possibility to be imagined. To decipher an archaic text therefore does not consist of identifying rules for a translation into readable text, as is the case of more developed writing systems. Rather, it consists of providing an understanding of the relation of the signs to specific objects and transactions recorded by scribes in their bureaucratic environment. To understand an archaic document entails knowing its economic and administrative function. Our understanding of the archaic texts, therefore, depends essentially on how much we know from later sources about the products and processes registered in these texts. This is the reason I shall begin with two examples dating from much later periods and then trace back the present theme from these understandable texts to their more difficult archaic precursors.

Labor in the Ur III Period

My first example is an accounting text (Englund 1991) written in the period of the third dynasty of Ur, dating about 1,000 years after the invention of writing. The text is typical for a certain subgroup of the administrative documents from this period, attesting a highly developed system of bookkeeping (Englund 1990a, 1990b: chap.1 and 2). The estimated number of texts from this period published up to now is about 30,000, which itself is only one-third of the texts from this period excavated legitimately and illicitly until now. The text which I have chosen is really only one small bit of the available information as a whole.

The text was written in the fourth year of the reign of the king Šu-sin, in the year 2034 B.C., according to the most commonly accepted chronology. It covers a period of exactly twelve months and contains the account of a foreman responsible for a crew of thirty-seven female workers of a cereal-production unit. The workers are titled "géme." This category of female workers corresponds to male workers called "guruš." Workers of this category were probably state property. They were, at least, assigned to production units for the full year as unskilled laborers. This is inferred from evidence that they were not installed in a specialized profession, although their work teams always specialized in narrowly defined activities, as in the present case. The entries in the text follow a well established scheme (see Figures 9.2 and 9.3). The text begins with a debit section consisting of a deficit transferred from the previous year and a precise calculation of the total labor expected from the crew of the foreman during the year, measured in work days.

The following credit section of the text contains a listing of all works performed by the workers during the year. We learn that the women were mainly occupied with the milling of various types of flour. All their activities were registered by the precise number of work days used. Generally these numbers were calculated figures. The amounts of grain products like flour, for instance, were converted into work days necessary for their production by means of certain standard coefficients. The female workers also had to undertake quite different tasks in addition to milling, performed under the supervision of other foremen in agricultural labor units. The final balance section gives the difference between the debit and the credit sections. We learn that the already very high deficit at the beginning of the year has again increased considerably. We know from other texts that deficits like the growing deficit in the present text had probably to be repaid at all costs. Upon the death of the foreman, for instance, the state had first rights to the valuables of his estate, including the family members, who themselves could be transferred to state ownership, that is into the status of a guruš or a géme.

Old Akkadian Account of Beer and Bread Production

My second example (Nissen et al. 1993: 48-49) is an Old Akkadian text, written some 200 years before the previous example. The tablet gives some indications of the mode of distribution of food such as cereals (Hrozny 1913) and particularly beer (Hartman and Oppenheim 1950; Röllig 1970; Stol 1971), products that were stored and controlled by centralized, hierarchical institutions. The text also shows how abbreviated information was coded for bookkeeping purposes. This was valuable information since, as noted above, bookkeeping was the main area of application of the early writing systems.

Figure 9.2 Account from the UR III period (approx. 2100-2000 B.C.) concerning female workers in a mill.

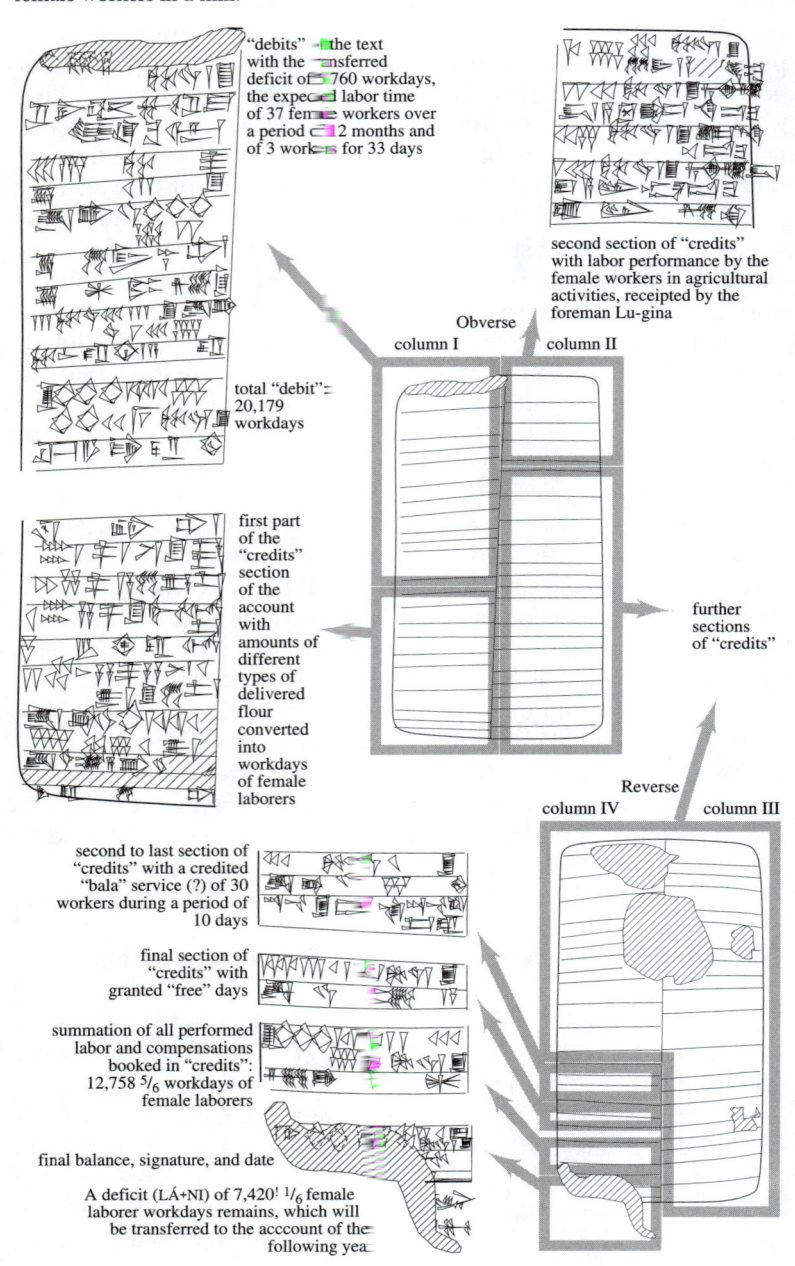

"debits" of the text with the transferred deficit of 5,760 workdays, the expected labor time of 37 female workers over a period of 12 months and of 3 workers for 33 days

second section of "credits" with labor performance by the female workers in agricultural activities, receipted by the foreman Lu-gina

Obverse column I / column II

total "debit": 20,179 workdays

first part of the "credits" section of the account with amounts of different types of delivered flour converted into workdays of female laborers

further sections of "credits"

Reverse column IV / column III

second to last section of "credits" with a credited "bala" service (?) of 30 workers during a period of 10 days

final section of "credits" with granted "free" days

summation of all performed labor and compensations booked in "credits": 12,758 5/6 workdays of female laborers

final balance, signature, and date

A deficit (LÁ+NI) of 7,420! 1/6 female laborer workdays remains, which will be transferred to the acccount of the following year

Figure 9.3 Flow chart revealing the structure of the account depicted in figure 1

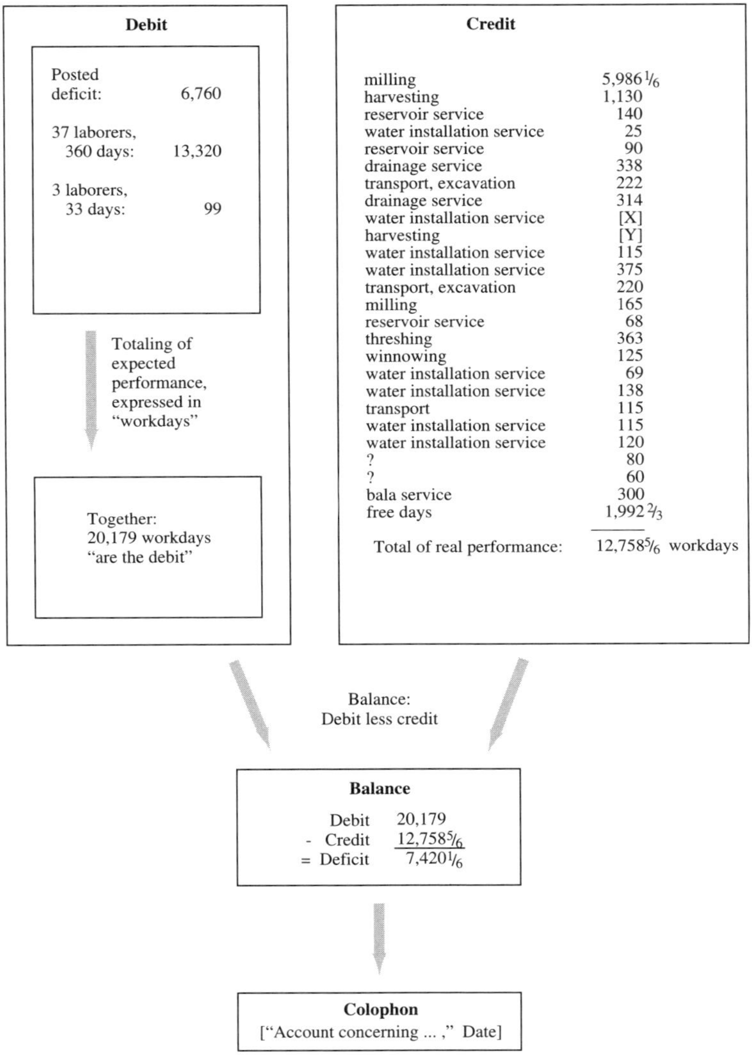

Debit		Credit	
Posted deficit:	6,760	milling	5,986 $\frac{1}{6}$
		harvesting	1,130
37 laborers,		reservoir service	140
360 days:	13,320	water installation service	25
		reservoir service	90
3 laborers,		drainage service	338
33 days:	99	transport, excavation	222
		drainage service	314
		water installation service	[X]
		harvesting	[Y]
		water installation service	115
		water installation service	375
		transport, excavation	220
		milling	165
		reservoir service	68
Totaling of expected performance, expressed in "workdays"		threshing	363
		winnowing	125
		water installation service	69
		water installation service	138
		transport	115
		water installation service	115
		water installation service	120
		?	80
		?	60
Together: 20,179 workdays "are the debit"		bala service	300
		free days	1,992 $\frac{2}{3}$
		Total of real performance:	12,758 $\frac{5}{6}$ workdays

Balance:
Debit less credit

Balance
Debit   20,179
− Credit   12,758 $\frac{5}{6}$
= Deficit   7,420 $\frac{1}{6}$

Colophon
["Account concerning ... ," Date]

Although we are still in the period of developed cuneiform writing, phonetic values of the signs were used only to register names.

The tablet contains fifteen entries recording the delivery of cereal products – i.e. bread and beer – to certain persons (see Figure 9.4). Each entry consists of two lines, always ending with a person's name. These persons were probably foremen who received these products for further distribution. At the end of the tablet the delivered amounts

Figure 9.4 Old Akkadian account of beer and bread production (approx. 2250 B.C.)

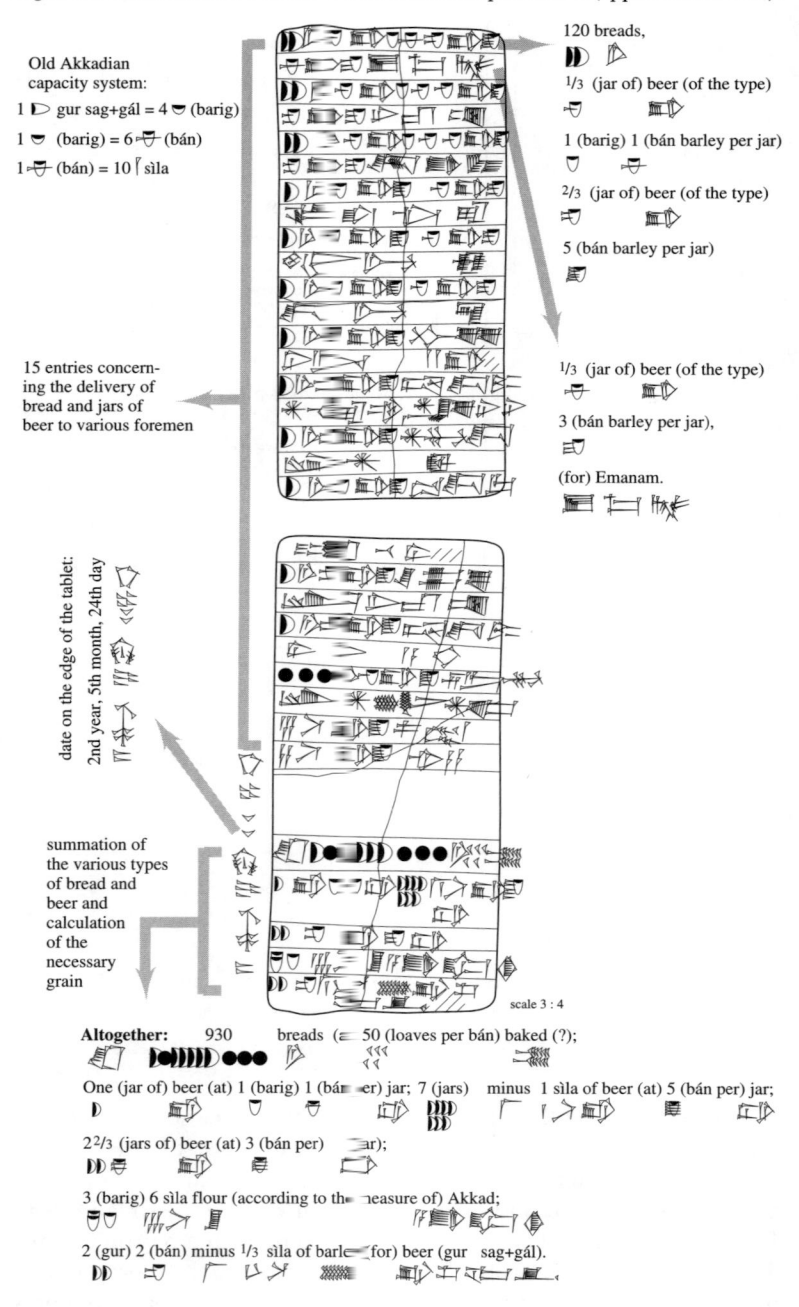

Old Akkadian capacity system:
1 gur sag+gál = 4 (barig)
1 (barig) = 6 (bán)
1 (bán) = 10 sìla

120 breads,

1/3 (jar of) beer (of the type)

1 (barig) 1 (bán barley per jar)

2/3 (jar of) beer (of the type)

5 (bán barley per jar)

15 entries concerning the delivery of bread and jars of beer to various foremen

1/3 (jar of) beer (of the type)

3 (bán barley per jar),

(for) Emanam.

date on the edge of the tablet: 2nd year, 5th month, 24th day

summation of the various types of bread and beer and calculation of the necessary grain

scale 3 : 4

Altogether: 930 breads (= 50 (loaves per bán) baked (?);

One (jar of) beer (at) 1 (barig) 1 (bán per) jar; 7 (jars) minus 1 sìla of beer (at) 5 (bán per) jar;

2 2/3 (jars of) beer (at) 3 (bán per) jar);

3 (barig) 6 sìla flour (according to the measure of) Akkad;

2 (gur) 2 (bán) minus 1/3 sìla of barley (for) beer (gur sag+gál).

were totaled separately for the different products. Finally, an amount of flour and an amount of grain were registered. These figures were apparently calculated estimates for the flour and barley necessary for the production of the bread and beer, respectively.

Archaic Accounts Signed by KU.ŠIM

I come now to the first archaic tablet (Nissen et al. 1993: 43-46). At first sight it seems very different from the previous examples, but a closer look shows that is is in fact the same sort of text. Several deliveries of various kinds of beer are registered. The amounts again are totaled separately and the totals are converted by simple coefficients into amounts of primary products – in this case malt and barley groats – necessary for their production (see Figure 9.5).

At the end of the text we find a combination of two signs that probably indicate the official who was responsible for the transactions. In the developed cuneiform script used to write the indigenous Sumerian language, these two signs were read KU and ŠIM, respectively. It is, however, unlikely that the signs were already used with phonetic values in the archaic period. Normally, it is difficult to say anything specific about persons like KU.ŠIM who signed such tablets. Fortunately, however, in the present case we know a little more about this person. The tablet belongs to an extraordinary group of over eighty-five well-preserved tablets that were obviously written at the time in the same context (Nissen, Damerow, and Englund 1991; Nissen et al. 1993; see the German edition for a complete photographic documentation of this text group). Some persons occur on these tablets several times and in different functions. We are therefore able to draw some conclusions about their status and responsibilities.

This is particularly true for the official KU.ŠIM, who signed the beer account. He was probably the chief administrator of a granary containing primary products for producing beer. Malt and barley groats were the main ingredients of beer at that time. One of the texts signed by him (see Figure 9.6) has an entry of about 1,800 liters of malt, which is the largest amount of malt attested on one text in the whole archaic text corpus. Another tablet with the sign combination KU.ŠIM in the subscript seems to be a kind of summary document. The tablet has only one entry, with a notation of about 135,000 liters of barley together with a notation for thirty-seven months (see Figure 9.7). This notation probably denotes a three-year time period consisting of two ordinary years of twelve months and one year with an extra month to adjust the lunar calendar to the solar year.

Figure 9.5 Proto-cuneiform accounting text (approx. 3000 B.C.) on barley groats and malt used in beer production

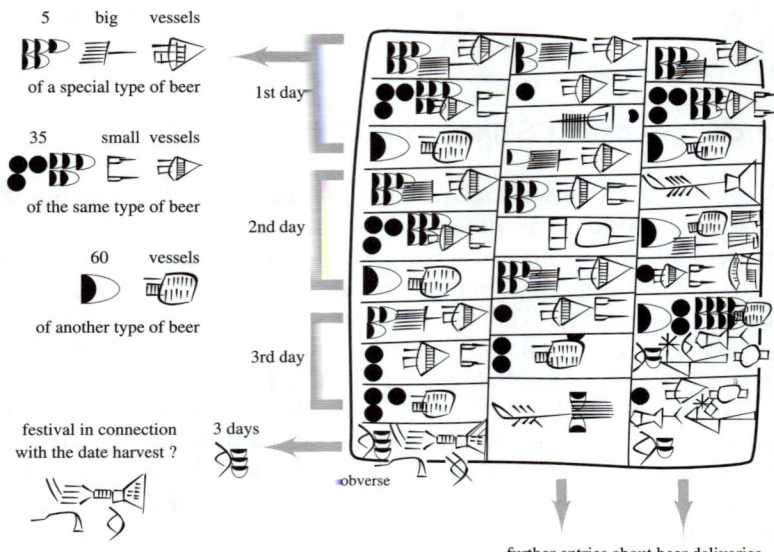

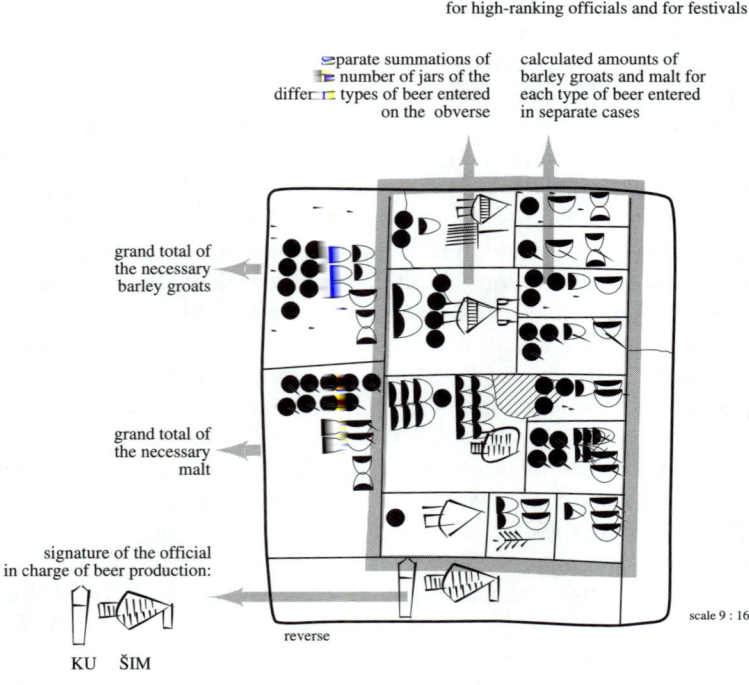

Figure 9.6 Archaic account on the ingredients needed to brew beer, i.e. barley groats and malt

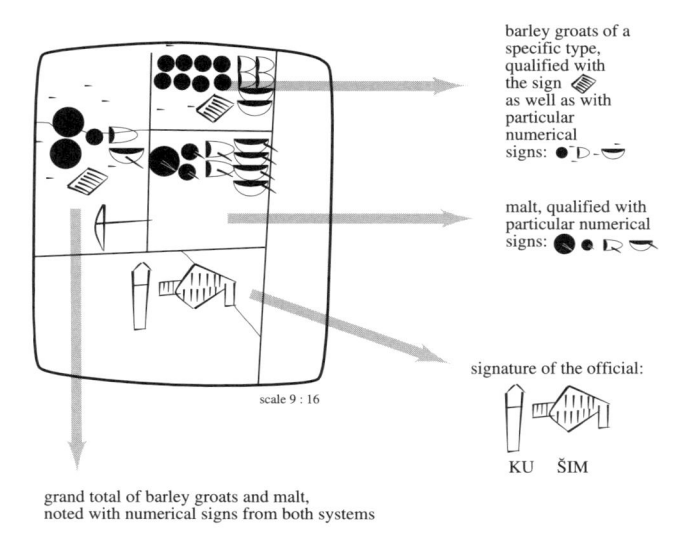

Figure 9.7 Archaic account on an amount of approx. 135,000 liters of barley

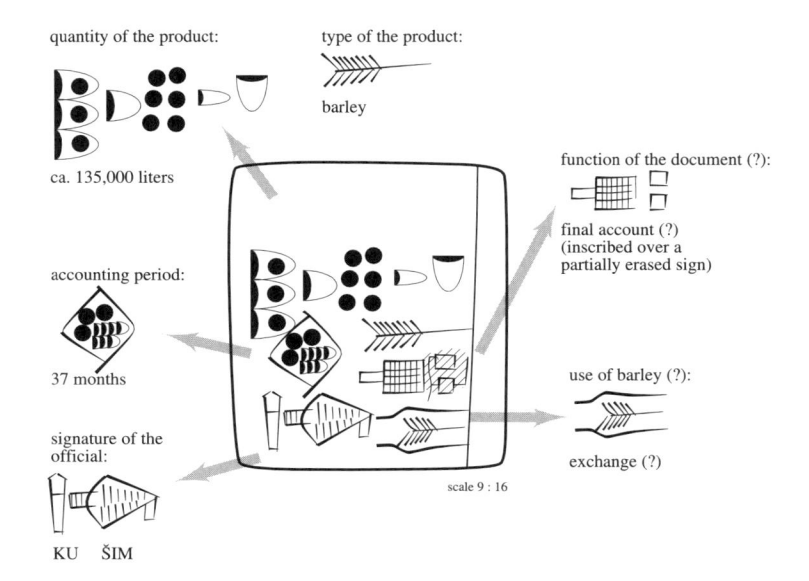

List of Officials

In summary, KU.ŠIM must have been an important person, although he probably did not belong to the small group of top-level administrators with standardized titles. Such titles are well known from a certain group of school texts that are commonly called lexical lists (Nissen and Englund 1993). Lexical lists consist of highly standardized sequences of signs and sign combinations ordered according to meaning. They probably served for the training of scribes, since they were copied over and over again. Some lists have copies recurring over a time span of over 1,000 years. In later times Akkadian translations or comments were added to the entries of such lists. They enhanced them to a sort of bilingual Sumerian-Akkadian dictionary.

Figure 9.8 Archaic list of officials

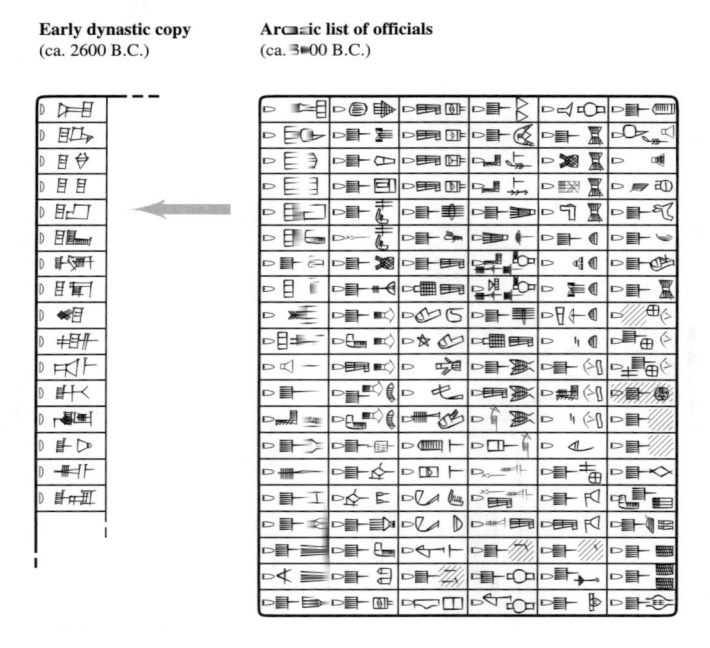

A special kind of lexical list is for officials (see Figure 9.8). The oldest copies of a major type of such lists come from the earliest stage of writing. They already show the canonical sequence of later sources. The most recent examples, which are still very similar in the sequence of entries, were written in the Old Babylonian Period, about 1,300 years later. In this period the list of officials was updated and afterwards again copied over and over again.

Can we get any information from such lists about functions and status of officials in the archaic period, when the oldest versions of those lists were probably composed? This is in fact possible, although the situation is a little complicated. Later versions of such lists are clearly related to the hierarchy of the administration. They start with the designation of the king and of some well-known high-ranking officials. However, the lists do not proceed strictly according to ranks in a hierarchical order. Successive entries often seem to represent certain subdivisions of the administration. Parts of such lists appear, therefore, to be enumerations of various professions on different levels of administrative status. Does the archaic list have the same or a similar structure? And if this is true, is it reasonable to assume that the canonical order of the entries reflects a real hierarchy at any other period than the time when the list was originally composed? There are strong indications that the entries in the archaic list of officials also corresponded somehow to high-ranking positions in the administration. Some sign combinations of this list occur in administrative texts either in the subscript or as qualifications of entries about receipts and expenditure (see Figure 9.9).

Comparing such entries with the two examples of deliveries of barley products to the aforementioned KU.ŠIM, we come to the conclusion that the first part of the list of officials in fact must contain denotations of persons or positions with a fairly high status. Most of these officials received between two and five times more barley and malt than KU.ŠIM did. This may be interpreted as indicating that they had control of more working personnel, for whose sustenance they were responsible. On the other hand, however, there are puzzling details of the relation between the list of officials and the appearance of these officials in administrative texts. The first entry of the list, for instance, in later lists representing the king, contains a sign combination representing a title without a similar prominent position in the administrative texts. For the time being we know for sure only that the persons in the archaic texts we are discussing here all belong to a group with a very high social status. This is in agreement with what is documented about them in the administrative texts; they had control over considerable amounts of produce.

Workers and Slaves

Let me turn now to the other end of the status hierarchy. In the first example we encountered low-ranking workers from the Ur III period (Gelb 1965; Struve 1969; Waetzoldt 1987, Waetzold 1988).

Figure 9.9 Archaic account documenting big amounts of barley distributed among high rank officials which are contained in the list of officials

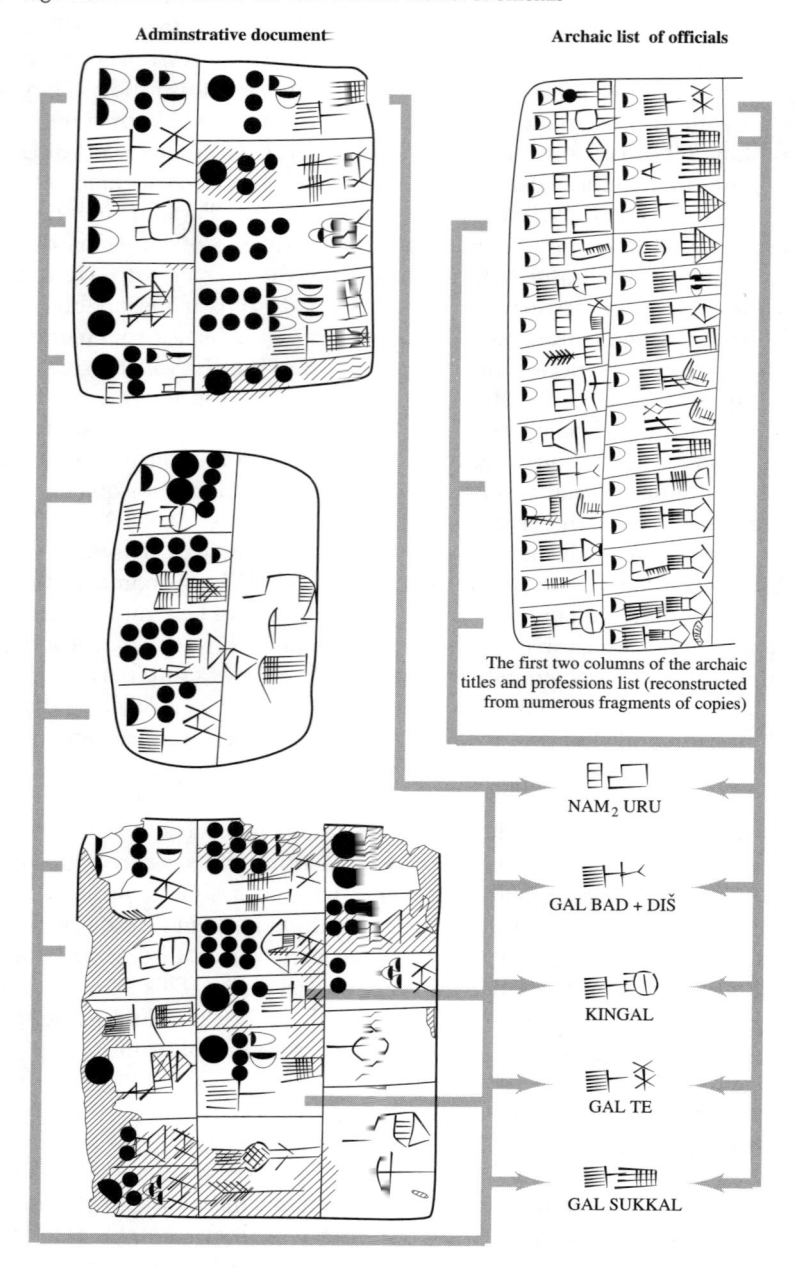

Are we able to identify individual workers of similar rank in the archaic texts? This is, in fact, possible, although mostly they are represented in the texts only by the rations they received. Some archaic tablets, however, provide direct information even about such workers (Nissen et al. 1993: chap. 11). The interpretation of such texts is based mainly on the identification of the archaic signs and sign combinations for male and female slaves, as I shall call them although we have no details about their living conditions. A small fragment of an originally much larger tablet, for instance, shows on one side some traces of entries about such people (Nissen et al. 1993: 74). On the reverse side, a total is partly preserved, the legible part indicating a minimum of 211 male and female slaves (see Figure 9.10).

Figure 9.10 Archaic account on slaves

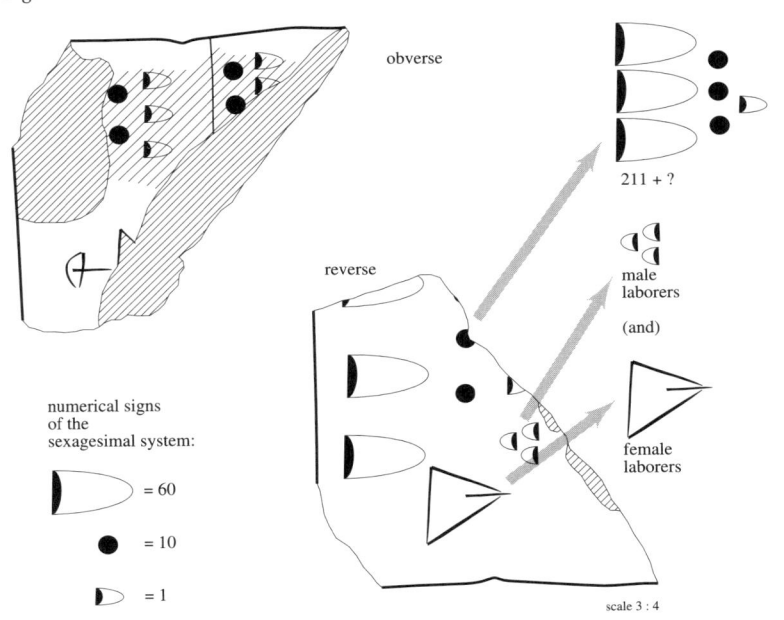

Another text of the archaic period may even provide us with some indirect information about the living conditions of such slaves (Cavigneaux, Finkbeiner, Seidel and Siewert 1991: no. 74). Some explanation is necessary before I come to the details of this text. Among the archaic texts that we understand almost completely is a group of some thirty texts and text fragments dealing with animal husbandry (Green 1980). They are yearly accounts of shepherds who were mostly responsible for small animals like sheep and goats. The herds normally numbered between 50 and 100 animals. Some texts deal with cattle. In this case the figures of registered animals are much smaller.

Besides shepherds' names, all of these texts contain figures about the number of adult animals in each individual's care, distinguishing males and females. Furthermore, there are figures of the male and the female offspring of the present year. The adult animals and the offspring were totaled separately. Finally, the amount of milk produce was calculated from the number of female animals and registered at the end of the tablet. This group of texts about animal husbandry includes two further texts showing the same format. These latter two come from a more recent excavation at the site of the ancient town of Uruk. One of these texts deals with pigs (Cavigneaux et al. 1991: no. 57), confirming that the scheme of the account previously reconstructed was commonly used for several types of domesticated animals. The second text (Cavigneaux et al. 1991: no. 74) also follows this scheme. This time, however, it is not animals that are registered on the tablets, but a number of human beings, qualified by the signs for male and female slaves (see Figure 9.11).

Finally, I want to present a proto-elamite example. The tablet was excavated at the beginning of the twentieth century in Susa in western Persia (Scheil 1905: no. 4997). At that time, however, the proto-elamite writing system was still so poorly understood that nobody paid special attention to this tablet, and for a long time its importance was not recognized. When we worked on a particular sign that we tentatively interpreted as the proto-elamite variant of the proto-cuneiform sign for male slaves (Damerow and Englund 1989: 55-60), we produced a plausible rendering of the text. It turned out that the text is a document about the distribution of grain rations for workers. The text is particularly important because it provides information about the size and the internal structure of organized groups of workers in the proto-elamite culture.

We learn from this text (see Figure 9.12) that a full brigade of 111 people, including the leader, consisted of ten subgroups. Each of the groups included ten workers and one foreman, altogether eleven people. Two such groups always formed a subunit receiving a particular ration of grain. On the tablet the monthly amounts of grain are recorded separately for each subunit of twenty-two persons. Assuming that the measurement units used in the proto-elamite culture are about the same as documented in the archaic texts from Mesopotamia, the daily rations must have been extremely low, namely less than half a liter of grain. This would be only half the amount documented in proto-cuneiform archaic documents. There are, however, some indications that the grain measures represented by corresponding signs in proto-elamite and proto-cuneiform texts were not identical.

Food Production and Social Status as Documented in Proto-Cuneiform Texts 165

Figure 9.11 Comparison of archaic accounts on pigs and slaves

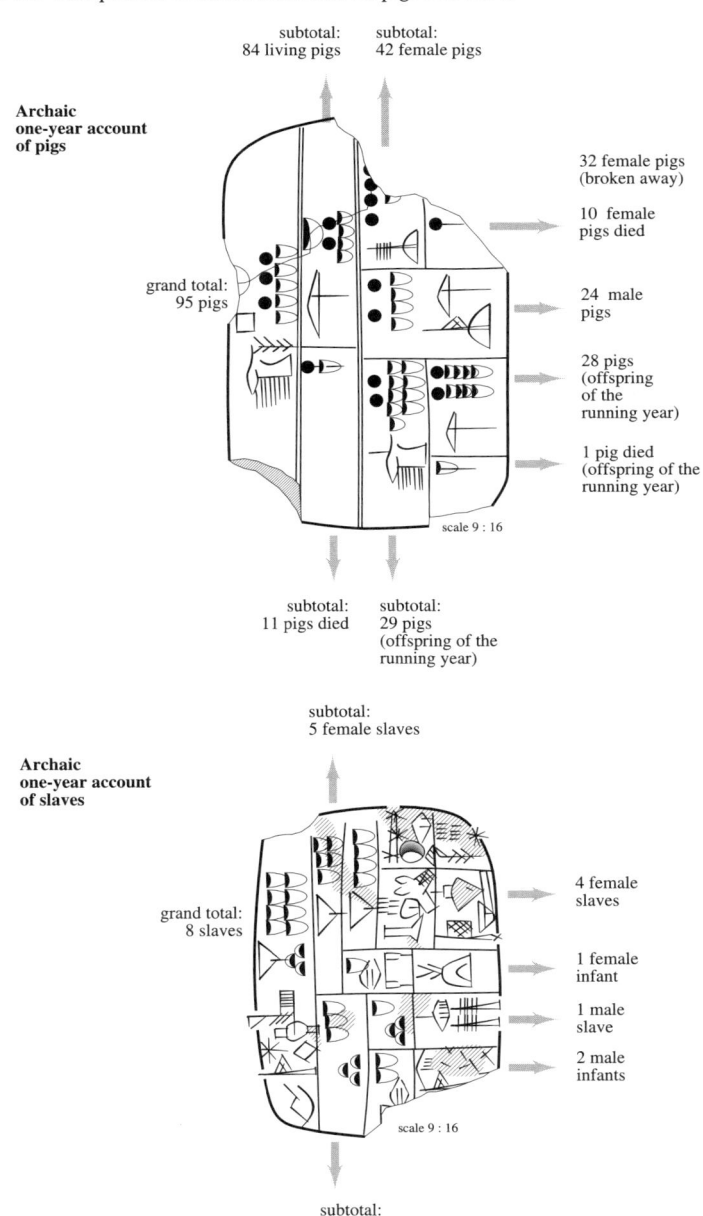

Archaic one-year account of pigs

subtotal: 84 living pigs
subtotal: 42 female pigs

32 female pigs (broken away)
10 female pigs died
24 male pigs
28 pigs (offspring of the running year)
1 pig died (offspring of the running year)

grand total: 95 pigs

scale 9 : 16

subtotal: 11 pigs died
subtotal: 29 pigs (offspring of the running year)

Archaic one-year account of slaves

subtotal: 5 female slaves

4 female slaves
1 female infant
1 male slave
2 male infants

grand total: 8 slaves

scale 9 : 16

subtotal: 3 male slaves

Peter Damerow

Figure 9.12 Proto-Ekamite tablet (approx. 3000 B.C.) containing an account of cereal rations for the labor gangs of two supervisors

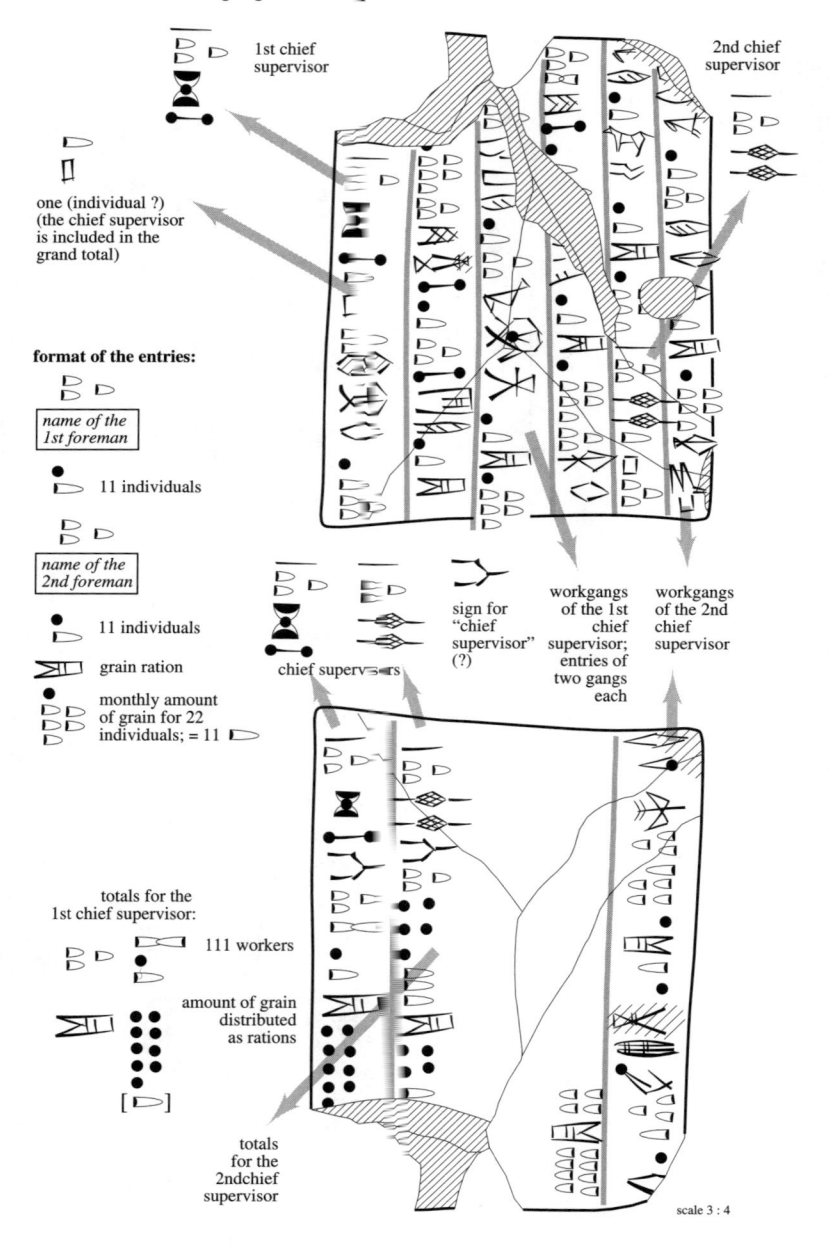

Summary

The examples I have presented show that in the archaic period around 3000 B.C. food production and distribution were no longer primarily matters of individual effort. They were already subject to a highly stratified social organization, which constituted huge differences in the social status of people. This social system was already fully developed when writing was invented as a major instrument for the control of economic transactions. It is reasonable to conclude that the rise of early civilizations depended on the establishment of such a system of social control of food and nutrition supply.

Within the realm of such a system, a person's status could no longer be significantly altered by his own initiative. For a considerable part of the population the status quest was, by definition of social role, in vain. This is remarkably different from the situation in so-called primitive societies. Whatever the phylogenetic roots of status may be, in the period of state formation and the invention of writing it was already a sociocultural phenomenon linked to the organization and exploitation of human labor. The access to resources, in particular the access to food supply, was largely dependent on one's position in the socially determined hierarchy. This system provided people – possibly for the first time in history – with a continuous abundance of resources. It was, however, probably a necessary condition of this continuity that only a minority was determined by status, itself defined within the social system. The ability to accumulate large food-producing resources was no longer a measure of an individual's ability to control the labor of others, but an attribute of the society as a whole. This, at least, we can learn from our present understanding of the archaic texts.

References

Adams, R.M. and H.J. Nissen. 1972. *The Uruk Countryside: The Natural Setting of Urban Societies.* Chicago: Chicago Univer. Press.

Algaze, G. 1989. The Uruk Expansion. *Current Anthropology* 30, no. 5: 571-608.

Cavigneaux, A., U. Finkbeiner, U. Seidel & H.H. Siewert. 1991. Uruk 33/34. *Baghdader Mitteilungen,* 22.

Damerow, P. and R.K. Englund. 1989. *The Proto-Elamite Texts from Tepe Yahya.* Cambridge Mass.: Harvard Univer. Press.

Damerow, P., R.K. Englund and H.J. Nissen. 1988a. Die Entstehung der Schrift. *Spektrum der Wissenchaft*, no. 2: 74-85.

Damerow, P., R.K. Englund & H.J. Nissen 1988b. Die ersten Zahldarstellungen und die Entwicklung des Zahlbegriffs. *Spektrum der Wissenschaft*, no. 3:46-55.

Englund, R.K. 1990a. Administrative timekeeping in ancient Mesopotamia. *Journal of the Economic and Social History of the Orient* 31: 121-85.

Englund, R.K. 1990b. *Organisation und Verwaltung der Ur III-Fischerei*. Berlin: Reimer.

Englund, R.K. 1991. Hard work—where will it get you? Labor management in Ur III Mesopotamia. *Journal of Near Eastern Studies* 50, no. 4: 255-80.

Falkenstein, A. 1936. *Archaische Texte aus Uruk*. Leipzig: Harrassowitz.

Gelb, I.J. 1965. The ancient Mesopotamian ration system. *Journal of Near Eastern Studies* 24: 230-43.

Green, M.W. 1980. Animal husbandry at Uruk in the archaic period. *Journal of Near Eastern Studies* 39: 1-35.

Hartman, L.F. & A.L. Oppenheim. 1950. On beer and brewing techniques in ancient Mesopotamia according to the XXIIIrd tablet of the series hAR.ra = *Hubullu*. *Journal of the American Oriental Society*, 10: Supplement.

Hrozny, F. 1913. *Das Getreide im alten Babylonien*. Sitzungsberichte der Kais. Akademie der Wissenschaften in Wien, Band 173 (1. Abhandlung). Wien: Hölder.

Langdon, S. 1928. *Pictographic Inscriptions from Jemdet Nasr*. Oxford: Oxford Univer. Press.

Nissen, H.J., P. Damerow and R.K. Englund 1991. *Frühe Schrift und Techniken der Wirtschaftsverwaltung im alten Vorderen Orient*, 2 ed. Bad Salzdetfurth: Franzbecker.

Nissen, H.J., P. Damerow and R.K. Englund. 1993. *Archaic Bookkeeping: Early Writing and Techniques of Economic Administration in the Ancient Near East*. Chicago: Chicago Univer. Press.

Nissen, H.J. and R.K. Englund. 1993. *Die Lexikalischen Listen der Archaischen Texte aus Uruk*. Ausgrabungen der Deutschen Forschungsgemeinschaft in Uruk-Warka, Band 13. Archaische Texte aus Uruk, Band 3. Berlin: Gebr. Mann.

Röllig, W. 1970. *Das Bier im Alten Mesopotamien*. Berlin: Gesellschaft für die Geschichte und Bibliografie des Brauwesens E.V., Institut für Gärungsgewerbe und Biotechnologie.

Scheil, V., ed. 1905. *Documents archaïques en écriture protó-élamite*. Mémoires de la Délégation en Perse, ed. V. Scheil, vol. 6. Paris: Geuthner.

Stol, M. 1971. Zur altmesopotamischen Bierbereitung. *Bibliotheca Orientalis* 28, no. 3/4): 167-71.

Struve, V.V. 1969. Some new data on the organization of labour and on social structure in Sumer during the reign of the IIIrd dynasty of Ur. In *Ancient Mesopotamia*, ed. I.M. Diakonoff, 127-72. Moskau: "Nauka" Publishing House.

Waetzoldt, H. 1987. Compensation of craft workers and officials in the Ur III period. In *Labor in the Ancient Near East.*, ed. M. Powell, 118-41. American Oriental Series 68. New Haven: American Oriental Society.

Waetzoldt, H. 1988. Die Situation der Frauen und Kinder anhand ihrer Einkommensverhältnisse zur Zeit der III. Dynastie von Ur. *Altorientalische Forschungen,* 15, no.1: 30-44.

10. LEVELING THE HUNTER
CONSTRAINTS ON THE STATUS QUEST IN FORAGING SOCIETIES

Polly Wiessner

Perhaps the most outstanding aspect of status among foragers is its obscurity, the way it lurks in the shadows of society. For many cultures it is possible to investigate how food is used to help create, support or challenge status distinctions, but for foragers it is necessary to turn in the opposite direction and consider how individuals are prevented from using food for the same ends. The prevalence and strength of such sanctions among foragers in and of itself attests to the potential of food accumulation, display, and distribution as a tool for manipulating status. If this potential were not so potent, such measures would hardly be necessary. In this paper I will (1) discuss the role of food, particularly meat, in status seeking in twenty-seven forager societies, (2) examine sanctions exerted to level those who seek status, and (3) try to elucidate why such measures are both prevalent and successful.

Foragers

It has been recognized in the last two decades that the category hunter-gatherer, although useful for some purposes, incorporates societies that exhibit a great deal of variation in many realms of life. As a result, several attempts have been made to subdivide hunter-gatherers according to their subsistence strategies and degree of social complexity. The critical variable on which most of these classifications have been based on the way hunter-gatherers deal with risk and uncertainty in their environments (Testart 1982; Wiessner 1977, 1982a, 1982b), that is, whether they use social techniques of risk sharing or rely heavily on storage. Woodburn (1982) has divided hunter-gatherers into two categories along similar lines: immediate-return and delayed-return systems. The former obtain direct and immediate returns for their labor; do not process and store food for significant periods of time; and use relatively portable, easily acquired, and replaceable tools that are made with skill but do not require a great deal of labor. The latter hold rights over valuable assets; use substantial technical facilities in production (boats, stockades, weirs etc.); process and store foods in fixed dwellings; improve or increase wild products by human labor; and hold assets in the form of rights over female kin given in marriage to other men. Binford (1980) has made a somewhat similar distinction, calling immediate-return systems "foragers" and delayed-return systems "collectors". The schemes of both Woodburn and Binford are most useful, but the terminology is somewhat misleading. On one hand, Woodburn's term "immediate-return systems" is inappropriate for hunter-gatherers who use sharing to pool risk, because reciprocation for goods or assistance given out is almost always delayed and may occur as long as years later. On the other hand, Binford's passive term "collectors" fails to convey the complexity of delayed-return systems. For want of better terms, sedentary hunter-gatherers who depend heavily on storage will be called "complex hunter-gatherers", following Hayden (1990), and those who rely heavily on sharing to pool risk will be called "foragers". Brian Hayden (this volume) deals with complex hunter-gatherers; here I will restrict my discussion to foragers.

Methodology

The forager literature is rich in information on food and status, though detailed information connecting both topics and the relation between the two often does not exist for a given society. Accordingly, twenty-seven foraging societies from different parts of the world were selected on the basis of the quality of information available in the literature and/or the possibility of checking up on certain points with the researchers (See Figure 10.1). Two qualifications need to be made. First, the line between foragers and complex hunter-gatherers is not always a clear one, particularly for Inuit groups. Second, the majority of the forager societies considered here do not live in a world of hunters, but have a long history of contact and exchange with surrounding, often dominant, agricultural populations that may have diminished the role of local leadership. All of those in tropical forests either exchange meat for carbohydrates with surrounding farmers or plant small gardens.

Figure 10.1 Foraging Societies Included in the Study

Australia	
Western Desert (general)	Sources
Pintupi	Gould 1980,1981
Gunwinggu	Myers 1988
	Altman and Peterson 1988
Asia	
Agta	Griffin 1984*
Batek (Semang)	Endicott 1988
Bihor	Williams 1974
Andamanese	Radcliffe-Brown 1964
Jahai (Semang)	van der Sluys 1993*; Schebesta 1954
Arctic	
Netsilik Inuit	Balikci 1970, 1971, 1984; Damas 1971
Copper Inuit	Damas 1972, 1984
Inuit of Quebec	Saladin d'Anglure 1984
West Greenland Inuit	Kleivan 1984
Iglulik Inuit	Damas 1971; Mary-Rousseliere 1984
Amassalik Inuit	Robbe 1989
North America	
Washo	Price 1975; Downs 1966
Cree	Rogers 1972; Scott 1988
Chipewyan	Sharp 1977, 1981
South American	
Guayaki/Ache	Clastres 1972; Kaplan 1983
Ayoréode	von Bremen 1991*
Ona	Lothrop 1928; Gusinde 1931
Kaingáng	Henry 1941
Africa	
Aka Pygmies	Bahuchet 1990
Mbuti Pygmies	Harako 1981;Turnbull 1965
Hadza	Woodburn 1982; Barnard and Woodburn 1988
!Kung San	Marshall 1976; Lee 1984; Wiessner 1977
G/wi San	Silberbauer 1981a,1981b; Tanaka 1980
!Ko San	Heinz 1966*

*plus personal communication

The focus will be on meat rather than vegetable foods for a purely practical reason: information on the procurement, consumption, and distribution of meat exists in most forager ethnographies, while comparable information on vegetable foods is relatively rare. It is worth mentioning, though, that a general rule of thumb does exist concerning the sharing of vegetable foods: staple foods that are widely available to all are usually distributed only within the household, to visitors or to closely related households whose members have not been able to gather that day. Only vegetable foods that are rare or highly variable in distribution, such as large roots among the Agta of the Philippines, are shared throughout the camp. It is unfortunate that there is not enough material in the literature to look at vegetable foods, because gathering provides the staple diet of most foragers, and some status appears to be accorded to good gatherers. Furthermore, because much competitive feasting involves vegetable foods or animals raised on them (Hayden 1990), a study of vegetable foods and status in foraging societies might provide valuable insights.

Status in Foraging Societies

Foragers are said to be some of the most fiercely egalitarian people in the world, tolerating no formalized differences in rank. It is necessary, then, to ask whether or not the concept of status exists at all among foragers, and if food could even be expected to be associated with status. The answer to this question is clearly affirmative: status, prestige, esteem, and high regard are terms that enter the ethnographies of most foraging societies, albeit with much qualification, even for societies that are considered the most egalitarian. It is mentioned in association with activities that benefit the group in some way: knowledge, ritual expertise, abilities in planning and organization, mediation, hunting skill, generosity, defense and interaction with outsiders. Ranking on the basis of high regard appears to begin at an early age in hunter-gatherers, as in other populations. For example, Hold (1980, [Hold-Cavell] this volume) found that children in G/wi San play groups form flexible hierarchies on the basis of focus of attention. Rank orders based on "high regard" are carried through until adulthood despite a strong socialization toward egalitarianism. When I asked about status, !Kung San of the community of /Xai/xai were able to readily classify men and women as individuals of great (social) strength, ordinary people, people with little strength, and people who were literally "nothing" respectively. Evaluations of status or influence showed an association with a number of variables, among them ability to maintain many exchange partnerships, power as healers, competence in hunting, and ability to deal effectively with outsiders.

Meat has the potential to be one of the best vehicles for obtaining status in forager societies because of attributes that draw attention. Meat is a desired and nutritious food, the only one that can satisfy what many hunter-gatherers experience as "meat hunger". On any given day, its availability is highly variable from household to household, so possession of meat can put the owner into the focus of attention. Furthermore, the appropriate distribution of meat has the potential to reaffirm social alliances, relieve tension, and demonstrate organizational abilities, activities that are all associated with high regard (Grammer, this volume). In theory, then, the procurement and distribution of meat should be expected to be widely used to gain status. Indeed, ethnographies indicate that this is often but not always the case (See Figure 10.2), because there is considerable intercultural variation regarding what attributes and abilities confer status.

Figure 10.2 Hunting Success and Status in Foraging Societies.

Good hunters receive:
Considerable status
West Greenland Inuit
Iglulik Inuit
Ona

Some status
Western Desert Aborigines
Inuit of Quebec
Mbuti Pygmies
Gunwinggu
!Ko San
G/wi San
!Kung San
Netsilik Inuit
Copper Inuit
Ammassalik Inuit
Ayoréode (high status for killing jaguar or men in warfare only)
Chipewyan

Generosity in sharing valued, but men do not gain high status through hunting
Washo
Guayaki/Ache
Batek
Pintupi
Hadza
Aka Pygmies
Andamanese
Agta
Jahai
Kaingáng

(insufficient information: Cree, Bihor)

Three out of twenty-five societies considered here grant prestige to good hunters. For twelve, hunters are allowed some acclaim, or, as Silberbauer (1981b: 235) describes it: "The G/wi do not make heros of their hunters, but hunting is nevertheless a prestigious activity." Not surprisingly, foragers who depend more heavily on hunting than gathering associate status with hunting. There are some suggestions in the literature that status provides an incentive for hunters, for instance Gusinde's remarks on Ona hunters (1931: 421 as translated in the Human Relations Area Files):

> Perhaps at the time he (the successful hunter) thinks that later on he himself will be permitted to share in a particularly productive hunt, and at the very least, something from the booty that his neighbor brings home. This matter-of-course mutual aid relieves everyone of worry about the future and of the bother of specially storing certain quantities of food. The Selk'nam actually does not need to fear serious times of need. To him it is a particular satisfaction ... to let the neighborhood share in his own pleasures: at the very least, pride drives him to do it, since a successful hunter is esteemed and loved by all, indeed, is even waited on and pampered.

In the remaining ten societies, generosity is praised, but successful hunting is not associated with high status. However, as we shall see later, such equality of hunters does not come by itself, but is strongly reinforced by ideology. This does not mean that status in these forager groups is not recognized at all; it is granted for other accomplishments such as ritual proficiency, defense, competence in dealing with outsiders or mediation.

When status is accorded to good hunters, its privileges are strictly curtailed to prevent it from being turned to dominance, defined as a relationship in which one individual continuously gains greater access to resources or has decisive influence over another in certain situations. In reviewing the literature on meat distribution, it appears that there are three ways of leveling the successful hunter, often used in combination: (1) removing the hunter from the focus of attention, (2) spreading the credit for the distribution among several individuals, and (3) erasing any concept of debt and obligation to the hunter and/or reversing the debt, so that sharing is seen as the hunter's debt to his society.

These sanctions begin when the ownership of the animal is first assigned after the kill, and continue until the last morsel of meat reaches its destination. Let us begin with how ownership of the carcass is assigned (See Figure 10.2).

Figure 10.3 Ownership of Animals Killed

Owned by hunter who made the first hit or demobilised animal
Copper Inuit
Netsilik Inuit
Inuit of Quebec
Inuit of West Greenland
Ona

Divided among members of hunting party or owned by hunter if hunting alone
Western Desert Aborigines
Agta
Ammassalik Inuit
Chipewyan
Washo

Owned by hunter, often given to another for distribution
Cree
Iglulik Inuit
Guayaki/Ache
Ayoréode
Chipewyan
Kaingáng

Divided between hunter and implement owner
Gunwinggu
G/wi San
Jahai

Owned by owner of the implement that inflicted first blow or demobilized the animal
Andamanese
Aka Pygmies
Mbuti Pygmies
Bihor
Pintupi
Batek
!Kung San

Ownership not clearly specified
Hadza

Ownership of Animals Killed and Hunter Etiquette

As is made clear in Figure 10.3, all foragers considered here assign ownership of the carcass to somebody (Dowling 1968) except for the Hadza. Ownership, however, means little more than having the right to distribute the meat or to decide who should do so, for all foragers have rules stipulating that meat must be widely shared. In only five out of twenty-seven societies is the ownership of the carcass and the right to distribute it assigned solely to the hunter who made the first hit or demobilized the animal. Four of these are Inuit groups for whom meat provides the bulk of the diet. In another five societies, the meat is either divided among members of a hunting party at the kill site or owned by the hunter if he is alone. Washo net hunting provides an exception. Here, the owner of the net or the drivers who captured individual rabbits have the right to keep them. Surplus rabbits are shared widely. The distinction between this category and the first is simply a matter of whether hunting is more often a group enterprise as opposed to an individual enterprise. For three societies, ownership of meat is divided between the hunter and implement owner, and in another six meat is owned by the hunter, but often given to others, such as elders or women in the camp, for distribution. Among the Hadza, who hunt large game almost exclusively, ownership is not clearly specified. Finally, in seven societies, the kill is considered to be the property of the person who owns the implement that inflicted the first hit or struck the blow that disabled the animal. This means, of course, that in most cases the carcass goes to the successful hunter, since the hunter who brought down the animal is usually the owner of the implement as well. Nonetheless, the potential of attributing the kill to the owner of the implement is significant – it can take the focus off the hunter and pass the obligation for the distribution to another who had not even participated in the hunt. For instance, Bahuchet (1990: 41) mentions that Aka elders who can no longer hunt loan weapons to younger men and in that way can still preside over the sharing, enter the exchange network and receive meat without losing dignity. Among the !Kung, the meat distribution can be a burden, particularly if the successful hunter is visiting another camp and "does not know the hearts of the people." He can then choose to hunt only with borrowed arrows, and thereby to pass the responsibility for distribution over to a senior member of the camp. Or, if a hunter is undergoing severe criticism for acting like a big shot, he can use a borrowed arrow and turn the carcass over to the owner as a sign that he is reforming his ways.

In societies where the hunter is given rights over distribution, extreme modesty is enforced. The !Kung provide an excellent example: when a hunter is successful, he does not stride into camp and announce his kill, but leaves the carcass in the bush, slips in from the back of the hut, and sits unobtrusively by his fire. Others approach him and ask if he had seen any animals during his hunt. Even if his kill is large, he replies that he saw nothing of consequence while out hunting or that he killed only a small, scrawny antelope. After low-key discussion, during which people display indifference or even negativity at the news of a kill, the meat is fetched for distribution. If the hunter is perceived as arrogant, the meat is insulted and his efforts are belittled (see Lee 1984 for a particularly good description). Among the Hadza, the successful hunter exercises similar restraint upon his return to the camp, sits down quietly and "allows the blood on the shaft to speak for him" (Woodburn 1982: 440). A successful Mbuti hunter speaks little of the kill or not at all and lets others give the details of the hunt (Harako 1981: 536). Similar modesty is imposed on the good hunter among the Guayaki, who is called "a man of good luck", (Clastres 1972), not a man of skill. Lothrop (1928: 422) gives the following description of the behavior of a successful Ona hunter:

> Returning to his windbreak the hunter would silently hand his bow to his wife to hang up and throw the meat on the ground near the fire or hang it on a tree. No one would pay attention to it, for it was considered bad manners to show elation at the success of the hunt or merriment at the prospect of food. After sitting around in a sullen silence for half an hour, the hunter would casually ask his wife why she did not cook some meat, and she would then do so. But until given leave she would not touch the meat, as it was his, but not her property.

The Meat Distribution

During the actual meat distribution the process of reversing the debt begins, that is, rather than allowing the hunter to place recipients in debt to him, efforts are made to downplay the hunter's merit and emphasize his duty to provide meat for others. For example, the belief that hunting success is an acceptance on the part of the game to let itself be captured (Downs 1966; Henry 1941; Robbe 1989; Saladin d'Anglure 1978; Sharp 1988), particularly by men who are generous in sharing, is widely held among foragers of North and South America and the Arctic. The Ammassalik Inuit say that each man is born with the quota of animals that he will kill in his life attached to him. Not every hunter, however, accepts this fate, and in the past murders have been committed or sorcery practiced to try to expropriate the quota of another (Robbe 1989: 370). The Hadza say that meat is "God's meat", to be brought back to the camp and shared by all (Barnard and Woodburn 1988: 18), and the Jahai consider whatever they procure in the forest to be gifts from the ancestors (van der Sluys 1993: 25). Attempts to avoid a sense of debt to the hunter are also evident in linguistic terms. The Aka Pygmies call what is received during sharing that "person's due" (Bahuchet 1990:

39); among the Batek, !Kung, Guayaki, and Jahai, and probably in most foraging societies, to say thank you is unheard of, for one's share is one's due. Van der Sluys (1993: 27) explains this lack of polite speech as follows:

> I argue that the absence of polite terms during Jahai social interactions indicates a tendency to avoid the idea of mutual obligation or reciprocity, which would interfere with the feeling of unconditional togetherness of social bonding. Creating debts in the form of reciprocity obligations which exists in many societies (Mauss 1923-4) is unthinkable among the Jahai.

Only for the G/wi San and Xo San is it mentioned that the receiver may return a small gift for the meat received (Heinz 1966; Silberbauer 1981b).

As the distribution of meat proceeds, the hunter is removed further and further from any possibility of amassing debts, and it becomes clear that, as Harako (1976: 78) states of the Mbuti Pygmies, "though ownership of game is formally expressed, the catch belongs to all members of the camp." In foraging societies, the successful hunter never divides the carcass up into numerous small pieces, publicly calling out the names of the receiver. Rather, the hunter or whoever is appointed to be in charge of the distribution cuts the animal into a number of large chunks and distributes them to a few other individuals, beginning two or three waves of sharing. The first generally involves the distribution of large portions of meat by the owner or owners to members of the hunting party and/or a number of others, such as in-laws, close consanguineous kin, exchange partners, or "name relatives". Although bridewealth is not paid in foraging societies, lifelong obligations to share meat with in-laws are usually stipulated (Marshall 1976; Lee 1979; Heinz 1966; Gould 1980; Altman and Peterson 1988). The recipients then subdivided their portions among their own kin, visitors or friends to begin the second wave of sharing. When this is complete, the meat is cooked and distributed within the household and to others in the camp who did not happen to receive meat in the first or second wave of the distribution. Figure 10.4 gives some idea of the nature of the first wave of distribution for larger game; small animals are often cooked at the fire of the hunter and shared with his family and visitors to their hearth.

One of the two most common forms of distribution found in ten out of twenty-seven societies is for the owner to divide the carcass among members of the hunting party, who in turn take their portions home and make their own distributions during the second wave of sharing. For nine, meat is distributed by the hunter according to set partnerships or kinship obligations, and in the case of certain animals, to co-hunters. The Copper and Netsilik Inuit butcher

Figure 10.4 Division of Game in First Wave of Sharing

Meat divided into large pieces and distributed relatively equally among party of hunters/helpers (often at kill site)
Western Desert Aborigines
Pintupi
Gunwinggu
Bihor
Mbuti Pygmies
Aka Pygmies
Washo
Inuit of Quebec
Inuit of West Greenland
Cree

Distributed by hunter according to set partnerships, name relatives and/or specific kinship obligations (for certain animals also with co-hunters)
Netsilik Inuit
Copper Inuit
!Kung San
!Ko San
Ayoréode
Jahai
Ammassalik Inuit
Ona
Kaingáng

Returned to camp, divided equally between all households
Andamanese
Guayaki/Ache
Agta
Batek

Other
Iglilik, Hadza, G/wi and Chipewyan (see text)

seals into fourteen parts and the distribution is made on the basis of a rigid system of meat-sharing partnerships (Damas 1972: 46-47). The !Kung also divide the carcass into large pieces and share the portions of meat according to kinship obligations and exchange partnerships, although rules governing the division are more flexible. Such distributions are followed by second and third waves of sharing. Among the Andamanese, Guayaki, Agta, and Batek, the meat is returned to camp and divided by the hunter and camp members into equal portions for each household in the camp, regardless of household size. The Agta strip the meat and fat from the carcass and meticulously measure out exactly equal shares for each household (Griffin 1984; Rai 1990). Household size is compensated for in the third wave of the distribution. The Hadza, G/wi, and Iglulik have other forms of distribution. A successful G/wi hunter, with or without his hunting partner, may decide to hold a men's feast (Silberbauer 1981a, 1981b). He issues invitations, and on the afternoon after the kill is made, the invited men gather to receive cooked pieces of meat. Toward the end of the feast, an enjoyable social occasion, families appear on the outskirts, and each guest is given a portion of raw meat to pass on to his family. When men's feasts are not held, raw meat is distributed directly by the owner or a senior man to fit household needs. Then second and third waves of sharing take place. The Hadza also hold a feast for initiated men, sending the rest of the carcass, "people's meat", to the camp, where shares are given to anybody who asks for them. Pregnant women are given priority. The Iglulik Inuit share villagewide and/or distribute meat as gifts. Among the Chipewyan (Sharp 1981: 238-39) to request meat degrades a man's reputation and thus is done via women:

> ... Since food procurement is, publicly, a male activity, any borrowing that males do (if it goes outside the boundaries of the restricted cognatic descent group) weighs heavily upon their reputation for power/knowledge. This is reflected in the preemptive claim men have over foodstuffs and the tendency to give ostentatiously far more than they are asked for. No matter how skilled the hunter, there are times when there is not enough food ...
> Borrowing, or rather the necessity to borrow, is in direct contravention of the symbolic values placed on males, since they are supposed to be competent and complete providers. By making this something that women do, and hence not really of notice, the public system and the male's position can be preserved ...
> ... The wife of a hunter receives a steady stream of visitors, each chatting for a while with the wife and other visitors, who await a piece of meat before starting home. If the pieces given are large they may be divided again at the woman's home and given to her female kin. Somehow the man who killed the animal seems to lurk, visibly but inconspicuously, in the background while the meat is shared.

As in the Chipewyan case, many foragers remove the hunter from the focus of attention during the second or third waves of the meat distribution either by delivering portions of meat via children or by handing the distribution over to the women (Damas 1972; Gusinde 1931: 398; Kaplan 1983: 67-68; Rokke 1989: 410; van der Sluys 1993).

The three waves of sharing thus create numerous donors and distribute gratitude for generosity over many in the exchange network. People are not only pleased with the hunters, but with all others who share with them. In the second and particularly in the third wave of distribution, women have considerable say over where the meat goes.

After the meat has gone through two or three waves of sharing, it is reasonable to ask what the hunter and his family gets out of it. The answer for most societies is "no more than an equal share", as can be seen in Figure 10.5. In only three out of twenty-five societies does the hunter get a greater share or preferred parts, and, for the Bihor, only in the case of net hunting. Although Pygmy, Agta, Bihor, and Batek hunters set aside portions of meat to trade with neighboring agriculturalists, the returns for these also are usually shared. In fifteen societies, the hunter gets a share that is roughly equal to that of other camp members, and usually the skin of the animal as well. In three, hunters get inferior shares, and in another four, the hunter is not allowed to partake of the meat from animals that he killed. As Clastres (1972: 168) explains for the Guayaki, this practice creates a total reciprocal interdependence of families: the hunter spends his life hunting for others, and others spend their lives hunting for him. Just as hunters in most foraging societies can not expect to get a greater than average proportion of their own kill, when others make kills, the former donors also can expect little more than an equal share.

Figure 10.5 Shares of Meat Received by the Hunter

Preferred parts or greater share of the kill
Inuit of Quebec
Bihor (in net hunting)
Chipewyan

Hunter receives share approximately equal to that of other group members
Washo (adult men)
Netsilik Inuit
Copper Inuit
Andamanese (distribution with respect to age)
Mbuti Pygmies
Agta
Pintupi
Gunwinggu
Batek
Hadza
G/wi
!Kung
Ona
Ammassalik
Jahai

Inferior parts or less meat than average
Western Desert
West Greenland Inuit
Ayoréode

Hunter not allowed to eat meat
Guayaki/Ache
Aka Pygmies
Washo (unmarried men)
Kaingáng (for pigs; only grown men can eat meat of tapirs that they have killed)

Insufficient information for Iglulik and Cree.

Discussion

To sum up, for all forager societies examined some concept of status is mentioned, although in only fourteen out of twenty-five is status associated with hunting. This indicates intercultural differences in valuing skills, which, in turn, have some correlation with natural environment, dependency on meat, cultural/symbolic evaluations of meat, and history of relations with surrounding populations. For all but one society, ownership of the carcass is established after a kill, and usually the successful hunter or hunters are designated. Meat of all but the smallest animals has to be shared, and in most cases the owners have some say over the first wave of the meat distribution or can elect somebody to do the job. For all societies, status is kept in check by ideologies and sharing practices that take the hunter out of the focus of attention and/or prevent him from turning success to dominance. This delicate balance is expressed in many ethnographies: Gould (1980: 85) writes for the Aborigines of the Western Desert that the hunter gets some social prestige, although there is no personal or family aggrandizement via foods or goods. Saladin d'Anglure (1984: 492) says of the Inuit of Quebec that the owner of an *umiak*, a large boat used for collective transport, had a certain recognized status, especially if he were also a good hunter, knew how to share his surplus and was a generous host. However, he could use his status only sparingly if he wished to preserve the cooperation and participation of other families in the collective activities of the band. Turnbull (1965: 183) describes a similar situation for the Mbuti Pygmies: "some men, because of exceptional hunting skill, may come to resent it when their views are disregarded, but if they try to force those views they are very promptly subjected to ridicule."

At least one of the following measures taken to keep successful hunters in check is found in every society considered: (1) demands for modest behavior that removes them from the focus of attention, (2) two or more waves of meat distribution that spread feelings of gratitude beyond the hunter to many in the exchange network, and (3) efforts to erase a sense of debt to the hunter. In other words, with a few exceptions, people try to prevent meat shared from becoming a "gift" in the sense used by Mauss 1950/1923-4) as something that compels a return due to a threefold obligation in humans to give, receive and reciprocate. To give in the context of Mauss' "gift", one must first possess. Though foragers initially recognize ownership of a kill, through cultural means they diffuse this concept in subsequent steps of the distribution and with it the necessity to directly reciprocate.

Despite this common core of leveling mechanisms, intercultural differences are substantial. Some social recognition for hunters is permitted for Inuit groups, who are highly dependent on meat, and in San groups. By contrast, status in general, and that associated with hunting in particular, is strongly downplayed among forest hunter-gatherers of Asia. Beliefs that remove credit from the successful hunter, i.e. the idea that animals give themselves over to hunters, are found in certain areas particularly North America, South America, and the Arctic. The view of the forest as a "giving environment" (Bird-David 1990, 1992) that provides food for people is prevalent in Asia and forest-living groups of Africa. Nonetheless, the prevalence of a strong common core of ideology and accompanying social sanctions to support equality in and of itself attests to the existence of an underlying predisposition for individuals to seek status. Although status distinctions can be greatly repressed, the quest for status on the part of individuals cannot be completely eradicated, and thus requires the regular applications of measures to keep it in check. These findings beg the question: "Why is the egalitarian ethic so strongly enforced in foraging societies, and why do the more able accept it?" After all, in many complex hunter-gatherer societies or agricultural ones, existing sharing practices for meat and other foods successfully reduce the risk, and yet people attain high status through food distribution (Hayden, this volume).

Here I propose that some insights can be found in the understandings of rank order that have come out of ethological studies: (1) although high status or a pronounced rank order gives greater access to resources to those on top, under certain circumstances it can be of benefit to those in lower positions who follow different strategies and (2) status in humans requires alliance and thus in part must be agreed upon (see chapters by Grammer and Hold-Cavell in this volume). In any society, success of one is relative to the achievements of others, and for every strategy there is a counterstrategy. Individuals can succeed relatively by achieving more themselves and/or by inhibiting the achievements of others. People are keenly aware the status of others and reluctant to let them get ahead unless they perceive that the advantages of having dominant leaders outweigh the disadvantages. However, if benefits of leadership are great, particularly in the face of intergroup competition, there are indications that people do indeed seek authority figures and readily accept a secondary position that is more secure (Eibl-Eibesfeldt 1989: 310-11).

In foraging societies of this century, where organized intergroup competition is infrequent partly due to the dominance of their neighbors, people have little to gain from having stronger leaders. Moreover, they even stand to lose, for dominance threatens the workings of social security networks. These exist in all forager societies and are geared to cover daily, weekly or monthly variations as well as what might be called the rare, definitive crunches – events that occur only a few times in a lifetime but bring death or disaster – whether they be caused by nutritional, medical or social/political factors. In societies with no storage, an extraordinarily wide range of risks must be pooled over the long term through reciprocal relationships that have very special conditions. The first condition is that the terms of the relationship must be that he who has food, goods or valuables gives to those in need, the need being relative to the means of both (Sahlins 1972). Second, returns for gifts of assistance cannot be stipulated by time, quantity or quality (Sahlins 1972) if they are to meet a wide variety of needs. In other words, the giver has no desire to receive an immediate and fixed return that would balance the relationship, but would rather wait for reciprocation until the situation of "have" and "have not" is reversed.

Relationships that pool risk are ideally balanced over a lifetime, if constantly controlled for cheating. For example, those who have things of value but do not give are subject to social control through gossip, ridicule or ostracism. Those who feel that they are being exploited may cease to produce for a while and force others to do their share. However, it is recognized that unpredictable events will make some people unable to reciprocate adequately even in the best of times, and, accordingly, a wide range of reciprocal ties are maintained so that people will win some times, lose other times, and break even in most. A one-way flow of food or assistance over a long period of time is mitigated by the fact that the cost of the assistance is often small for the donor in relation to its value to the recipient: to host a family in one's camp and give it permission to forage on one's land for six months is little in comparison to the fact that this may save the family from starvation. The irritations caused by a one-way flow of goods or the effort of maintaining a relationship over a considerable distance are not buffered by intellectual or economic considerations, but by emotional ones; the determining factor in the survival of relationships over time and distance is friendship and affection (Wiessner 1981, 1982a, 1986).

Sharing of meat from successful hunts is only one aspect in this broader system of reciprocal relationships to reduce risk, a system on which every individual depends (Bahuchet 1990; Barnard and Woodburn 1988; Wiessner 1981).[1] Any success in gaining status and converting this to dominance that would allow certain individuals greater access to natural or human resources, impose indebtedness or attain authority is structurally incompatible with the terms of such social means of risk reduction. Greater access to resources would make one party permanently a "have" and the other a "have not", requiring the "have" to close himself off from exploitation. Inflicting a debt on another destroys the loose terms of the relationship in which returns are not stipulated by time, quantity or quality. Finally, relations of dominance would adversely affect the emotional ties that are so critical to the maintenance of relationships over long periods of time. Accordingly, the less productive people keep the status of the more able or motivated people in check to prevent them from disrupting the risk-sharing system that is so essential to their well-being. The most productive, although economically able to break out of the system in the short run (if not morally and emotionally), cannot afford to do so in the longer run, a fact stated in many ethnographies.

In closing, it should be noted that the fierce equality enforced in forager societies can pose an obstacle to current development, for strong leadership from within greatly facilitates organization and the power of a group to make its demands heard. It will continue to be so until: (1) abundant resources are available that permit individuals to cover risks through means other than pooling, such as storage that reduces fluctuations in subsistence income and finances payments to deal with social or political problems (i.e. bridewealth or compensation/fines) and (2) intergroup competition imposes a need for organization and/or representation by a dominant leader. There is, however, no reason to believe that status differences and more pronounced leadership will not ultimately come about with social and economic change, even though egalitarian ideologies stubbornly resist. As the many leveling mechanisms in forager societies imply, the tendency of individuals to seek status and influence is a current that runs through all societies.

Notes

I would like to thank Bion Griffin, Volker von Bremen, Serge Bahuchet, Pierre Robbe, Cory van der Sluys for most helpful discussions and providing additional information.

1. Numerous studies have demonstrated the effectiveness of sharing in reducing interhousehold variation in meat consumption (Bailey 1991; Kaplan et al. 1984, 1985a, 1985b; Griffin 1984; Smith 1988; Speth and Spielmann 1983; Tanaka 1980; Wilmsen 1989). The benefits of sharing, both nutritional and social, for the average household have been established, although these may not always show up in short-term studies (Hawkes 1993).

References

Altman, J. and N. Peterson. 1988. Rights to game and rights to cash among contemporary Australian hunter-gatherers. In *Hunters and Gatherers: Property, Power and Ideology*, ed. T. Ingold, D. Riches and J. Woodburn 75-94. Oxford: Berg.

Bahuchet, S. 1990. Food sharing among the pygmies of Central Africa. *African Study Monographs* 11: 27-53.

Bailey, R. 1991. *The Behavioral Ecology of Efe Pygmy Men in the Ituri Forest, Zaire*. Museum of Anthropology. Ann Arbor: Univer. of Michigan.

Balikci, A. 1970. *The Netsilik Eskimos*. Garden City, N.J.: Natural History Press.

Balikci, A. 1971. The structure of Central Eskimo associations. In *Alliance in Eskimo Society*, ed. L. Guemple, 40-55. Seattle: Univer. of Washington Press.

Balikci, A. 1984. Netsilik. In *Handbook of American Indians*, vol. 5, ed. D. Damas. Washington, D.C.: Smithsonian Institution.

Barnard, A. and J. Woodburn 1988. Property, power and ideology in hunting-gathering societies: An introduction. In *Hunters and Gatherers: Property, Power and Ideology*, ed. T. Ingold, D. Riches and J. Woodburn, 4-31. Oxford: Berg.

Binford, L. R. 1980. Willow smoke and dogs' tails: hunter-gatherer setttlement systems and archaeological site information. *American Antiquity* 45: 4-20.

Bird-David, N. 1990. The giving environment: Another perspective on the economic system of hunter-gatherers. *Current Anthropology* 13: 189-95.

Bird-David, N. 1992. Beyond "the original affluent society": A culturalist revision. *Current Anthropology* 33: 25-47.

Cashdan, E. 1985. Coping with risk: reciprocity among the Basarwa of northern Botswana. *Man*, 20: 454-76.

Clastres, P. 1972. The Guayaki. In *Hunters and Gatherers Today*, ed. M. G. Bicchieri, 138-174. New York: Holt, Rinehart and Winston.

Damas, D. 1972. The Copper Eskimo. In *Hunters and Gatherers Today*, ed. M. G. Bicchieri. New York: Holt, Rinehart and Winston.

Damas, D. 1984. Copper Eskimo. In *Handbook of North American Indians*, vol. 5, ed. D. Damas, 387-41. Washington, D.C.: Smithsonian Institution.

Dowling, J. 1968. Individual ownership and the sharing of game in hunting societies. *American Anthropologist* 70: 502-7.

Downs, J.F. 1966. *The Two Worlds of the Washo*. New York: Holt, Rinehart and Winston.

Eibl-Eibesfeldt, I. 1989. *Human Ethology*. New York: Aldine.

Endicott, K. 1988. Property, power and conflict among the Batek of Malaysia. In *Hunters and Gatherers: Property, Power and Ideology*, ed. T. Ingold, D. Riches and J. Woodburn, 110-28. Oxford: Berg.

Gould, R. A. 1980. *Living Archaeology*. Cambridge: Cambridge Univer. Press.

Gould, R. A. 1981. Comparative ecology of food-sharing in Australia and northwest California. In *Omnivorous Primates*, ed. R. Harding and G. Teleki, 422-54. New York: Columbia Univer. Press.

Griffin, P. B. 1984. All food is shared: Agta forager acquisition, distribution and consumption of meat and plant resources. Paper presented at conference on The Sharing of Food: from Phylogeny to History, Bad Homburg, Germany.

Gusinde, M. 1931. *Die Feuerland Indianer. Die Selk'nam: Vom Leben und Denken eines Jägervolkes auf der grossen Feuerlandinsel.* Mödling bei Wien: Verlag International Zeitschrift Anthropos.

Harako, R. 1976. The Mbuti as hunters. A study of ecological anthropology of the Mbuti Pygmies (Ituri, Zaire). *Kyoto University African Studies* 10: 37-99.

Harako, R. 1981. The cultural ecology of hunting behavior among the Mbuti Pygmies of the Ituri forest, Zaire. In *Omnivorous Primates*, ed. R. H. and G. Teleki, 499-555. .New York: Columbia Univer. Press.

Hawkes, K. 1993. Why hunter-gatherers work: an ancient version of the problem of public goods. *Current Anthropology* 14: 341-61.

Hayden, B. 1990. Nimrods, piscators, pluckers and planters: The emergence of food production. *Journal of Anthropological Archaeology* 9: 31-69.

Heinz, H.J. 1966. The social organization of the !Ko Bushmen. Unpublished M.A. thesis, Univer. of South Africa.

Henry, J. 1941. *Jungle People: a Kaingáng Tribe of the Highlands of Brazil.* New York: J.J. Augustin.

Hold, B. 1974. Attention structure and rank specific behavior in pre-school children. In *The Social Structure of Attention*, ed. M. Chance and R. Larsen, 177-201. London: Wiley.

Hold, B. 1980. Attention-structure and behavior in G/wi San children. *Ethology and Sociobiology* 1: 275-90.

Kaplan, H. 1983. *The Evolution of Food Sharing among Adult Conspecifics: Research with Ache Hunter-Gatherers of Eastern Paraguay.* Ann Arbor: University Microfilms International.

Kaplan, H., K. Hill, K. Hawkes and A. Hurtado. 1984. Food sharing among the Ache hunter-gatherers of Eastern Paraguay. *Current Anthropology* 25: 113-14.

Kaplan, H., K. Hill, K. Hawkes and A. Hurtado. 1985a. Hunting ability and reproductive success among male Ache foragers: preliminary results. *Current Anthropology* 26: 131-33.

Kaplan, H., K. Hill, K. and A. Hawkes and A. Hurtado. 1985b. Food sharing among Ache foragers: tests of explanatory hypotheses. *Current Anthropology* 26: 223-46.

Kleivan, I. 1984. West Greenland before 1950. In *Handbook of North American Indians*, vol. 5, ed. D. Damas, 595-621. Washington, D.C.: Smithsonian Institution.

Lee, R. B. 1979. *The !Kung San: Men, Women and Work in a Foraging Society.* Cambridge: Cambridge Univer. Press.

Lee, R. B. 1984. *The Dobe !Kung*. New York: Holt, Rinehart and Winston.
Lothrop, S. K. 1928. *The Indians of Tierra del Fuego*. New York: Museum of American Indians.
Marshall, L. 1976. *The !Kung of Nyae Nyae*. Cambridge, Ma.: Harvard Univer. Press.
Mary-Rousseliere, G. 1984. Iglulik. In *Handbook of North American Indians*, ed. D. Damas, 431-46. Washington, D.C.: Smithsonian Institution.
Mauss, M. 1950 (1923-4). *Essai sur le Don*. Paris: Presses Universitaires de France. (First published in L'Annee Sociologique 1923-4).
Meggitt, M. 1962. *Desert People*. Sydney: Angus and Robertson.
Myers, F. 1988. Burning the truck and holding the country: property, time and the negotiation of identity among Pintupi Aborigines. In *Hunters and Gatherers: Property, Power and Ideology*, ed. T. Ingold, J. Riches and J. Woodburn, 52-74. Oxford: Berg.
Price, J. A. 1975. Sharing: the integration of intimate economics. *Anthropologica* 17:2-27.
Radcliffe-Brown, A. 1964. *The Andaman Islanders*. New York: Free Press of Glencoe.
Rai, N. K. 1990. *Living in a Lean-to: Philippine Negrito Foragers in Transition*. Museum of Anthropology Ann Arbor, Michigan, Univer. of Michigan.
Robbe, P. 1989. Le chasseur arctique et son milieu: strategies individuelles et collectives des Inuit d'Ammassalik. Unpublished Doctorat D'État ès-sciences thesis. Université Pierre et Marie Curie, Paris.
Rogers, E. S. 1972. The Mistassini Cree. In *Hunters and Gatherers Today*, ed. M. G. Bicchieri, 90-137. New York: Holt, Rinehart and Winston.
Sahlins, M. 1972. *Stone Age Economics*. Chicago: Aldine.
Saladin d'Anglure, B. 1984. Inuit of Quebec. In *Handbook of North American Indians*, ed. D. Damas, 476-507. Washington, D.C.: Smithsonian Institution.
Saladin d'Anglure, B. 1978. L'Homme (*angut*), le Fils (*irniq*), et la Lumiére (*qau*) ou le cercle du pouvoir masculin chez les Inuit de l'Arctique Central. *Anthropologica* 20: 101-44.
Schebesta, P. 1954. *Die Negrito Asiens: Wirtschaft und Soziologie*. Vienna-Mödling: St. Gabriel Verlag.
Scott, C. 1988. Property, practice and aboriginal rights among Quebec Cree hunters. In *Hunters and Gatherers: Property, Power and Ideology*, ed. T. Ingold, D. Riches and J. Woodburn, 35-51. Oxford: Berg.
Sharp, H. 1977. The Chipewyan hunting unit. *American Ethnologist* 4: 377-93.
Sharp, H. 1981. The null case: The Chipewyan. In *Woman the Gatherer*, ed. F. Dahlberg, 221-224. New Haven: Yale Univer. Press.
Sharp, H. 1988. Dry meat and gender: the absence of Chipewyan ritual for the regulation of hunting and animal numbers. In *Hunters and Gatherers: Property, Power and Ideology*, ed. T. Ingold, D. Riches and J. Woodburn, 183-202. Oxford: Berg.
Silberbauer, G. 1981a. *Hunter and Habitat in the Central Kalahari Desert*. Cambridge: Cambridge Univer. Press.

Silberbauer, G. 1981b. Hunter/Gatherers of the Central Kalahari. In *Omnivorous Primates*, ed. R. Harding and G. Teleki, 455-98. New York: Columbia Univer. Press.

Smith, E. A. 1988. Risk and uncertainty in the 'original affluent society': Evolutionary ecology of resource-sharing and land tenure. In *Hunters and Gatherers: Property, Power and Ideology*, ed. T. Ingold, D. Riches and J. Woodburn, 222-51. Oxford: Berg.

Speth, J. and K. Spielmann. 1983. Energy source, protein metabolism, and hunter-gatherer subsistence strategies. *Journal of Anthropological Archaeology* 2: 1-31.

Tanaka, J. 1980. *The San Hunter-Gatherers of the Kalahari*. Tokyo: Univer. of Tokyo Press.

Testart, A. 1982. The significance of food storage among hunter-gatherers: residence patterns, population densities, and social inequalities. *Current Anthropology* 23: 253-530.

Turnbull, C. M. 1965. *Wayward Servants: The Two Worlds of the African Pygmies*. London: Eyre and Spottiswoode.

van der Sluys, C. 1993. The dynamics of Jahai worldview. Seventh International Congress on Hunting and Gathering Societies, Moscow.

von Bremen, V. 1991. *Zwischen Anpassung und Aneignung: Zur Problematik von Wildbeuter-Gesellschaften im modernen Weltsystem am Beispiel der Ayoreode*. Munich: Anacon.

Wiessner, P. 1977. *Hxaro: A Regional System of Reciprocity for Reducing Risk among the !Kung San*. University Microfilms: Ann Arbor, Michigan.

Wiessner, P. 1981. Measuring the impact of social ties on nutritional status among the !Kung San. *Social Science Information* 20: 641-78.

Wiessner, P. 1982a. Risk, reciprocity and social influences on !Kung San economics. In *Politics and History in Band Societies*, ed. E. Leacock & R. B. Lee, 61-84. Cambridge: Cambridge Univer. Press.

Wiessner, P. 1982b. Beyond willow smoke and dog's tails: a comment on Binford's analysis of hunter-gatherer settlement systems. *American Antiquity* 57: 171-8.

Wiessner, P. 1986. !Kung San networks in a generational perspective. In *The Past and Future of !Kung Ethnography: Essays on Honor of Lorna Marshall*, ed. M. Biesele, R. Gordon and R. Lee, 103-36. Hamburg: Helmut Buske.

Williams, B. J. 1974. A model of band society. *American Antiquity*, Memoir 29.

Wilmsen, E. 1989. *Land Filled with Flies*. Chicago: Univer. of Chicago Press.

Winterhalter, B. 1986. Diet choice, risk and food sharing in a stochastic environment. *Journal of Anthropological Archaeology* 5: 369-92.

Woodburn, J. 1982. Egalitarian societies. *Man* 17: 431-51.

11. FOOD AND THE STATUS QUEST IN FIVE AFRICAN CULTURES

Igor de Garine

Like other social mammals, humans generate status differences that are based, among other things, on access to food among individuals of the same group or the same society. Such discrepancies, which tend to become institutionalized, can, of course, be analyzed in terms of Darwinian adaptation and biological success, but they have other functions specific to human beings. Within a society, these discrepancies help to establish communication between individuals who would, if they were totally equivalent, have no reason to interact and might remain isolated monads. Status differences are linked to social structure and social dynamics. The quest for food and the quest for sex both correspond to the fulfillment of primary needs – and humans spend more effort on the former. As Levi-Strauss (1949: 40) puts it, in human societies not only women but also food are part of the scarce commodities system (initiated by the incest taboo) through which society establishes its control over individuals.

Sharing systems, which are usually nonegalitarian, operate among some nonhuman primates, as demonstrated, for instance, among baboons, vervets, and purple-faced langurs (Oates 1987: 205; Harding 1975: 249-50; Hladik 1975: 6). They also exist in human societies between males and females, young and old, but humans are the only creatures that purposely create discrepancies in access to food in order to achieve dominance. A couple of centuries ago the shogun Leyasu Tokukawa wrote of Japanese peasants: "So that they live, so that they die, feed them just enough so that they survive and are able to work for us. Deny them with judicious forethought what they are asking for, so that they never become too powerful and rebel against us" (Mitra 1982: 1).

Socioeconomic factors are most often referred to as creating and illustrating status differences between individuals and between groups. They are often of a symbolic order. They may actually result in permanent differences in nutritional status that affect performance and survival. On one hand, populations living "below the poverty line" that have not achieved their genetic potentialities are a conspicuous feature of our modern world. On the other, permanent overeating, as observed in the Western world, has negative biological consequences. Status through food can be obtained in many ways; there is more to it than potlatch-like competitions. As illustrated by Hinduism, it may even be achieved through dieting or fasting to the limits of starvation, as done by the Sadus.

Conceptually, there are two aspects to social status: a static one, that is, ascribed status, such as that of an Indian Brahmin, and a dynamic one, that is, achieved status, which is established through individual efforts such as those of a successful businessman. However, the notions of ascribed and achieved status constantly overlap, and one can talk about status achieved in the framework of ascribed status. Power goes to the well-fed; fat is, to a large extent, "beautiful". Nahoum (1979: 22-32) points out that in Italy during the Middle Ages, the nobles were called *popolo grosso* and the serfs *popolo magro*. An African chief has to be fat since he is the symbol of the prosperity of his people. The same situation existed in Calabria, where starved peasants were proud of the plumpness of their lord (Teti 1976: 91). Conversely, as described by Misasi, (1976: 121), the mountain bandit who rebelled against the system was thought of as strong, stalwart, handsome, avid for good food and beautiful women. Today this image applies to the "Americans" (the term used for Sicilians who have emigrated to the U.S.), occasionally members of the Drangheta, the Calabrian Mafia (Teti 1995:23).

Food is a constant counterpoint to social events and may appear as a status symbol of the privileged. A hundred years ago Brillat Savarin (1885: 1) wrote, *"Dis-moi ce que tu manges, je te dirai ce que tu es"* (Tell me what you eat, I'll tell you what you are). He was the inventor of the *éprouvettes gastronomiques* (gastronomical tests) that assessed the social status of individuals – what Bourdieu (1979) calls their "distinction" – by the way they reacted to various types of meals.

There are at least three ways of gaining status through food:

1. by displaying and consuming prestigious foods on specific conspicuous consumption opportunities. This "fighting with food,"

appropriately termed by Young (1971), to enhance one's position (as in the potlatch) is well documented.
2. by having permanent access, quantitatively and qualitatively, to the best foods, according to prevailing cultural standards. This may have nothing at all to do with dietetic aspects and be purely symbolic, a criterion for class stratification. As remarked by Bourdieu (1979: 209-10), in present-day France, the highest levels of distinction illustrated by academics and artists are illustrated when individuals moving up the social ladder stop eating large amounts of the food of their previous diet (often very nutritious) and adopt very different and sophisticated items, which are often less nourishing. In a totally different environment, Gopaldas remarks that in Gujarat, India, the segment of the Rathwakoli tribals (the Baghats) trying to climb in the caste system through *sanskritisation*, discard meat and alcohol from their regime, thus diminishing the variety in their diet. This results in "obtaining social benefits but suffering from a higher prevalence of specific nutritional disorders" (Gopaldas, Gupta, and Saxena 1983: 217). As we shall see, permanent access to alcoholic drinks may also be a token of "distinction".
3. One of the populations we shall be dealing with, the Massa, offer an intermediate situation: status is displayed and gained by allowing certain biological groups of the society (adult men, usually young) periodically to have a greater access to valued foods and to become fat, handsome, and prestigious.

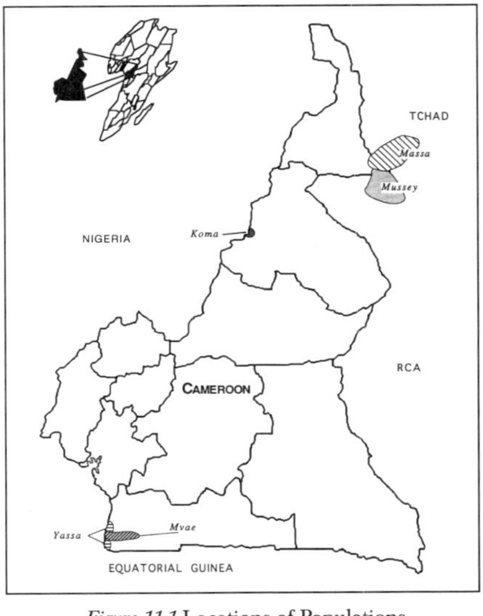

Figure 11.1 Locations of Populations

The purpose of this paper is to examine different types of status quests and how food is used to pursue these in five Cameroonian populations: the Massa, the Mussey, the Koma, the Yassa, and the Mvae; to find out what they have in common; and to ask ourselves if food in the status quest can be interpreted in terms of maximization of inclusive fitness and in terms of improvement of psychosocial well-being.

The Massa

The quest for status can be understood only against the background of the general food system. Massa country, located along the banks of the Logone River some 250 kilometers south of N'jamena, the capital of Chad, is characterized by climatic hazards, especially irregular rainfall and flooding, which affect food production. This leads to food uncertainty and a constant seasonal shortage of cereals, which in former times caused severe famines. As acknowledged by interviews with informants and by oral literature, food anxiety is present, with the consequence that abundant food supplies and fatness are appreciated.

Figure 11.2 Food Calendar in a Tropical Savanna Environment Population – The Massa (Cameroon)

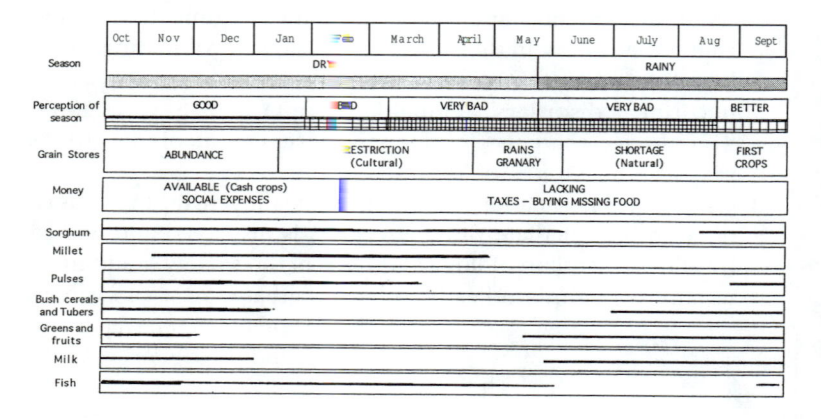

Month	Oct	Nov	Dec	Jan	Feb	March	April	May	June	July	Aug	Sept
Season	DRY								RAINY			
Perception of season	GOOD				BAD	VERY BAD			VERY BAD			BETTER
Grain Stores	ABUNDANCE				RESTRICTION (Cultural)			RAINS GRANARY		SHORTAGE (Natural)		FIRST CROPS
Money	AVAILABLE (Cash crops) SOCIAL EXPENSES					LACKING TAXES – BUYING MISSING FOOD						

Sorghum
Millet
Pulses
Bush cereals and Tubers
Greens and fruits
Milk
Fish

The Traditional System

The Massa, who number 200,000 individuals equally distributed in Cameroon and Chad, have a mixed type of economy; they are farmers, herdsmen (cows, sheep, goats), and fishermen. They value three main food items: red sorghum *(Sorghum caudatum)*, fish, and the milk of their cows. They are, however, reluctant cultivators. Being a successful fisherman, although appreciated, does not bring much fame. Herding is their most prestigious activity, and milk is the most favored item in the diet. This is understandable since cattle ownership constitutes the avenue to social success. Cattle compose the bridewealth (a minimum of ten heads of cattle are necessary to obtain a wife) and allow a network of durable social bonds to be established through a cattle-lending system, the *golla,* which is described by the Massa as "allowing one's partner to drink one's cows' milk" *(ci mbira).* Among the Massa, the most envied role is that of a *sa ma fareyna,* "a man with cattle", who is, as such, surrounded by many child-bearing wives. Herding has also generated a complex status-enhancing institution, the *guru.*

The *Guru*

At different periods of the year, men spend most of their time taking care of the cattle, the most valued asset in the culture. They live with the herd, drink its milk, and receive a more abundant diet than the rest of the villagers. They dance and wrestle to display their own strength and beauty, and to affirm the affluence of their village.

There are two kinds of *guru.* One is individual, the *guru walla.* During sessions the participant remains secluded and ingests very large quantities of food, mostly milk and red sorghum. Over a period of two months, he consumes daily about 7 kg. of food, i.e. around 13,000 kilocalories, which is a world record for daily consumption over such a long period in a nonexperimental situation (Sims, Goldman, Gluck, Morton, Kelleher, and Rowe 1968; Garine and Koppert 1991: 9; Pasquet, Brigant, Froment, Bard, Garine, and Apfelbaum, 1992). After two months of a very sedentary life, the participant has made spectacular progress and gained about 20 kg.

Figure 11.3. Weight of Food Consumed by S. During One-Week Fattening Session. Village of Kogoyna, September 1976 (in grams).

Day	Sorghum flour	Milk	Fresh fish	Dried fish	Fresh vegetables	Butter	Food energy (Kcal)
1st	2,655	3,446	0	87	158	0	12,188
2nd	2,687	2,924	41	0	178	0	11,565
3rd	2,525	3,169	123	0	0	0	11,183
4th	2,914	2,908	0	0	238	0	12,317
5th	3,391	3,171	0	0	195	0	14,166
6th	3,852	3,251	0	0	204	0	15,749
7th	3,927	3,913	0	0	191	42	16,823
Average	3,136	3,255	23	12	166	6	13,422

He is now ready to resume normal life or, most often, to join the second kind of fattening session, the collective *guru.* Only about 5 percent of the male population participate in the *guru walla,* but most men take part several times during their lives in the collective *guru.*

There are various types of collective *guru,* of which the most common is the *guru sarmana* ("the *guru* of the new grass") that takes place from September to January. In the collective *guru,* the participants

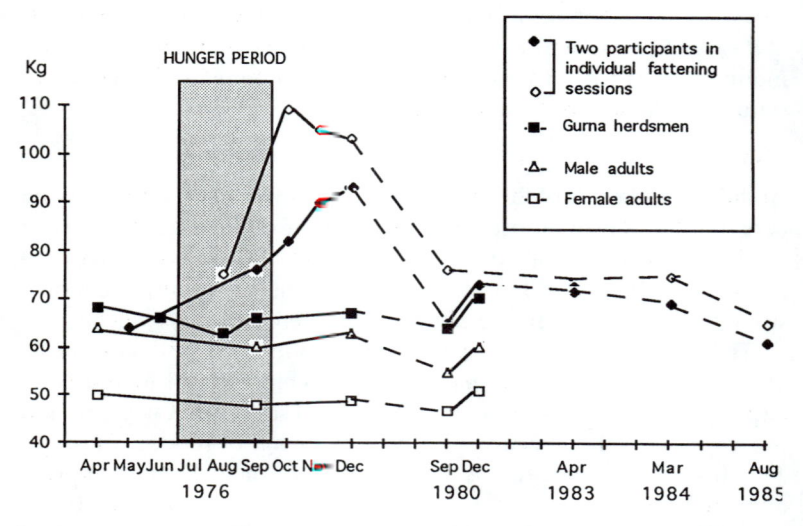

Figure 11.4 Seasonal Weight Fluctuations in a Tropical Savanna Population – the Massa (Cameroon)

(whom we shall call *gurna*[1] from now on) lead a more active life. They take care of the cattle and participate in the seasonal activities of the village. They demonstrate their physical fitness and their skill in dancing, singing, and wrestling, and are a credit to their village, whose dynamism and prosperity has enabled them to achieve such fitness. They consume mostly cows' milk and sorghum porridge and receive about 4,000 kilocalories daily (about 1,000 more than the villagers) and a larger amount of animal proteins and lipids. They appear in all seasons to be taller and heavier than the other villagers (Garine and Koppert 1991: 21).

Cultural views

What are cultural views with regard to this institution? Men are supposed to enter the *guru* (literally to "eat *(ti)* the *guru*) in order to drink milk *(ci mira)*, to become beautiful *(naa,* meaning both good and beautiful), and to grow *(nya,* meaning to increase, grow [for animals, plants, and objects]).

Beauty

If we skim through the tales, we can quote a few examples concerning beauty and desirability.

> Three brothers decided to go out to choose a wife. Two were twins, the other a single child. The latter decided to drink milk beforehand. He drank milk for a long time and grew fat. He put on a leopard loinskin, one

Figure 11.5 Comparison of the Diet of the Gurna and the Adult Male Villagers, Kogyna 1976

	Feb-May kilo-calories	Feb-May animal proteins (gr)	June-Aug kilo-calories	June-Aug animal proteins (gr)	Sept-Dec kilo-calories	Sept-Dec animal proteins (gr)
Gurna n = 17	3,828	63.3	3,224	74.0	5,323	110.0
Adult male villagers n = 27	3,090	57.6	2,970	30.0	3,090	47.3
Gurna advantage	738	5.7	254	44.0	2,235	63.6

Nutritional Advantage of the *Gurna* in 1976 (yearly average)

	kilocalories	animal proteins (gr)
Gurna n = 17	4,126	82.7
Adult male villagers n = 27	3,050	44.9
Gurna advantage	1,076	37.8

Amount of Milk Drunk by the *Gurna* As Compared To the Male Adult Villagers Kogoyna, 1976 (gr per capita per day)

	Dry season February-March Milk (gr)	Rainy season June-September Milk (gr)	Harvest season October-December Milk (gr)
Adult male villagers n = 2	66	124	46
Gurna n = 17	1,027	1,669	1,781

Figure 11.6 Anthropometry of the Massa as Compared to the Neighbouring Mussey* 1980

	Massa Men n=24	*Massa* Women n=50	*Massa* Gurna** n=12	*Mussey* Men n=29	*Mussey* Women n=45
Sept., end of shortage period					
Height – cm.	172.8	160.7	178.7	175.5	163.9
Weight – kg.	53.1	43.5	67.0	56.8	49.5
Arm circumference – cm.	25.2	23.2	27.5	24.9	24.8
Tricipital skinfold – mm.	27.0	23.4	30.0	28.1	29.3
Subscapular skinfold – mm.	62.5	79.0	76.0	65.4	81.2
Dec., full crop period	n=24	n=50	n=10	n=29	n=45
Height – cm.	173.1	161.0	179.7	175.6	164.1
Weight – kg.	58.3	47.8	69.2	61.3	53.3
Arm circumference – cm.	26.3	24.6	28.1	26.5	26.2
Tricipital skinfold – mm.	29.2	26.4	34.1	30.2	33.7
Subscapular skinfold – mm.	65.2	84.0	83.5	69.1	87.8

*Massa village of Kogoyna, Mussey villages of Gulmunta and Bigui.
**after participating in the *Guru* for 20 days.

of his brothers a gazelle skin and the other that of a bush antelope. After walking for a long time, they came across a group of women. 'Ladies, tell us which of us is the most beautiful.' They answered, 'You are all beautiful but the one with the leopard skin is the most handsome!' The twins thought it was because of the leopard skin and stripped their brother of it, but it was just the same, he was still declared the most attractive.

In a previous paper (de Garine 1987) I documented the grooming, singing, and dancing activities and their focus on women, ranging from a highly romantic to a very crude approach.

Milk drinking is also related to becoming strong, heavy, and powerful, and to wrestling. The tales are full of examples: "A chief put his daughter in a hut in the *guru walla* to drink milk. The girl said that she would marry the man who was strong enough to throw her in wrestling. The lion tried his chance and, at first, was unsuccessful. He then also went to the *guru*, won the contest, and married the girl."

It appears from the analysis of the oral literature and from informal interviews with informants that fatness is linked to strength and makes men desirable to women.

Testing Attitudes Toward Body Shape

We have studied the Massa opinion regarding the body shape of the two types of *gurna* compared to that of thin and undernourished adult males (Garine 1995). We used a set of nine photographs showing various types of Massa body build. The photographs were shown to twenty-two men and seven women. They were asked to indicate which individuals they preferred and those they disliked most, and to say why. Then they were asked to comment on the rest of the photos. Thin individuals were the most often rejected. Men considered them as poor and "too weak to work in the sun." Women thought they were ugly and disproportioned. From our previous work we expected that the fattened *gor walla* would be selected unanimously, but this was not the case.

The three very fat *gor walla* were chosen as frequently in a negative way as in a positive one. Favorable comments referred to the fact that they were ideal *gor walla*, having consumed much milk and sorghum porridge. The men, especially those who had undergone the same experience, considered them as being attractive to women and strong for wrestling. But, as noted by Fallon and Rozin (1985) with regard to U.S. students, the evaluation differed according to the sexes. The women found them too heavy, easily out of breath and consequently bad lovers, probably difficult to feed, and "poor workers in the sun." They appreciated them as sons, not as lovers or husbands.

A prestigious aspect in relation to fat body shape is having been provided with good food: "That man, he certainly has drunk milk and sorghum porridge!"; "That one, he is well taken care of by his parents!"; etc. Fatness means affluence. Strength is considered to go together with size; being big, and heavy but firm is valued. The wrestler type belongs to the collective *guru*, "upright in his footsteps, with thighs like millet stalks." Finally, the type selected as being the best – handsome, functional and well-to-do – was a slightly plump athlete who made the most of every occasion outside the community to demonstrate his efficiency as a dancer, singer, wrestler, and lover. He can also be a hard worker who can stand the heat of the sun, and he has cows available to him.

Role of the Collective Guru

The role of the *gurna* is rather transparent; they act as the "warriors" of their kinship group and, through their physical fitness, their beauty, their mock aggressive behavior toward men and seductiveness toward women, they demonstrate the power of their clan. Their way of "fighting with food" is by overeating choice food in order to become sociometric stars, thus accumulating prestige for the group, for their fathers and for themselves, and they may use this for their own economic and matrimonial strategy. They travel outside their territorial community and, being sexually attractive, spread their genes and secure wives from other genetic groups. Their role in taking care of the cattle with which the bridewealth is paid and the active way in which they seduce women may be regarded as contributing to the expansion of the population to which they belong. The stores of fat they accumulate afford them a better resistance to periods of food shortage than the rest of the group. They also keep a permanent supply of energy in reserve, eventually for heavy tasks. This is in line with biological adaptation.

On the negative side, their privileged use of milk may be seen as jeopardizing the access by the women and children to one of the best protein-rich foods available in the Massa diet. Women are remarkably thin compared with men, much more so than among a neighboring population, the Mussey (Garine and Koppert 1991: 22) (see Figure II.6). Since milk is almost the only source of protein during the rainy season, when food shortages occur, the *gurna* may contribute indirectly to the level of sickness and death in women and children during that period. Spreading their genes but restricting food for mothers and offspring is hardly adaptive in the Darwinian sense. Social prestige and biological rewards may lie on different grounds.

Conspicuous Consumption

The *guru walla* takes place at a time when milk is available but when the cereal shortage is at its peak. It is a typical case of conspicuous consumption: the *gor walla* puts on weight at the time when everybody else is on a restricted diet. Perhaps we are witnessing here some sort of "prosperity magic": the *gor walla* is fattening at the same time as the sorghum crop is growing. The symbolic link is corroborated by the fact that a *guru walla* session can never go on after the sorghum canes are cut in the field after the harvest. This would mean the death of the participant. He could be considered as filling an ambiguous function at the level of his community: demonstrating by his fatness during the seasonal shortage period that there is no lack of food, that the group nourishing him has things under control and has the power to defy the seasonal hardships. In this way, the *gor walla* is rather like the symbol of his kinship group's material success and of the favor bestowed on the group by the supernatural powers that allowed its fulfillment. He may therefore contribute to the general psychosocial well-being of the group that has helped him to achieve his envied status.

It should be added that with the Massa we are witnessing a very egalitarian type of society: most of the men have their time of fame. Only 5 percent of the men go through the *guru walla*, which implies being linked to a wealthy cattle owner as well as being a popular character, but most men have attended the collective *guru* and have been praised for their skill and beauty. This has helped them to get a wife, enabled them to start a family, and given them access to the envied condition of *sa far-yna*, a family head able to take part in the matrimonial strategies.

Aggressive display of wealth is not tolerated and would rapidly result in witchcraft being performed on the arrogant individual. He would also run the risk of being accused of sorcery.

Other Associations of Food and Status

The Massa have other more classical ways of using food in order to enhance their status. As in other African societies, most religious and social occasions are accompanied by feasts, especially funerals of elderly people, where cattle must be slaughtered. Domestic meat is always available during rituals, as is sorghum porridge. Guests have to be "full" *(hop hoiya)* at the end of the day if their host is to maintain a good image.

Food can also be linked with status but without the conferring of social prestige by merely demonstrating the niche a person occupies in the social network. This is the case of foods associated with women's prescriptions and women's avoidances. Children, who are immature and irresponsible members of the community, are entitled to consume a broad range of vegetable and animal products gathered from the bush and which no self-respecting adult would openly touch.

Numerous foods are thus specific to children and constitute one of the privileges of their age bracket. It should be noted that certain foods are also social symbols of poverty and dearth. Foods for the poor and famine foods, which encompass many of the children's range, are also status markers that display the opposite of abundance and affluence. Similarly, a number of smelly and dirty preparations or dishes are the privilege of the very old, whose time is spent, who no longer expect any sexual satisfaction, and who have lost their social responsibility and become like children while waiting for death.

In addition to participant observation and key informant interviews, we have used questionnaires to determine the rating obtained by different foods among the traditional Massa, such as: (1) What do you eat most often? (2) What do you prefer eating? (3) What do you dislike? (4) Which foods do you offer to guests to demonstrate that you are rich? (5) Which foods would you eat if you had no financial restrictions? (6) Which foods are eaten by the poor? The data are not yet fully analyzed but general trends appear in relation to foods regarded as status symbols in comparison to the Mussey, the traditional Massa, the urbanized Massa, and the Fulani trend setters.

Paradoxically, milk is never selected, although it is the most valued item of the diet. The probable reason is that it is not conceived as a food, but as a beverage consumed near the cattle, which confers fatness and mirth. People in mourning should abstain from drinking it since they should not be merry; they must consume bitter foods.

Red sorghum has an ambiguous position. Eaten most frequently, it is both preferred and disliked, and does not figure among prestigious items. It is probably a "superfood" (Jelliffe 1967: 273-81) that traditionally provides most of the calories in the diet, and is usually present in rituals to which individuals are linked emotionally. However, it is progressively losing its importance. Fish is esteemed by all and is frequently consumed. It has to be fresh and large to be prestigious. Domestic meat is also appreciated by everyone, while staples such as rice and late pricked sorghum (*S. durrah*) are prestigious but not necessarily liked. Another white cereal, bulrush millet *(Pennisetum sp.)*, is disliked, probably because of its taste.

All vegetable products from the bush, wild leaves, and cereals appear as symbols of poverty and hunger. A general term used to designate them is *sangawna,* "it grows in the bush, in hunger time and does not fill the stomach." Prestige through food implies a feeling of repletion. This is a characteristic of the *guru* institution, but it applies also to daily life: good food has to be filling. This is why red sorghum, which is not sieved and is difficult to digest, is still preferred to white rice, which is "like water."

Table 11.7 Frequency of Consumption, Preferences and Dislikes Among the Massa, Mussey, and Foulbe of Mayo Danaye (Cameroon)

	Mussey (Gobo)	**Traditional Massa** (Bougoudoum)	**Urbanised Massa** (Yagoua)	**Urbanised Foulbe** (Yagoua)
Frequently consumed	Early red sorghum Bulrush millet Late red sorghum Pulses Cucumbers Traditional vegetables	Early red sorghum Fish Okra Traditional drinks	Rice Early red sorghum White pricked sorghum Fish, pasta Doughnuts Traditional and imported Syrups Coffee and tea	Rice White sorghums Meat, fish and meat preserves Okra, doughnuts Carbonated drinks
Preferences	Bulrush millet Rice, white sorghum White pricked sorghum Chicken, meat, fish Sesame, fat foods Soft and alcoholic drinks	Early red sorghum Rice, meat Large fresh fish All alcoholic drinks	Early red sorghum Rice, meat Fish Soft drinks	Same as above plus fresh meat
Dislikes	Early red sorghum Bulrush millet Groundnuts Traditional dishes with an unpleasant smell	Bulrush millet Pricked sorghum Rice Early red sorghum Cassava Wild cereals, wild leaves Some	Bulrush millet Pricked sorghum Early red sorghum Traditional drinks	Red sorghum Alcohol Pork
Prestige, wealth	White sorghum Rice, meat, fish Fatty and sweet foods Manufactured drinks and alcohol	Rice, pricked white sorghum, meat Fresh fish, fatty and sweet foods Manufactured drinks and alcohol	Rice, pasta Meat, large fish European food Manufactured drinks and alcohol	Rice Meat

Food preferences and the prestige linked to consumption of alcohol are an outstanding feature. The drinking pattern has changed from the times when most rituals were accompanied by sorghum beer brewing. Pasta and manufactured drinks from the market are beginning to appear as luxury foods; they may be offered to guests by the members of the salaried classes and civil servants. Here "fighting with food" means competition between bottled beer and local alcohol, *arki*. Social status is achieved by being able to drink and offering rounds. This pattern determines prestige according to negro-urban values influenced by European models. Distilling has become the best way for women to obtain money.

Another trend-setting group for the Massa and other neighboring "heathens" is the Fulani, who are both hated and envied. This Muslim group invaded northern Cameroon in the nineteenth century and militarily dominated most of the local populations. Today the

Fulani retain most of the political and economic power. Notwithstanding the ambiguous attitudes they elicit, they act as trend setters. In the field of food they are notable for their preference for white-colored staples, the prestige they confer on rice and meat, and their avoidance of alcohol and pork.

Food consumption is a marker of more comprehensive lifestyles. Three life styles operate among the Massa, each with its own scale of values.

1. The traditional way of life: recognition is gained from being a *sa fareyna* (cattle man) rich in cattle and wives, and the sponsor of *gurna*. He does not suffer from food shortages. His granaries are full, he can practise food hospitality and be lavish on ritual occasions.
2. The negro-urban (southern Cameroon) lifestyle: a high-protein diet can be attained thanks to an income from salaried work and administrative power. Meat, large fish, and sugary goods are valued, as are consuming snack foods, barbecued meats, attending bars, drinking beer and alcohol, and liberally offering rounds of drinks.
3. The Fulani pattern of life: prestige is displayed through choice daily food, white staples, meat, milk. Sweet foods and snacking are valued. Food is given away as alms to the poor, and religious events, which imply fasting during the day, are lavishly celebrated at night.

The competition between the negro-urban and the Fulani style continues as the traditional way of life is slowly vanishing.

The Mussey

Food and the status quest points to a quite different picture among the Mussey, a population neighboring the Massa on the south and numbering 200,000 individuals; 10,000 dwell in Cameroon, the rest in Chad. The Mussey are sorghum and millet cultivators who also raise ponies and goats. They were efficient warriors and proud hunters and they still announce themselves at social gatherings by loudly calling out their mottos, most of which refer to hunting: "My name is Corporal. I am a true male. I kill game for my father!"

Here status is displayed on ritual occasions, as among the Massa, by slaughtering chickens and goats for almost any event and cattle at the funerals of important people, up to ten head or more (each representing about one year of cash income). Today sons are still expected to slaughter at least one head of cattle at their father's funeral; they "lose face" if they do not comply and earn recognition if they are generous. Two village rituals per month added to individual celebrations of family events together amount to an average of four occasions for display per month.

The Mussey also have a specific institution to gain status: economic and political dominance is attained through the acquisition of magico-religious powers. When an evil event, such as repeated sickness or death in the family, strikes an individual, he first consults a diviner to determine the origin of the evil and offers a sacrifice to placate the supernatural power involved. If the disequilibrium continues, he may go through a psychopathological bout involving prostration, getting lost in the bush, having spells of violence, talking incessantly, etc., all of which are signs that he is possessed and about to become a *sa fuliana* "man of the spirits." He is then taken to the head of a possession college, a *sa billa* (the man of the throwing knife), who treats him and finally gets him to "spill out" the name of the deity involved. From then on the patient knows whom to placate and, incidentally, can act as an intermediary between his possessing spirit and other sick individuals. This allows him to receive gifts, mostly chickens, goats or cattle from people who come to consult him. He himself is obliged to give away part of what he has received to his own healer. Heads of possession colleges are frequently given animals to increase their herd, which they slaughter during rituals, eating much of the meat themselves. They are constantly organizing ritual feasts, of which the members of their college partake. Many elderly people, especially old women, join these associations specifically in order to "eat meat."

Impersonating supernatural beings, they are allowed to adopt very gluttonous or eccentric behavior toward food. Many cynically admit that they became a member of a college for the meat it provides. The magical powers of college members and especially of the college chiefs are very much dreaded by ordinary people whom they can bewitch, using the influence of the spirits they control. The *sa billa* are very powerful indeed since they can extort ordinary villagers or practise witchcraft on them to obtain cattle, domestic animals, and, nowadays, money.

One of the possession colleges, that of the *Fulisu bagayna* (spirits of the bush) has evolved into a youth-into-manhood initiation group. The members formerly helped with the social control of the community by punishing offenders, but also constantly took valuables from the villagers. Today the role of head of a possession college is very much sought after. Ambitious and wealthy individuals are ready to give away considerable riches to obtain from a high-ranking college leader the throwing knife and the various magic plants that will allow them to start a college of their own and accumulate wealth in the form of cattle, money, sheep, goats, and chickens. These are abundantly consumed on the ritual occasions decided by the college chief and also those occurring during the general ritual cycle. College members act, to a certain extent, as a gourmet club, acquiring prestige by partaking in these feasts.

In order to escape from the influence and the demands of these associations, which are feared for their witchcraft, many villagers join the Christian missions. Among the Mussey the status quest favors mature adult males, individuals with psychopathological problems, and elderly people, mostly old women who, having fulfilled their duties as wives and mothers, are beyond restraint and allow themselves to behave in an outrageous way – hardly characters on whom the future of the group depends. This is not especially in line with the arguments of those who bluntly apply Darwinian theory to cultural practices.

The Mussey's *fulina* system also appears among the southern Massa, but the Mussey most frequently are adopting the *guru* system of the Massa. The Massa appear to them as trend setters enjoying an enviable style of life; the Mussey are thus implicitly admitting their own inferiority.

Figure 11.8 Trend-Setting System in Mayo Danaye Populations

Primary Trend Setters in Life Styles	Secondary Trend Setters in Prestigious Occasions	Tertiary Trend Setters in Prestigious Occasions	Hardly Civilized
Muslim Fulani : permanent food choice. Christian, Muslim, national festivals, individual occasions	Massa, Guru Traditional ritual occasions	Mussey, possession. Traditional ritual occasions	"Kirdi"
Urbanites SCORN from the Muslim to →	"Heatens" (Kirdi) from the Massa to →	"Slaves" (Misna) from the Mussey to →	"Barbarians" (Kado)*
ENVIED STATUS ←			

* In this case the term is applied to a specific population South West of the Musey

The Mussey have been Christians for many years and are little influenced by the Muslim style of life. Today they grow cotton and are involved in the cash economy. The tendency of their food consumption is similar to that of the urbanized Massa: attending markets, consuming snack foods and barbecued meat, drinking local alcohol, and being generous with food on all festive occasions.

The Koma

The Koma are a population of mountain cultivators numbering 1,500 and dwelling in the Alantika range of northern Cameroon, on the Nigerian border. They are shrewd savanna agriculturalists who grow sorghum, millet, yams and who gather much of their food from their environment. Although they raise cattle (zebu and dwarf humpless cows) meat is conspicuously absent from their daily diet, coming only from small game, rodents, insects. Small fish from brooks are also consumed.

Beer brewing and cattle slaughtering on ceremonial occasions allow individuals to improve their status and move up an intricate age grade system that leads the way to becoming high-ranking initiates and respected policy makers at village level. This applies to both sexes. The avenue to social success is through millet and sorghum growing. It appears as a status achievement in its own right, but mostly it provides the basic ingredients for the beer brewing that is a compulsory part of any ritual and status-enhancing event as well as the main incentive to collective work parties. Van Beek (1978) was so impressed that he entitled his book on a similar group *Beer Brewers in the Mandara Mountains*.

Among the Koma, status is achieved through the slaughtering of cattle on ritual occasions, e.g. the *Nagë Napo* (the cattle dance) offered by a man to honor his wife's qualities as a mother and her hard work in the fields. On each occasion the meat is ceremoniously distributed to all categories of kin, including affines, and to the religious leaders of the community. While strengthening the ties with his in-laws and honoring his own kin and high-ranking initiates, a man climbs up in the age grade system, which results in more information being disclosed to him about the sacra upon which the magico-religious life rests. A man can slaughter cattle only after he has asked permisson from his father, through whom the opinion of the elders will be expressed. Permission will be granted only if the community acknowledges that he has reached the rank to which he aspires both economically and in his daily behavior. He is allowed to demonstrate his newly-achieved status only in the framework of the position ascribed to him by his fellow villagers; without their consensus he would not be allowed to hold the *Nagë Napo* feast.

The cattle dance can be performed up to six or seven times in a life span, the slaughtering of traditional dwarf cattle being compulsory on the last occasion. The grantee is then at the top of the social scale; he knows everything about the secret rituals and the places where the sacra are hidden. He is able to drink his own beer out of his own pot without sharing it. He will be entitled to a prestigious burial during which the horns of all the animals he has slaughtered will be tied to his chest; he can then leave his earthly condition to join the friendly spirits that protect the village.

Figure 11.9 Prestige Through Food Among the Koma

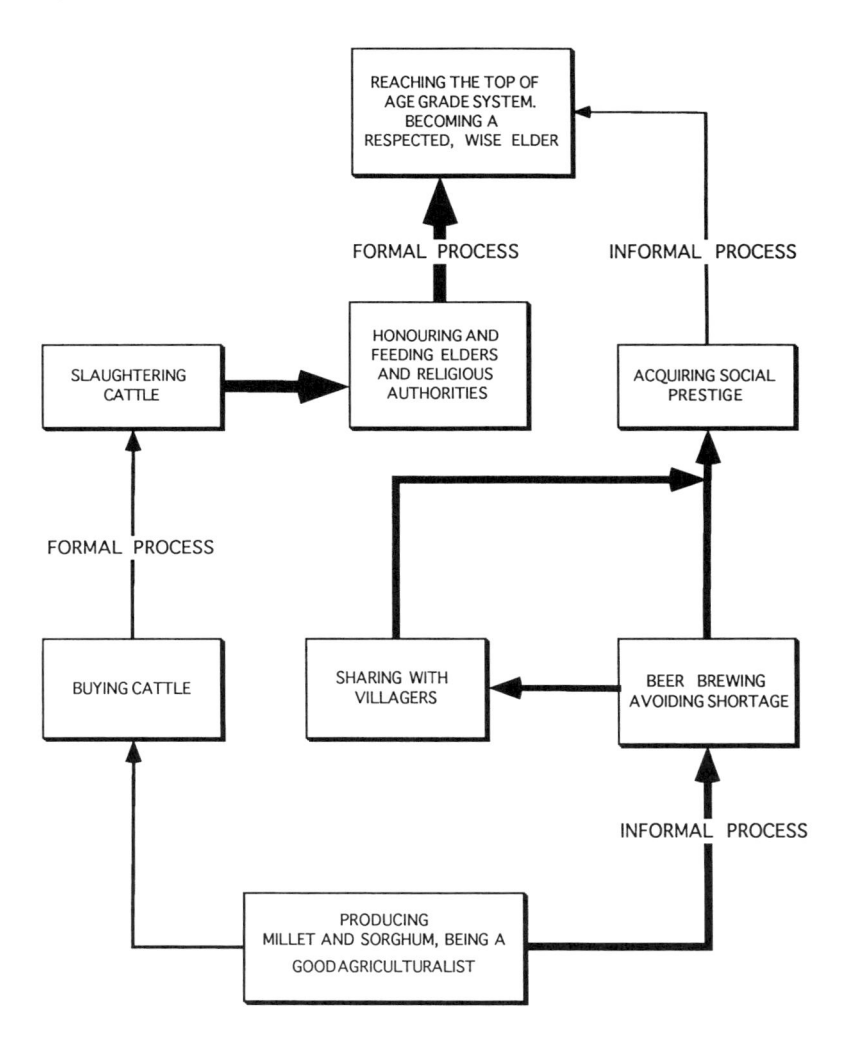

```
                    ┌─────────────────────┐
                    │ REACHING THE TOP OF │
                    │  AGE GRADE SYSTEM.  │
                    │     BECOMING A      │
                    │ RESPECTED, WISE ELDER│
                    └─────────────────────┘
                              ▲
                    FORMAL PROCESS   INFORMAL PROCESS
                    
    ┌──────────┐   ┌──────────────┐   ┌──────────────┐
    │SLAUGHTERING│─▶│ HONOURING AND│   │ACQUIRING SOCIAL│
    │   CATTLE  │  │FEEDING ELDERS│   │   PRESTIGE    │
    │           │  │ AND RELIGIOUS│   │               │
    │           │  │ AUTHORITIES  │   │               │
    └──────────┘   └──────────────┘   └──────────────┘
         ▲
    FORMAL PROCESS
    
    ┌──────────┐   ┌──────────────┐   ┌──────────────┐
    │  BUYING  │   │ SHARING WITH │◀──│ BEER BREWING │
    │  CATTLE  │   │  VILLAGERS   │   │AVOIDING SHORTAGE│
    └──────────┘   └──────────────┘   └──────────────┘
         ▲                                    ▲
         │                            INFORMAL PROCESS
    ┌──────────────────────────┐
    │        PRODUCING         │
    │ MILLET AND SORGHUM, BEING A │
    │    GOOD AGRICULTURALIST  │
    └──────────────────────────┘
```

Outside of these rather rare occasions, market days allow the display of convivial drinking. All collective work parties and ritual activities offer the opportunity to gain personal prestige through brewing beer and offering pots of it to members of the assembly according to precise rules and intricate strategies.

The harvest period, which celebrates the merits of successful agriculture, is an especially auspicious period for offering beer and food to the invited threshing party. From December to February, the family chiefs thresh their millet one after the other, which means that many men consume little other than millet beer and remain drunk most of the time. Sorghum beer provides one-third of the total energy consumed throughout the year. Public drinking reveals age sets and displays the ranking of each one. Within each set, mock fighting and what I would call "antagonistic drinking" takes place, especially between individuals who have been circumcised together. This mock violence accompanies the display of prosperity and eases the tension and the jealousy of evil supernatural influences.

Climbing in the age grade system implies heavy economic costs. Fulani cattle range from $60 (U.S) to $200 but local dwarf cattle can reach $400. It is compulsory to slaughter one in order to reach the last step. Providing beer, also a heavy burden for the age grade ceremony, involves the sacrifice of a bird, the Adamawan violet plantain eater *(Musophaga rossae savannicola),* 70 pots of beer (490 litres, representing about 100 kilograms of cereals), and 24 porridge balls (representing 50 kilograms of sorghum flour). For a *Nagë Napo* (prestigious cattle slaughtering), 75 pots of beer and 20 porridge balls are necessary; for a *nisuka* (the coming back of the cow's skull), 7 pots and food; for the burial of a woman, 37 pots of beer.

This system is similar to other well-known competitive eating and drinking institutions. One of its specific features among the Koma is that it is totally devoid of real hostility and violence, which would demonstrate loss of face.

The Yassa and the Mvae

The Yassa, who are 1,500 in number, live on the coast of southern Cameroon near Campo, next to the Equatorial Guinea border. They have a totally different type of culture: they are sea fishermen and cassava growers. They are literate and have been active in a cash economy for many years. Most of them are familiar with the large Cameroonian cities, and many have worked in Duala. The Yassa grow most of their staple (cassava) and vegetable products. Fish appears daily in the diet and is their main source of income. From outside they buy salt, sugar, wheat flour, and snack foods. They have been Catholics for many decades and, except for possession rituals *(mindi* and *ekong),* have lost their traditional magico-religious beliefs. Feasts are therefore those of the Catholic calendar, and Sunday provides the opportunity of a good meal and day-long heavy drinking.

Their neighbors, the Mvae (about 2,000 individuals), live inland from the Yassa. They are traditional forest cultivators and are clever at trapping game. They share the same modern features as the Yassa except that they are Protestants. They cultivate all the vegetable products they need, and are efficient agriculturists, growing a broad range of tubers, vegetables, pulses, fruit, and even producing surpluses to sell to the Yassa. Game meat appears daily in their diet. From the outside market they buy the same items as the Yassa and, of course, soft and alcoholic drinks. Like the Yassa, they have lost their traditional magico-religious beliefs. They no longer engage in conspicuous consumption contests, as existed in the neighboring Fang tribe. As among the Yassa, festive occasions are those of the Christian and national calendar. In both groups, other opportunities for festivity are offered by events in the family calendar such as funerals and especially weddings. On these occasions maternal and paternal kin as well as affines make contributions of food and display their affluence. Specific foods are consumed, e.g., domestic animals, sheep, game, and, where the Yassa are involved, large smoked snappers *(Lutjanus)*. In both cases plantain bananas and drinks including beer, red wine, cognac, and whisky are a must. A "demijohn with earrings" means a container of 20 litres of red wine onto which two bottles of whisky are tied with a piece of printed cloth.

A specific food item is especially status-conferring among the Yassa, as in many other forest populations of Cameroon: the Gabonese viper, *Bitis gabonica*. It is very dangerous and only elderly men are considered strong enough magically to ingest it. To be permitted to consume it means one has reached the top policymaking strata of the society.

Status is demonstrated in daily meals, where the valued dishes of elaborate gastronomy should appear. Proteins particularly should be present. Mvae women, speaking of themselves, say, "Here in the village, if you are successful, you have many plantations and much food: peanuts, cassava and will be much honoured. They are the activities which bring us honour. When you hold *tontines* [monthly feasts] around, you are honoured, but the basis of all that is work!" (Bouly de Lesdain 1991).

Among men, however, the discriminating factor is the ability to consume manufactured drinks: beer, wine, whisky, cognac. Palm wine, which is abundantly consumed, is not a prestigious item. Although the taste is appreciated, drinking it demonstrates that one cannot afford to buy manufactured drinks. Being able to offer drinks every evening to friends and guests, to provide alcoholic beverages galore on Sundays and choice foods and dishes on Christian festive days displays the family's affluence. This is not very different to what can be observed in Western cultures.

A final aspect of the quest for status through food and drinks is demonstrated by *tontines* monthly feasts organized by age classes, based on a compulsory subscription, and held in turn in the home of each member. Large amounts of barbecued fish, meat and drinks are consumed on these occasions. Keeping up with the other members of the age set appears essential.

If we look into the food frequency and attitudes towards food, we find that both groups are basically happy with their diet and draw on an elaborate cuisine to make it palatable. The tuberous basic foods, especially cassava *(Manihot)* are valued. For the Yassa as well as for the Mvae, the plantain banana is a prestigious food. Conversely, breadfruit, although palatable, is looked down upon since it does not involve work and is a "lazy farmer's diet." The Mvae appreciate a broader range of tubers, e.g., cocoyams *(Xanthosoma)*, yams *(Dioscorea)*, groundnuts *(Voandzeia)* and a wide selection of vegetables and fruit, all of which they grow. Although rice is acknowledged as a prestige food, it is not yet widely used, as is the case for other manufactured products such as tinned food, salt, and sugar. The popular status-enhancing foods are meat and, to a certain extent, fish.

Figure 11.10 Attitudes Toward Foods (% of the total number of answers : Yassa N = 146, Mvae N = 114)*

	Frequency Y	M	Affluence, Hospitality Y	M	Unlimited Wealth Y	M	Shortage, Poverty Y	M
Cassava Sticks	54	47	40	12	0	0	34	32
Smoked Cassava Balls	21	6	64	0	88	20	0	0
Vegetables, Leaves	17	28	0	0	0	0	8	76
Plantain Banana	3	9	90	62	77	20	0	0
Green Banana	1	0	0	0	0	0	40	31
Coco Yam	1	-	12	39	69	14	38	10
Breadfruit	3	-	0	0	0	0	85	19
Rice	3	-	35	42	3	19	0	0
Meat in General (game)	8	34	83	95	5	14	3	34
Chicken	1	-	78	50	0	22	0	0
Mutton	0	0	13	46	1	18	0	0
Fish in General	74	24	75	41	0	24	88	32
Red Wine	32	13	87	69	0	38	0	0
Beer	48	15	73	27	10	24	0	0
Manufactured Alcohol	-	-	47	68	3	25	0	0
Sweet Drinks	4	3	0	0	0	0	0	0
Palm Wine	14	57	7	12			100	58

*NB. Each question may have received several answers

The Yassa, who eat fish at 74 percent of their meals, would also offer it to guests (75 percent of the respondents). However, since it is readily available, they also consider it a shortage food. Conversely, they would would serve meat, which is scarce, to guests (83 percent of the cases). The Mvae, who consume meat at 35 percent of their meals, would offer it to their guests in 95 percent of the cases. At the same time it appears as a shortage food in 34 percent of the responses. Fish, on the other hand, appears to demonstrate affluence in 41 percent of the answers. It would seem that rarity has an influence on food status.

Alcoholic beverages such as beer, wine, and spirits also appear among the most prestigious items. Apart from drinks, it is quite apparent that, although these two groups have been in a monetary economy and exposed for a long time to Christian and negro-urban influences, their prestige foods (cassava, plantain bananas, fish, and meat) are still very traditional.

Discussion

We have described five cases of the use of food in the status quest, four of which are very different. In various societies there are indeed many ways of acquiring status through the use of food. Displaying one's status through the food one consumes and acquiring a status position through its convivial distribution are complementary activities. Ascribed and achieved status constantly merge. There are also several scales of value within a same society, according to which one might seek recognition through fasting just as well as through ostentatious display.

In all five societies we have observed three main approaches:

(1) seeking a privileged access to food and, as among nonhuman primates, obtaining both nutritional and social benefits, (2) feasting with food and drinks on specific, ritualized occasions, (3) displaying permanently one's status through the consumption of food and drink, both quantitatively and qualitatively.

What do these five societies have in common? There is no evidence of institutionalized antagonistic opportunities of fighting with food, as in the western British Columbian or Melanesian fashion, no potlatch-like contests. Here, there are no problems of shame or publicly losing face; people are expected to fill the rank designated by the community. Here status is situated somewhere between ascribed and achieved status. Prestige through food use is displayed on specific festive occasions, and the rest of the time people are expected to maintain modest daily fare. If we look into the prestige foods of all five groups, only a few of them come from the Western world. The valued items belong mostly to the domesticated range, which might mean that the status value of food is related to the work involved in its production: "You will earn your bread with the sweat of your brow." This is why tasty breadfruit, for instance, which does not require agricultural skill, is scorned by the Yassa and the Mvae. A notable aspect is that none of the vegetable resources from the wild appear as prestige or wealth foods, but rather as the symbol of poverty and dearth so that these five groups are all shifting away from wild food. Meat and, to a certain extent, large fish appear as the highest status-conferring foods. This includes meat from both domestic animals (involving work, although not as much as the hand-fed pigs of Melanesia), and from game.

The craze for game meat pervades most of the rain forest areas of Africa. For villagers as well as for sophisticated Duala businessmen or tourists dwelling in luxurious hotels, game is a necessary item for many status-conferring occasions. Food habits are known to be changing according to the behavior of higher-ranking trend setters whose lifestyle appears rewarding (Omololu 1971: 166). It is paradoxical that most of the affluent groups of Cameroon have a craving for game, which is consumed daily and obtained mainly from the Pygmies, a population that is scorned by everyone as being uncivilised (Kazadi 1981: 237; Grinker 1990: 112). Why is it that game caught by the Pygmies is appreciated even by neighboring villagers who are actually very clever at catching it themselves? Is it the fact that it is obtained through the genuine forest population, which has thereby privileged its magical relation with the wild?

To varying degrees, traditional status-seeking is becoming affected by outside influences and enviable lifestyles. As we have seen, Western models may be dominant, but we also must look for other local trend-setting influences, such as those exerted by the Fulani on many traditional groups of northern Cameroon, or the influence of the Massa *guru* institution on their Mussey neighbors.

Obtaining prestige through food and drinks on an individual basis is becoming more and more common. In all populations, alcoholic drinks rate highly among the prestigious items of the diet. This was already the case when drinking accompanied traditional rituals. It is today increasingly carried out on a daily basis. Among groups that are moving up the socioeconomic ladder and have cash at their disposal, using alcoholic drinks and lavishly sharing them is a good way of informally asserting oneself. People are very tolerant towards drunkards, and the prestige of the intoxication progresses upward from traditionally brewed beer to traditionally distilled alcohol to manufactured alcohols bought on the market. Can we follow Yudkin (1978: 4) when he insists on the dissociation operating between biological food needs and hedonistic social food wants? He stresses the importance of alcohol and its ability to reduce anxiety and self-criticism. Could we suggest that this operates in a modernizing world where traditional groups have lost faith in themselves, are suffering from anomy, and are longing for a social position they will never attain? Could they be seeking recognition and status in face-to-face closed groups through drinking and offering drinks?

As suggested by Rappaport (1968: 67-85), prestigious pig slaughtering may contribute to biological adaptation. Among the Massa, the *guru* institution has consequences that affect fitness, but mostly for the masculine population. As we have seen among the Mussey, access to meat through taking part in the feasts organized by the *fulina* possession groups benefits mainly the mature adults, elderly women, and misfits.

Among the Koma, sorghum beer reaches 5 percent alcohol content and represents a one-third of the calories ingested in that group. Seeking recognition through beer brewing and drinking has few positive results. It may be richer in vitamins PP and B-12, phosphorous and calcium than sorghum porridge, but it contains only half the calories, one-quarter of the proteins and no glucids (Adrian and Sayerse 1954: 136; Pele and Le Berre 1966). It is more nutritious to eat one's millet crop than to drink it! It is unnecessary to expand on the consequences of gulping down badly distilled local alcohol, as the Massa and the Mussey do, or to search for a positive biological role derived from displaying and seeking status through absorbing manufactured beverages and standing rounds of drinks, as is the case among the Yassa, the Mvae, and many other populations undergoing Westernization (Chhabra, Ramesh, and Metha 1991: 56). From concrete behavior in which the relation between social and biological aspects appears rather obvious, we have reached a situation where symbolic advantages may be sought even at the expense of biological fitness and where psychocultural well-being might be pursued over inclusive fitness.

The observation of these five African populations suggests that cultural uses of food in the status quest is not necessarily attuned to optimal biological adaptation in Darwinian terms. Are we witnessing here a specific tendency of humanity, which is to fiddle around with its biological fitness, coming close to jeopardizing it, in order to satisfy psychocultural wants of a totally different order and that might utimately lead to its extinction?

Notes

1. *guru* = collective fattening session
   gurna = participant in the collective fattening session
   guru walla = individual fattening session
   gor walla = participant in the individual fattening session. The same word designates both singular and plural forms.

References

Adrian, J. and C. Sayerse. 1954. *Les plantes alimentaires de l'ouest africain. I. Les mils et les sorgho du Sénégal*, Dakar: Organisme de Recherche sur l'Alimentation et la Nutrition africaines, Gouvernment général de l' Afrique occidentale francaise, Direction générale de la Santé publique.

Bouly de Lesdain, S. 1991. La femme mvae face à son environnement: Célibat ou union matrimoniale. Mémoire de Magistère/Rapport de l'Office de la Recherche Scientifique et Technique Outremer (ORSTOM). Université René Descartes, Sorbonne, Paris V.

Bourdieu, P. 1979. *La Distinction: Critique Sociale du Jugement*. Paris: Editions de Minuit.

Brillat-Savarin, A. 1885. *La Physiologie du Goût*, tome I. Paris: Bibliothèque Nationale.

Chhabra, K.B., P. Ramesh, and U. Metha. 1991. Food and nutrient intake of alcoholic labourers. *Ecology of Food and Nutrition* 25, no 1: 51-7.

De Garine, I. 1987. Massa e Moussey: la question de l'embonpoint. *Autrement: Fatale Beauté*, 1: 104-15.

De Garine, I. 1995. Cultural aspects of the male fattening sessions among the Massa of Northern Cameroon. In *Social Aspects of Fatness and Obesity*, ed. N.J. Pollock and I. de Garine. Amsterdam, Gordon, and Breach: 45-70.

De Garine, I. and G. Koppert. 1991. Guru: fattening sessions among the Massa. *Ecology of Food and Nutrition* 24, no. 1: 2-29.

Fallon, A.E. and P. Rozin. 1985. Sex differences in perception of desirable body shape. *Journal of Abnormal Psychol.* 94, no. 1:102-5.

Gopaldas, T., A. Gupta, and K. Saxena. 1983. The phenomenon of Sanskritisation in a forest dwelling tribe of Gujarat: Ecology, food consumption pattern, nutrition intake, anthropometric, clinical and hematological status. *Ecology of Food and Nutrition* 12: 217-27.

Grinker, R.R. 1990. Image of denigration: structuring inequality between foragers and farmers in the Ituri forest, Zaïre. *American Ethnologist* 17, no. 1: 111-30.

Harding, R.S.O. 1975. Meat-eating and hunting in baboons. In *Socio-ecology and psychology of primates*, ed. R.H. Tuttle. The Hague: Mouton.

Hladik, C.M. 1975. Ecology, diet and social patterning in monkeys and apes. In *Socio-Ecology and Psychology of Primates*, ed. R.H. Tuttle, 3-36. The Hague, Paris: Mouton.

Jelliffe, D.B. 1967. Parallel food classifications in developing and industrialised countries. *American Journal of Nutrition* 2, no. 3: 273-81.
Kazadi, N. 1981. Méprisés et admirés: l'ambivalence des relations entre les Bacwa (Pygmées) et les Bahemba (Bantu). *Africa* 51, no. 4: 835-47.
Levi-Strauss, C. 1949. *Les Structures Elémentaires de la Parenté.* Paris: Presses Universitaires de France.
Misasi, N. 1976. In Magna Sila. In *Calabria,* con introduzione di P. Crupi. Cozenza: Pellegrini.
Mitra, A. 1982. Malnutrition, illness and society. *Food and Nutrition Bulletin of the United Nations University* 4, no. 3: 1-2.
Nahoum, V. 1979. La Belle Femme. *Communications* 31: 22-32.
Oates, J.F. 1987. *Food distribution and foraging behavior in primate societies,* eds. B.B. Smuts, D.L. Cheney, R.M. Seyfarth, R.W. Wrangham, T.T. Strusaker, 197-209. Chicago, London: Univer. of Chicago Press.
Omolulu, A. 1971. Changing Food Habits in Africa. *Ecology of Food and Nutrition* 1: 165-68.
Pasquet, P., L. Brigant, A. Froment, D. Bard, I. de Garine, and M. Apfelbaum. (1992). Massive overfeeding and energy balance in man: The Guru walla model. *Americal Journal of Clinical Nutrition* 56:483-90.
Pele, J. and S. Le Berre. 1966. Les aliments d'origine végétale au Cameroun. Yaoundé, Cameroun, Office de la Recherche Scientifique et Technique Outre-Mer.
Rappaport, R. 1968. *Pigs for the Ancestors – Ritual in the Ecology of a New Guinean People.* New Haven, London: Yale Univer. Press.
Sims, E.A.H., R.F. Goldman, C.M. Gluck, E.S. Horton, P.C. Kelleher, and D.W. Rowe. 1968. Experimental Obesity in Mass. *Trans. Ass. Amer. Physicians J.* 81: 153-70.
Teti, V. 1976. *Il Pane, la Beffa e la Festa.* Rimini, Florence: Guaraldi Editore.
Teti, V. 1995. Food and Fatness in Calabria. In *Social Aspects of Fatness and Obesity,* ed. N.J. Pollock and I. de Garine. Amsterdam, Gordon, and Breach: 3-30.
Van Beek, W.E.A. 1978. Bierbrouwers in de Bergen, ICAU Mededeling 12, Utrecht, Instituut voor Culturele Antropologie.
Young, M.W. 1971. *Fighting with Food. Leadership, Values and Social Control in a Massim Society.* Cambridge: Cambridge Univer. Press.
Yudkin, J. 1978. Physiological determinants of food choice. In *Diet of Man: Needs and Wants,* 243-60. London: Applied Science Publishers.

12. FOOD, COMPETITION, AND THE STATUS OF FOOD IN NEW GUINEA

Pierre Lemonnier

In New Guinea, food, status, and competition can be linked in at least three ways. In addition to success in war and the ability to control the spiritual world, organizing distributions of food is another prominent avenue to political power, and by far the best-documented in the anthropological literature. Because ceremonial exchanges of pigs or pork and/or vegetal products are often linked to intergroup competition, these can be regarded more or less as a secondary result of peacemaking procedures. In turn, the symbolic values attributed to different kinds of food – notably to pork – can be related to particular social functions of food exchanges, and therefore, as we shall see, to extremely contrasting types of socioeconomic organization.

Whereas the main feast giver, the "Big man", is a well-known figure whose role, status, and socioeconomic functions I shall recapitulate with the help of some classic examples from anthropology, the link between war, peace, and ceremonial exchanges of food has to be demonstrated. Finally, I shall argue that among other cultural values embodied in pigs (or pork), their role as a possible substitute for human life may be a crucial and powerful variable for the comparison and understanding of New Guinea societies in general. For this purpose, my analysis will focus on three sets of societies: two in the Highlands of Papua New Guinea, and one in the southern part of the island straddling the border between Irian Jaya and Papua New Guinea.

Competitive Ceremonial Exchanges of Food

Giving and receiving food is an everyday occurrence in New Guinea. Visitors are given a meal; an individual must share his snack with friends and kin encountered on the road; he must provide food to whomever helps with a task. Furthermore, at a more ritualized level, the giving or sharing of food is an important medium of sociality that accompanies many life events such as birth and death, initiations, marriage, etc.

Moreover, in many societies large-scale gifts of food are also a key medium of intergroup relationships, and sometimes the main focus of communal life. Months and years in advance, members of a village, a clan or even a whole tribe clear and plant new gardens, and escalate their hunting or pig-raising activities with the intent of presenting huge quantities of food to visitors. Frequently, items of "wealth" (shells, feathers, etc.) also are included in these exchanges; depending on the occasion, food itself may or may not be regarded as "wealth".[1]

Quite often, but by no means always, these events are competitive. Piles of yams, pyramids of coconuts, rows of live pigs or carcasses are displayed before the guests. Frequently the hosts make speeches boasting of their own generosity and achievement. The guests may also be reminded of their comparatively poor performance at a previous feast, or be challenged to repay their hosts with equal munificence in the future. Competition does not imply that one side must give more than the other; challenging an exchange partner to match your own achievement is quite sufficient to initiate rivalry between individuals or groups.

Even though both female and male labor are necessary for the preparation of such feasts, which I shall call "ceremonial exchanges", in accordance with the literature, the main organizers are men. They initiate the event, they set the date, they coordinate the production of a surplus of food so that it will be ready in time. When the feast is a success, they gain "prestige" and "influence;" part of this prestige goes to members of the group they represent.

This is the general picture; the particulars vary considerably. For instance, sometimes competition takes place only among groups; sometimes the intergroup event is friendly and seen as an opportunity to share common wealth, but within each group, clans and their leaders compete among themselves in the organization of the feast. In other cases, rivalry takes place both within and among groups. Above all, it is the status achieved by feast organizers as well as the complex of social relations emphasized or reproduced in feast giving that differ tremendously from one part of New Guinea to the next.

The Big-Man Complex

The most famous organizers of ceremonial exchanges on the island are the Big men of the western part of the Papua New Guinea Highlands. Instead of accumulating wealth (pigs and other items of wealth), they manipulate it, and their prestige derives as much from their skill at manipulating things and social relations while assembling wealth as from the way they handle ceremonial distribution. The prestige they gain in the course of ceremonial exchanges raises their status in either their hamlet, clan, or tribe, depending on their place in the ever-changing hierarchy of Big men. As a rule, a Big man speaks for his group, advises on local affairs (especially on war and peace), looks after refugees, helps young men accumulate the bridewealth they need to get married, etc. He usually has more wives, more gardens, and more pigs than ordinary people. But just as important as the size of the labor force he recruits is the range and scope of his network of social relations, in particular those he maintains with his many affines.

Whereas warfare (and often male initiation) is the main social institution in some of the other Highland societies of New Guinea, it is the organization of these exchanges of food and wealth that commands energy as well as endless social strategies in Big-man societies. On a given day, 40 to 600 pigs may be distributed, dead or alive, to visiting groups, sometimes along with hundreds of shells (which are mutually exchangeable with pigs). The Melpa *moka* or the Enga *tee*,[2] for instance, are cycles of intergroup ceremonial exchanges of pigs and other kinds of wealth (shells, cassowaries, cosmetic oils, etc.). In addition to expressing rivalry, these gatherings are also a time for various social events. Within these group events, individuals have their own partners from whom they receive or to whom they give. People also use these occasions to fulfill many social obligations related to marriage, age-grade ceremonies, and homicide compensations. In particular, individual gifts to affines and to maternal kin are often an integral part of the intergroup ceremonial exchange.

As Strathern (1969, 1971) has shown, the fact that various social "logics"[3] are embedded in the preparations and the actual ceremony of exchange is a crucial feature of Big-man societies. At the heart of this embedding, wealth items that are used as competitive gifts, particularly pigs, are not only re-exchangeable, but also are commonly used in bridewealth and all kind of compensations, particularly death compensations (Godelier 1986; Modjeska 1982; Strathern 1982). I have tried to demonstrate elsewhere (Lemonnier 1990, 1991) that peace ceremonies may be the link between marriage, warfare, competitive exchanges, *and* the use of the same kinds of "wealth items" in these three sets of social relations. My model can be summed up as follows:

1. In this part of New Guinea, the pig or at least its fat or blood is viewed and used as a life-giving substance.
2. Highland cultures admit to varying degrees of specificity the possibility that a pig, or pork, can be a formal substitute for human life, i.e. can be used both to compensate a homicide and to obtain a wife.
3. Making peace implies paying compensation for the dead warriors, and, more often than not, strengthening friendly ties by an exchange of women.
4. Furthermore, exchanging pigs (or pork) and women gives people an opportunity for future peaceful encounters.

This model has proved to be plausible when confronted with ethnographic data. In most Big-man societies, as well as among other Highland societies that had large exchanges of pigs or pork, intergroup ceremonial exchanges often contain some reference to previous compensation for the life of enemies or allies.[4] The literature also shows cases in which the alternative between peace ceremonies and ceremonial exchange is explicit (Sorenson 1972: 358-61), and cases in which gifts between recent enemy groups are subsequently transformed into regular exchanges between individuals (Boyd 1984: 33). Moreover, small-scale ceremonial exchanges of pigs exist in many Highland societies in which warfare and male initiations are the main social institutions (and daily preoccupation); in these cases, the leaders are first of all great warriors, but they are also the ones who organize the "pig festival", so they can also be seen as incipient Big men (Lemonnier 1990: 23-27).

Substitution, Competition, "Finance" and the Pig

At the core of what can be called the "Big-man complex" lies, at least formally, the pig-as-life-substitute. Two reasons suit the pig to this function. In the first place, it is the basis of that set of social strategies and technoeconomic practices of the Big-man society that Strathern (1969, 1978) has called "finance". In the second place, the cultural value locally attributed to the animal allows people to use it as a substitute for life, as a means of compensation; as we shall soon see, it happens that substitution and competition are logically linked. Let us start with "finance".

Whether he represents his clan as a whole or some smaller group of people, a Big man needs the help of others in order to muster pigs and wealth for a ceremonial exchange. Some of these others are the members of his own household, or of his brother(s)'s or son(s)'s families, etc. He also relies on non-kin followers who are dependent on him, such as bachelors for whom he will pay bridewealth, refugees to whom he has given land, and one or two of those unfortunates known in New Guinea as "rubbishmen". But a Big man also needs to use the wealth and pigs of people outside his own family or community because to successfully compete with rivals he needs to assemble and give away more pigs than he can muster locally. Additionally, by using pigs raised in other communities, he reduces the risks of epizootic outbreaks. [5] Collaborators outside the clan, usually affinal and maternal kin, help a Big man in two ways. They raise some of his pigs and give them back when needed, that is, a few days before an intergroup exchange, and they give him their own wealth and pig(s) so that he will give the wealth away in their names as well as in his own. Months or years later he will repay his followers and collaborators what he received from another Big man (and group) in a subsequent exchange.

It sometimes happens that a Big man's follower does not obtain his due share in repayment for his help to that Big man in a previous exchange. Instead of receiving wealth items, such a "little man" may even be threatened with a beating by some *protégés* of the Big man (Meggitt 1974: 190-91). In other words, in Big-man societies there exists some exploitation of other people's work, sometimes by pressure. Although this is only an incipient form of exploitation, the possibility creates a striking difference with some so-called egalitarian Highland groups, notably Great-man societies (see next section).

In short, a Big man is a strategist who calculates where and when to "invest", either in a social relation – e.g. by helping someone to meet a particular social obligation by supplying him or her with some shells or pigs – or in an ongoing exchange partnership. In the latter case, the Big man will try to receive the return goods before the event for which he needs pigs. At some point, several competing Big men may have the same potential collaborators, and this complicates the game. Finally, the "bigger" a Big man, the more collaborators he attracts, because his success is considered proof that he is a worthy partner.

Two key points here, which, taken together, make finance and Bigmanship work, are: (1) You can "invest" a pig in some other social transaction long before you actually give the return for that pig to the original donor; that is, you can profit from a gift before you must return it; if all of a Big man's "creditors" called in their "debts" at the same time, he would be in a tight spot; (2) A sow can give birth to several piglets that, in turn, grow up, thereby transforming work into wealth.

In addition to its role in "finance" the pig is a necessary part of the Big-man complex because it is viewed as a substitute for human life,[6] or at least a token of life, both in the context of marriage and of death compensation. As soon as two groups share the same idea of substitution, i.e. replacing a human being by a "thing", they can indemnify each other by a gift, rather than fighting until the losses are evenly divided. However, substituting things for life or death[7] opens up a completely new realm of competition. The goods (pigs and other items of wealth) offered as compensation for death are the same as those used for bridewealth. Above all, these goods can be used in peaceful rivalry; thus, rather than comparing blows and casualties, groups and people can compete by comparing the respective quantities of similar items of wealth they manage to amass.

The key role of the pig as a substitute for life in Big-man societies can also be demonstrated in two other ways. First, by looking at those rare Highland societies that do not have any kind of intergroup pig exchanges, e.g., the "Great-man" societies analyzed by Godelier (1986); and then by considering ceremonial exchanges of yams in several South New Guinea societies.

Great-Man Societies: Ceremonial Exchanges Within the Group and the Principle of Equivalence

Great-man societies are found in the eastern part of the Highlands, mainly among the Anga tribes. With the exception of an overwhelming male domination over females, these are largely egalitarian societies. Status is not based on the manipulation or accumulation of wealth. Some Great men, such as those in charge of male initiations, inherit their positions; others, such as the great warrior, the saltmaker and the cassowary hunter in the Baruya studied by Godelier,[8] achieve their status through their success in particular spheres. But in all cases, the power of Great men is not permanent and, unlike that of Big men, it is restricted to these domains.

In Great-man societies, the only large-scale ceremonial exchanges take place *within* the tribe itself when the entire community gives food to the young male initiates. Among the Baruya the idea of substitution barely exists. Principles of equivalence and reciprocity underlie exchanges of women, and sister exchange is the basic marriage rule; there is little that resembles bridewealth (even though the concept does exist: Baruya sometimes give bridewealth to obtain wives from foreign tribes, and small gifts of pork are given to matrilineal kin). A woman is given for a woman. Similarly, the death of a warrior is compensated for primarily by the killing of another warrior. Shells and vegetal salt are given as homicide compensation, but this happens only after the score has been more or less evened out by fighting. As one can see, the important difference between Big-man societies and Great-man societies is that among the Baruya, marriage, life-event, and homicide compensations have no common medium of exchange.

Although pigs are raised in Great-man societies, they play no role in homicide compensations or in peacemaking ceremonies, and are rarely a component of marriage exchanges.[9] Vegetal salt, considered to be a symbolic equivalent of semen, is the main item used in compensation, but its manufacture and manipulation involve no particular social strategies. Whereas in Big-man societies producing and manipulating wealth opens up a wide range of compensation exchanges (bridewealth, homicide compensations or payments to maternal parties upon death) and accompanying social relations, in Great-man societies the range of substitutions, such as woman for woman, death for death, is extremely limited. This gives little incentive to place emphasis on wealth; the role of Big man never emerges. As for intergroup exchanges, they are seldom, with the exception of warfare, and characterized by the exchange of items of different nature, particularly in intertribal trade.

One must also note that warfare is continuous and peace infrequent among the Baruya. Unlike the peace ceremonies that might have been the starting point of the Big-man system, when peacemaking does occur, peace ceremonies between the Baruya and their enemies are not followed by regular exchanges.[10] Furthermore, the Baruya are the one group that have a monopoly on the production of the salt used locally in compensation. Their enemies produce no salt, or no salt that matches the quality and value ascribed to Baruya salt. Unlike pigs, though, salt bars do not bear young, which make them poor candidates for any process of finance.

In the final analysis, the two social landscapes differ widely. In Great-man societies, warfare and male initiations are the main focus of interest of the group as a whole; regular intergroup exchange is unknown, and pigs are barely present in exchanges. Status has nothing to do with the manipulation of wealth, and the very idea of exploiting someone else's work, as Big men sometimes do, is totally unthinkable here.

Competitive Exchange of Food Without Big Men: Coastal South New Guinea

The key role of the pig as a substitute for life can be further appreciated in an indirect way by analysing the case of several coastal societies in South New Guinea as reported in the ethnographic literature.[11] Although they resemble Big-man societies in some aspects, these societies have quite a different socioeconomic organization. As we shall see, this can be related to the cultural values they attribute – or rather do not attribute – to the pig. To summarize, in these societies:

1. Huge intergroup exchanges of food are common and often strongly competitive. Among the Keraki, for instance, witnesses have seen up to five rows of fences, each several hundred yards long, on which yams – "probably millions" – were displayed (Williams 1936: 232-33). But pigs and wealth are totally absent from these competitive exchanges.
2. These ceremonial gifts of food are often an explicit substitute for fighting, including internal feuding and external warfare; people agree to compete by displaying and giving yams (or coconuts, sago, grubs, etc.) rather than by exchanging blows. These competitive ceremonial exchanges are thus often linked to peacemaking procedures (for instance, people will discuss peace at such a meeting), but it should be noted that peacemaking *is not* associated with the exchange of food itself. Unlike Big-man feasts, this is not a time for compensation for homicide or marriage.
3. In order to conclude a peacemaking ceremony, people first try to equalize the casualties as in Big-man and Great-man societies. Then they give their enemies women (as spouses) or children with the idea of replacing the dead warriors. Yet, these cultures also compensate homicides and war losses with wealth; they give necklaces of dog's teeth, shells, canoes, but *no pigs or pork*.
4. Pigs are used in various ceremonial contexts, particularly in male initiations and rituals of growth. It is only when a rite of passage is associated with a ceremonial distribution of vegetal products that pigs can also be killed; nonetheless, the distribution of pork is seldom a part of the ceremony.

Another key difference with respect to Big-man societies in South New Guinea is that the basic marriage rule is sister exchange. There is no bridewealth, but there is some possibility that a woman may be indirectly equated with wealth. For instance, among the Keraki, a man who has no sister "buys" a woman, who is then considered his sister and can be exchanged for a wife. Similarly, a sisterless Jaqaj gives some items of wealth to his affines, but this wealth is returned to him when he finally finds a woman to give in return. In all cases, it is noteworthy that the "wealth" in question comprises no pigs or pork.

5. There are no Big men here, at least none of the Enga or Melpa type. The most "powerful" leaders (all things being relative) are great warriors, and their influence is far greater than that of Highlands Great men. They have more wives (and young wives) than ordinary men, and in some cases they have a claim to the products of other people's work. Among the Kiwai, for instance, "certain great leaders of the past had acquired such an influence over the people that they could at times induce or compel these people to bring them game and fish and make their gardens, while the headman himself did nothing" (Landtman 1927 169).

Conversely, one finds no such privileges in South New Guinea groups (Kimam, Keraki) in which "influence" goes primarily to feast-organizers who are, first and foremost, renowned gardeners. At any rate they are *primus inter pares* and they must share prestige and influence with other figures, great warriors, great gardeners, and sorcerers, whereas Big men are the prominent figures in their groups. Of course, prestige is also gained by organizing ceremonial exchanges of food, but because these exchanges do not involve wealth in the form of pigs, their preparation entails far less complex social strategies than in Big-man societies. "Finance" does not occur, and there is no basis for anything like a Big-man complex.

In short, all the ingredients found in Big-man societies are present in South New Guinea, but in a different order. The fundamental difference here is that in South New Guinea *there are no links between compensation, competition and pigs*. As I have mentioned, compensations for life (marriage) and death (homicide) do not include pigs or pork. Also, whereas in the Highlands gifts related to past compensations make up an important part of most ceremonial exchanges, in South New Guinea the display and distribution of food have nothing to do with such compensations. Not only do these coastal societies radically separate the means by which they compete and the means by which they compensate, but they also keep the pig outside these two domains. I maintain that the crucial point here is that they do not consider the pig as a possible substitute for human life. The problem is now to try to explain why this is so.

Pigs vs. Women; Pigs and Women

Pigs are found in South New Guinea, but in the great majority of cases these are wild pigs captured in the forest as piglets and tamed.

They can grow "big and fat" and become "monsters" that can no longer stand on their legs, but the actual raising of pigs in captivity is almost nonexistent. Williams (1936), for instance, a keen ethnographer, never saw a litter. We have no indication of the pig-per-capita ratio, but, at least in certain cases, the number of pigs killed during a feast can be as high as that in some Big-man societies. For instance, for a Marind-anim feast, a noncompetitive feast focused on age-grade rites, the figure can reach thirty to fifty pigs (van Baal 1966: 408, 842). The animals used in a ritual context are first and foremost wild boars, and when it happens that wild sows are tamed, they are not used in the rituals linked with the boys' growth nor in male initiations.

In short, in South New Guinea, even when it is tamed the pig is considered a wild animal, a symbol of zeal and bravery, associated with head-hunting. Its role in ritual is most important, but the restricted range of its social uses is striking when compared to Big-man societies. Moreover, an in-depth comparative study shows that in Big-man societies, pigs fulfill many of the functions played by women in South New Guinea societies.

As already mentioned, in South New Guinea marriage is basically the exchange of a woman for another woman; in peacemaking, women are an explicit replacement for dead warriors. Women also have two more social functions in these societies: their role as a means of compensation for ordinary services and grievances, and their place in fertility rites.

In South New Guinea societies, the lending of one's wife for the night to another man, i.e. lending her "sexual services", not procreative powers, is a form of repayment for various services rendered by this man. Hired killers, magicians, and sorcerers are paid in this way, as are men who help with work or even loan a tool. Similarly, a thief can indemnify his victim in this manner. Women in this specific context as sexual objects are reusable and re-exchangeable. In a case described by Boelaars (1981: 98), a Jaqaj prostitute "might be taken to another settlement, which has paid for her, and killed and eaten like a pig." In these particular contexts it appears that women are regarded as items of wealth, although we have absolutely no information as to whether members of South New Guinea societies see it this way.

Regarding fertility rites, in Big-man societies pig fat and blood are connected with the cyclic reproduction of humans, animals, and plants (Brown 1972: 49; Strathern 1982: 119; Tumu et al. 1989: 35-36). But the pig has no such function in South New Guinea. There, general fertility depends on warfare, which provides enemy heads associated with the reproduction of coconuts, and on heterosexuality. Female and male sexual fluids are collected after intercourse and used to restore the fertility of humans as well as that of all things, in particular that of gardens. I tried unsuccessfully to determine the respective roles of man and woman in these rites. However, a comparison of fertility rites with rites to make boys grow shows that female fluids have some importance in fertility rites, whereas only semen is used in male initiations. Finally, it is clear that the symbolic system of these cultures of South New Guinea assigns to women many of the functions that Big-man societies attribute to pigs.

At this point, it seems impossible to determine why different New Guinea societies combine pigs, women, intergroup competition, compensation, fertility, etc. in such contrasting ways. However, as a result of this comparative study we do see that in New Guinea pigs and women in some way fulfill the same functions. In South New Guinea, women and pigs are kept separate, which might be linked to the observation that in South New Guinea the pig is never a substitute for life. This raises another question: "Is there anything in women's gender roles that can be linked with the possible attribution of life-giving powers to pigs?"

As a pure hypothesis, I will suggest that the answer to this question might lie in one of the salient features of "domesticated" pigs in South New Guinea, that is, they are tamed wild pigs. Generally speaking, if one considers New Guinea as a whole, the intensity of the use of pigs in ceremonial exchanges seems to be correlated with the amount of work, notably female work, invested in the animal (Feil 1985: 98; Lemonnier 1990: 139-43). In the case of South New Guinea societies, it is true that women do most of the work related to pigs, both in agriculture and in animal husbandry, but the total amount of work devoted to the animals is far less than in Big-man societies. Furthermore – and this may be the key to the problem – the piglets are not born in captivity. The difference between South New Guinea and the Highlands, then, is that South New Guinea women are not associated with the reproduction of pigs. It appears that in the Highlands, where pigs are not of wild origin, more female work must be devoted to pig husbandry, and the more work invested, the more the pig will be valued and used in ceremonial exchanges, many of which are linked with compensation procedures.[12]

Here again, the ethnography of South New Guinea seems to support this hypothesis, because in the very few cases where pigs are exchanged for some kind of wealth, not only is this wealth used in affinal payments, but the pigs are also involved in children's growth rites. In other words, when South New Guinea cultures link pigs and wealth (albeit in a highly marginal way), this occurs in a context of affinal payments – and therefore compensation for life – and human growth. Moreover, it is possible to show that in this case, it is clearly the female work involved in the care of the animal that is paid for. If, as I think, this proximity of the raising of pigs and that of children is not simply fortuitous, one may postulate that we have here the beginnings of the idea that the fecundity of women can be transferred to pigs through the labor and care they expend on them.

For want of comparative data on the local representations of pigs in various New Guinea societies, this remains a hypothesis. Nevertheless, there are indications that the way women are or are not associated with pigs is a key variable in our understanding of food exchanges in New Guinea cultures and societies, and their accompanying economic and political aspects

Notes

1. As we shall see, the eventual re-exchangeability of the items is an important criterion to distinguish if these should be regarded as food or wealth.
2. Mention of only those particular tribes in which ceremonial exchanges have been described at length in the literature (includes Bulmer 1960; Elkin 1953; Feil 1984; Meggitt 1967, 1974, 1977; Strathern 1971); but see also Brown (1964, 1972, 1978) for the Chimbu and Lederman (1986) for the Mendi.
3. By social "logic" I mean what appears to the analyst as the functional or symbolic issue of a particular set of social relations, behaviors, and representations that are interconnected, derived from one another or at least compatible.
4. This might not be the case in the contemporary Papua New Guinea Highlands. Concerning the Enga and the *Tee*, both D.K.Feil (personal communication) and P. Wiessner (personal communication) deny that a pig can be a substitute for life. My hypothesis seems nevertheless well-documented in Brown (1964: 246, 335-36; 1972: 32, 49-50; 1978: 220; Elkin (1953: 183-84, 199), Lederman (1986: 149, 162-63), and Strathern (1971: 1–96, 121-22, 219; 1981: 210). As for the *Tee*, as historically reconstructed by P. Wiessner and A. Tumu (*Historical Vines: The Formation of Regional Networks of Exchange, Ritual and Warfare Among the Enga of Papua New Guinea*. forthcoming), war reparations, particularly those to allies, were important factors in its development.
5. On the logic of "finance" cf. Lederman (1986: 211) for an opposite view.
6. Strathern (personal communication) has pointed out that substitution can have a number of submeanings i.e., (1) as a means of replacing, (2) as a symbolic replacement, (3) as an equivalent or means of obtaining something in return, as in bridewealth. Until more information is available, I would suggest that it can take on all three meanings.

7. By giving some items as a "payment" for an enemy warrior that has been killed, those who give them potentially save the life of one of their own warriors, who could have been killed in payback. This is true even when compensation is paid to allies; in that case, it is feared that dissatisfied friends would attack their former allies.
8. See also Bonnemère (1991, 1996) for the Ankave, Fischer (1968) for the Yagwoya, Herdt (1981, 1987) for the Sambia, and Mimica (1981) for the Iqwaye.
9. Among the Baruya, pieces of pork are reciprocally exchanged as gifts marking the betrothal of two men with each other's "sister"; gifts of pork are also made to the maternal kin of a newborn baby, but in no way does this resemble bridewealth.
10. Godelier (1989) has shown that by marrying enemy women as a part of peace-making procedures, Baruya and their foes are perpetuating conflict rather than consolidating peace. In effect, the solidarity between brothers-in-law is stronger than that between a man and his paternal kin. As a result, intermarrying with the enemy leads to betrayal and to internal conflicts that are a burden on the unity and strength of a given group. Giving a wife to an enemy group is a *cadeau empoisoné*, or poisoned gift.
11. For a more detailed analysis of the South New Guinea case, see Lemonnier (1992, 1993). The ethnography under consideration here is that of the Marind-anim (van Baal 1966, 1984; Vertenten 1923), Jaqaj (Boelaars 1981), Kimam (Serpenti 1968, 1972, 1977, 1984), Keraki (Williams 1936), Kiwai (Landtman 1927), and Asmat (Trenkenschuh 1970; Zegwaard and Boelaars 1955; Zegwaard 1959; van Amelsvoort 1975). These six groups I shall hereafter call "South New Guinea societies". Since these lines have been written, Knauft (1993) has published an important synthesis on this part of New Guinea. See also Lemonnier 1995.
12. We should not overlook Kelly's (1988) hypothesis that pigs raised primarily by foraging are prone to run away from all humans except those who raise them, which makes the exchange of live pigs impossible.

References

Barth, F. 1975. *Ritual and Knowledge among the Baktaman of New Guinea*. Oslo: Yale Univer. Press.

Boelaars, J.H.M.C. 1981. *Head-Hunters About Themselves. An Ethnographic Report from Irian Jaya, Indonesia*. The Hague: Martinus Nijhoff.

Bonnemère, P. 1991. Constitution and treatment of the human body among the Ankave-Anga of Papua New Guinea: The making of a sociality through female links? Paper presented to the workshop "Embodiment and Sociality: a Melanesianist perspective", Manchester, England, 16-17 July.

Bonnemère, P. 1996. *Le pandanus rouge. Corps, différence des sexes et parenté chez les Ankave-Anga (Papouasie Nouvelle-Guinée)*. Paris: CNRS Editions/Editions de la Maison des Sciences de l'Homme.

Boyd, D.J. 1984. The production and management of pigs: Husbandry option and demographic patterns in Eastern Highlands herd. *Oceania* 55, no.1: 27-49.

Brown, P. 1964. Enemies and affines. *Ethnology* 3, no.4: 335-356.

Brown P. 1972. *The Chimbu. A Study of Change in the New Guinea Highlands.* Cambridge, Mass.: Schenkman Publishing Company.

Brown P. 1978. *Highland Peoples of New Guinea.* Cambridge, London, New York: Cambridge Univer. Press.

Bulmer, R. 1960. Political aspects of the Moka ceremonial exchange system among the Kyaka people of the Western Highlands of New Guinea. *Oceania* 31, no.1: 1-13.

Elkin, A.P. 1953. Delayed exchange in Wabag sub-district, Central Highlands of New Guinea, with notes on the social organization. *Oceania* 23, no.3: 161-201.

Feil, D.K. 1984. *Ways of Exchange. The Enga Tee of Papua New Guinea.* St. Lucia: Univer. of Queensland Press.

Feil, D.K. 1985. Configuration of intensity in the New Guinea Highlands. *Mankind* 15, no.2: 87-100.

Fischer, H. 1968. *Negwa. Eine Papua Gruppe im Wandel,* München: Klaus Renner.

Godelier, M. 1986. *The Making of Big men. Male Domination and Power among the New Guinea Baruya,* transl. Rupert Swyer, Cambridge, Paris: Cambridge Univer. Press/Editions de la Maison des Sciences de l'Homme.

Godelier, M. 1989. Betrayal a key moment in the dynamic of segmentary tribal societies. *Oceania* 59: 165-180.

Herdt, G. 1981. *Guardians of the Flute. Idioms of Masculinity.* New York: McGraw-Hill.

Herdt, G. 1987. *The Sambia. Ritual and Gender in New Guinea.* New York: Holt, Rinehart and Winston.

Kelly, R.C. 1988. Etoro suidology. A reassessment of pig's role in the prehistory and comparative ethnology of New Guinea. In *Mountain Papuans. Historical and Comparative Perspective from New Guinea Fringe Highlands Societies,* ed. J.F. Weiner, 111-86. Ann Arbor: Univer. of Michigan Press.

Knauft, B. 1993. *South Coast New Guinea Cultures. History, comparison, dialectic.* Cambridge: Cambridge Univer. Press.

Landtman, G. 1927. *The Kiwai Papuans of British New Guinea.* London: Macmillan and Co.

Lederman, R. 1986. *What Gifts Engender. Social Relations and Politics in Mendi, Highlands Papua New Guinea.* Cambridge: Cambridge Univer. Press.

Lemonnier, P. 1990. *Guerres et Festins. Paix, Échanges et Compétition dans les Highlands de Nouvelle-Guinée.* Paris: Editions de la Maison des sciences de l'Homme.

Lemonnier, P. 1991. From Big men to Great men. Peace, substitution and competition in the Highlands of New Guinea. In *Big men and Great men. Personifications of power in Melanesia,* ed. M. Strathern and M. Godelier, 7-27. Cambridge: Cambridge Univer. Press.

Lemonnier, P. 1992. Le porc comme substitut de vie: formes de compensation et échanges en Nouvelle-Guinée. *Social Anthropology* 1: 33-55.

Lemonnier, P. 1993. Pigs as ordinary wealth. Technical logic, exchange and leadership in New Guinea. In *Technological Choices. Transformations in*

Material Cultures since the Neolithic, ed. P. Lemonnier. London: Routledge.
Lemonnier, P. 1995. Fertile chimeras. *Pacific Studies* 18, n°4: forthcoming.
Meggitt, M.J. 1967. The pattern of leadership among the Mae-Enga. *Anthropological Forum* 2, no.1: 20-35.
Meggitt, M.J. 1974. Pigs are our hearts. The Te exchange cycle among the Mae-Enga of New Guinea. *Oceania* 44: 165-203.
Meggitt, M.J. 1977. *Blood is their Argument. Warfare among the Mae-Enga of the New Guinea Highlands.* Palo Alto: Mayfield.
Mimica, J. 1981. Omalyce. An ethnography of the Ikwaye view of cosmos. Ph. D. dissertation, Australian National Univer., Canberra.
Modjeska, C.N. 1982. Production and inequality: perspectives from Central New Guinea. In *Inequality in the New Guinea Highlands Societies,* ed. A. Strathern, 50-108. Cambridge: Cambridge Univer. Press.
Serpenti, L. 1968. Headhunting and magic on Kolepom. *Tropical Man* 1: 116-39.
Serpenti, L. 1972. Ndambu, the feast of competitive growth, *Tropical Man* 5: 162-187.
Serpenti, L. 1977. *Cultivators in the Swamps. Social Structure and Horticulture in a New Guinea Society (Frederik-Hendrik Island West New Guinea).* Assen, Amsterdam: van Gorgum.
Serpenti, L. 1984. The ritual meaning of homosexuality and paedophilia among the Kimam-Papuans of South Irian Jaya. In *Ritualized Homosexuality in Melanesia.*, ed. G. Herdt, 292-336. Berkeley: Univer. of California Press.
Sorenson, E.R. 1972. Socio-ecological exchange among the Fore of New Guinea. *Current Anthropology* 13: 349-83.
Strathern, A.J. 1969. Finance and production: two strategies in New Guinea exchange systems. *Oceania* 40: 42-67.
Strathern, A.J. 1971. *The Rope of Moka. Big men and Ceremonial Exchange in Mount Hagen, New Guinea.* Cambridge: Cambridge Univer. Press.
Strathern, A.J. 1978. Finance and production revisited: in pursuit of a comparison. *Research in Economic Anthropology* 1: 73-104.
Strathern, A.J. 1981. Death as exchange: two Melanesian cases. In *Mortality and immortality: The Anthropology and Archaeology of Death.*, ed. S. Humfries and H. King, 205-223. London: Academic Press.
Strathern, A.J. 1982. Witchcraft, greed, cannibalism, and death. Some related themes from the New Guinea Highlands. In *Death and the Regeneration of Life,* ed. M. Bloch and J. Parry, 111-33. New York: Pergamon.
Trenkenschuh, F. 1970. *An Asmat Sketch Book: Handbook for Missionaries to Asmat, Irian Jaya.* Djajapura: The Franciscan Press.
Tumu, A., P. Munini, A. Kyangali and P. Wiessner. 1989. *A View at Enga Culture.* Madang: KPI Production for the Department of Enga.
van Amelsvoort, V.F.P.M. 1964. *Culture, Stone-Age and Modern Medicine.* Assen: van Gorgum and Co. N.V.
van Baal, J. 1966. *Dema. Description and Analysis of Marind-anim Culture (South New Guinea).* The Hague: Martinus Nijhoff.

van Baal, J. 1984. The dialectic of sex in Marind-anim culture. In Ritualized Homosexuality in Melanesia, ed. G. Herdt, 128-66. Berkeley: Univer. of California Press.

Vertenten, P. 1923. Het Koppensnellen in Zuid Nieuw-Guinea [Headtaking in South New Guinea]. *Bijdragen Tot de Taal-, Land- en Volkenkunde* 79: 45-72.

Wiessner, P. and A. Tumu, forthcoming. *Historical Vines: The Formation of Regional Networks of Exchange, Ritual and Warfare Among the Enga of Papua New Guinea.*

Williams, F.E. 1936. *Papuans of the Trans-Fly*. Oxford: Clarendon Press.

Zegwaard, G. 1959. Headhunting practices of the Asmat of Netherlands New Guinea. *American Anthropologist* 61: 1020-41.

Zegwaard, G. and J.H.M.C. Boelaars 1955. De sociale structuur van de Asmat-stam [Asmat Social Organization]. *Adatrechtbundels*, 45 (serie S. Nieuw-Guinea, n°53): 244-301.

13. OF HARVESTS AND HIERARCHIES
SECURING STAPLE FOOD AND SOCIAL POSITION IN THE TROBRIAND ISLANDS

Wulf Schiefenhövel & Ingrid Bell-Krannhals

There does not seem to be any other society where the bulk of the harvest, the yield of a family's hard work throughout the year, is given away. The Trobrianders do just that. Their harvest gifts (*uligubu*) consist of yam (*tetu, Dioscorea alata*), the staple food. After careful, strategic decisions, the harvest gifts are channeled to various recipients, who are mostly but not necessarily members of the nuclear or extended family. People who have been working together, preparing the soil by slash-and-burn technique, erecting elaborate fences as protection against feral pigs, and doing the time-consuming and demanding tasks of planting, weeding, and harvesting will live on yam they receive from other families. Why does this tradition exist? Why do the Trobrianders not follow common patterns of taking what they have harvested and then, as need or custom may make necessary, sharing portions of the supplies from time to time?

The Austronesian-speaking Trobrianders are unique in a number of ways, some of which were well portrayed by Malinowski (1922, 1929, 1935) after he had shifted his fieldwork from the small island of Mailu off the southeastern coast of mainland New Guinea to the inhabitants of the Trobriand group of islands in the Solomon Sea. The people there are proud of their very developed and sophisticated traditions, the spectacular elements of their culture like the *kula* with its many splendid events, the competitive harvest (*kayasa*), their success in the carving and other businesses, their provincial and national politics (the Papua New Guinea ambassador to the European Community, for instance, is a Trobriander), and their strong chiefs (*gweguyau*), who still hold the reins in their hands, much to the dismay of the national administration and missions. Important things have changed since Malinowski's days, but in many respects the Trobrianders of today seem to have stepped from the pages of their famous ethnography. This chapter attempts to put the findings of our ongoing fieldwork, which we began in 1982, into the frame of reference provided by this book.

Social Hierarchy of the Trobrianders of Tawema Village

Kaileuna, with a surface area of roughly 50 square kilometers, containing seven villages and approximately 1,500 inhabitants, lies west of the main island Kiriwina, the administrational center of the Trobriand group. By far the majority of the inhabitants of the Trobriand Islands are still horticulturists and gatherers of marine resources. Due to the geographical location of Kaileuna, the people there are out of the main stream of acculturation and in many ways closer to traditional life than their neighbors on Kiriwina. Tawema had 240 inhabitants when we began fieldwork in 1982; it has grown since then. This has led to the addition of a new cluster of houses at the former periphery in the west (see Figure 13.1). At this site the several consecutive church buildings have been erected. It seems possible that this new "suburb" is gaining political importance, because a number of high-ranking men have shifted their houses here. In 1992 a clearing was made for another cluster of houses further to the west. The originally circular shape of the village may at one stage be given up in favour of a more rectangular one.

The Trobrianders speak an Austronesian language and seem to be a mix between people of Papuan origin and newcomers. Early Austronesian seafarers introduced some 4,000 years ago a sophisticated technique to build and sail outrigger boats, their language, and probably other items. The history of this cultural contact and influx of genes is still largely unknown (Bellwood 1989 for anthropological and linguistic features; Serjeantson and Hill 1989 for genetic features). The Trobrianders, like various other ethnic groups in this area (usually called Massim and classified according to the particular "curvilinear" style of carvings) have a matrilineal descent system. The children of a couple belong to the clan of their mother, and through this clan they receive certain rights, especially eligibility for

Figure 13.1 Tawema Village, Kaileuna, Trobriand Islands, 1992

liku owner

B: Mwasai   E: Motaesa   F: Mounaki   G: Tokunupei   H: Vapalaguyau   I: Topiesi

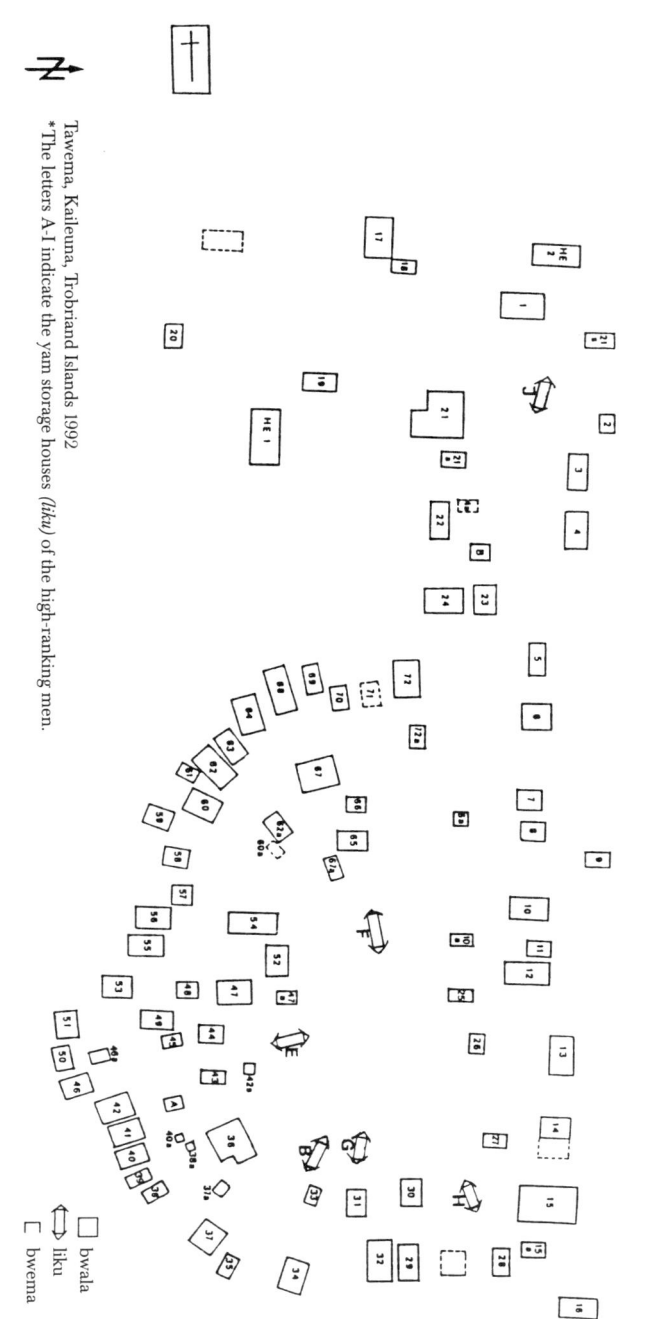

Tawema, Kaileuna, Trobriand Islands 1992

*The letters A-I indicate the yam storage houses (*liku*) of the high-ranking men.

chieftainship. Despite matrilineality, this position is held exclusively by men, some of whom are very influential indeed. In Tawema the position of the village chief is more that of a *primus inter pares* than that of a powerful political leader. This is of relevance for the rank hierarchy to be discussed later. In Kiriwina, however, some chiefs, above all the paramount chief representing the whole group of islands, still have substantial power. It may be added here that rights connected to land and gardens do not follow the matriline but are usually inherited from the father (Weiner 1976; Bell-Krannhals 1990).

Figure 13.2 Tawema Village, Kaileuna, Trobriand Islands, 1983

liku **owner**
A: Bwegima   B: Mwasai   Yauratila I.   D: Kilagola   E: Motaesa   F: Mounaki

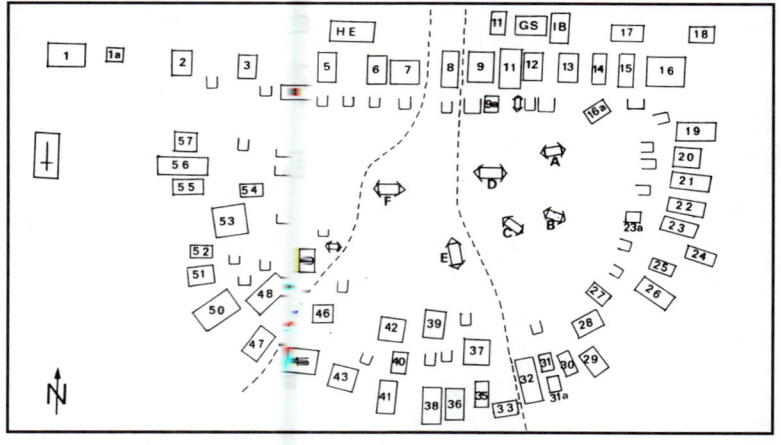

Tawema, Kaileuna, Trobriand Island 1983
*The letters A-I indicate the yam storage houses *(liku)* of the high-ranking men.

☐ bwala
⇦ liku
☐ bwema

The old village plan of Tawema (see Figures 13.2 and 13.3) conveys elements of Trobriand social ideology. The living houses (*bwala*) are arranged in a circle-like ring, while the thatched verandas (*bwema*) with storage space under the roofs form a second ring. Toward the middle, on the village ground proper, stand the slim and high *liku*, the yam storage houses of the men of high rank (see Fig. 13.4) in a somewhat irregular third ring. They point, with one of the gables, towards a small innermost circle. This is the real center of the society, it becomes alive during important ceremonies.

In Tawema and other villages this inner center of the settlement is where institutionalized chiefs may have their *liku* (see *liku* D of Figures 13.2 and 13.3 and Figure 13.5; the new chief of Tawema has, however, not shifted his *liku* E there, Figure 13.1).

Figure 13.3 Tawema Village, Kaileuna, Trobriand Islands, 1987

liku owner
A: Bwegima   B: Mwasai   Yaurabina I.   D: Kilagola   E: Motaesa   F: Mounaki   G: Tokunupei

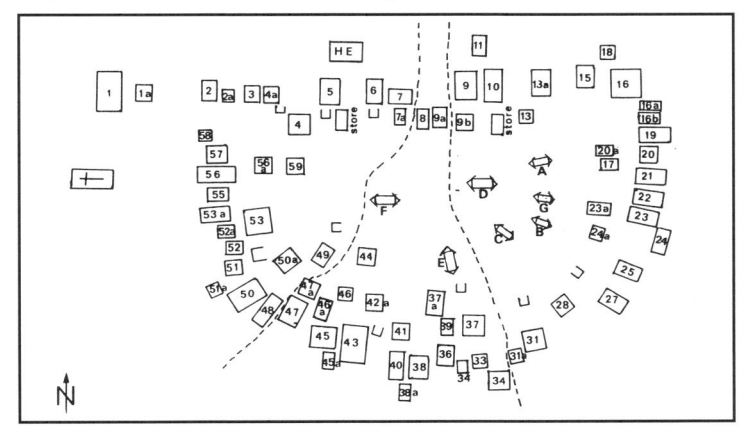

Tawema, Kaileuna, Trobriand Islands 1987
*The letters A-I indicate the yam storage houses *(liku)* of the high-ranking men.

☐ bwala
⇔ liku
⌐ bwema

The circular configuration of the village betrays the ideal of Trobriand society: the backs of the houses are, as it were, shielding the community against the "outside"; the "inside" orientation of the *bwala* entrances toward the center results in everybody facing everybody, permitting social control but, at the same time, presumably creating the feeling of a bonded group. In the discussion we will analyze the village layouts in the years 1983, 1987, and 1992 and the corresponding sociopolitical changes in Tawema, which are correlated to the quest for status.

Trobriand traditions often contain ritualized elements of competition. This becomes particularly obvious during the *kayasa*, a contest among the men of a village for producing, displaying, distributing, and receiving the largest amount of harvested yam. An

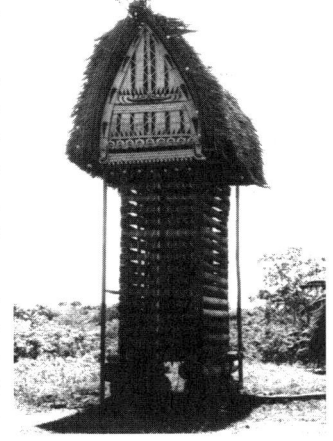

Figure 13.4 A Typical *Liku* yam house of a high-ranked man

Figure 13.5 Plan of Omarakana Village, Kiriwina, Trobriand Islands, Papua New Guinea (after Malinowski 1929)

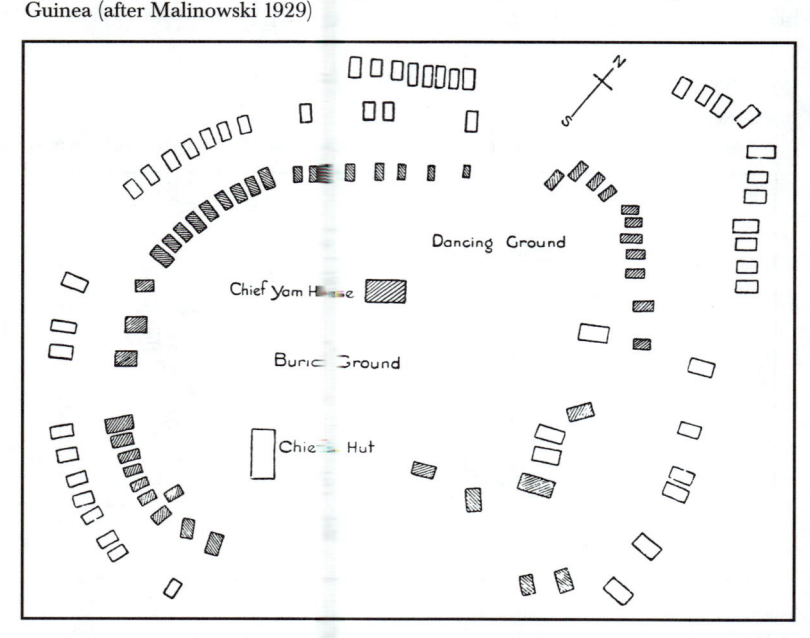

ambitious male family head who has gathered enough valuables of various kinds to host the costly ceremony starts the process with a speech to the village community in which he, with the rhetorical eloquence and wit typical of Trobriand orators, challenges the others to win the prize money he is offering. In Tawema the first prizes are, as in former times, the valued *kena* earthenware pots from the Amphlett Islands; they have to be imported because the coral atolls of Kiriwina and Kaileuna do not offer suitable clay for their manufacture. Everybody participating in the *kayasa* receives a prize, nowadays often accompanied by sums of money. Those who finish last get small tokens for their participation but are often subject to friendly ridicule by the spectators. The organizer of such a contest, called *toli kayasa*, may have to put up the equivalent of US$ 1,000 or even considerably more.

In 1982, Topiyesi, the eldest son of chief Kilagola, acted as *toli kayasa*. Everybody, including the visitors from other villages who regularly attend the final stages of the *kayasa*, agreed that the contest led by Topiyesi was quite spectacular and successful. He is a physically very powerful, intelligent, and a socially skillful man. He was born around 1951 and was only thirty-one years old or so when he took over the role as initiator and organizer of the contest. He was supported by unusually numerous and active siblings, including five brothers and two sisters who live in Tawema and one brother in a well-paid position on a cruise boat for wealthy tourists. Between 1990 and 1992 a *liku* was built for Topiyesi right next to his *bwala*. It is further from the center of the village than other storage houses (see Figure 13.1). Its oblique position in comparison with the row of *bwala* around it indicates how important it is to orient all *liku* toward the inner circle. By 1990 Topiyesi had risen to be one of the three most high-ranking men in Tawema. His position was also shown by the fact that he had a new spacious fiberglass dinghy at his disposal, which was loaned to him by an influential man from the main island. With this boat and his own outboard motor Topiyesi conducts economically successful fishing, marketing, and passenger transport.

In 1984, Vapalaguyau, then approximately fourty-four years old, took over the role as *toli kayasa* for a harvest competition in 1985, calling the village community to compete for the prizes he had accumulated. Shortly afterwards, however, the wife of the chief died and the *kayasa* had to be called off. In November 1991 Vapalaguyau's own wife died, and he had to remain in the state of mourning until the *sagali* ceremony in July 1992 relieved him of his withdrawn existence. He is one of the respected traditional healers and has specialized in helping women in childbirth. Like Topiyesi, he is vital, intelligent, socially competent, and one of the high-ranking men. It is no happenstance that a *liku* was also built for him; it is, as seems to be the rule for the first such storage houses, rather inconspicuous and does not protrude into the open village space (see Figure 13.1).

Clinical Aspects

From 1982 to 1992 approximately 1,500 patients received medical treatment from our team. Else, the only medical post accessible to the inhabitants of Tawema is located in the village of Kaduwaga and is usually not equipped with enough effective medicines nor with skilled and motivated personnel. Except in one case where an infant could not be sufficiently breastfed and in a few others where dysentery and/or helminthic infestation caused health problems in infants, there is no malnutrition in Tawema or in the neighboring villages. This is not surprising given the favorable conditions with fertile coral gardens and plentiful marine resources. It is, however, interesting to note that infants and children are small for their age when compared with European cohorts (see Figure 13.6).

The ratio of weight to height, on the other hand, results in completely normal figures. As can be seen from Figure 13.7, the values of virtually all infants and children fall within the 97.5 percentile in which the German counterparts would also be represented.

Figure 13.6 Height for Age of Trobriand Children Compared to German Children

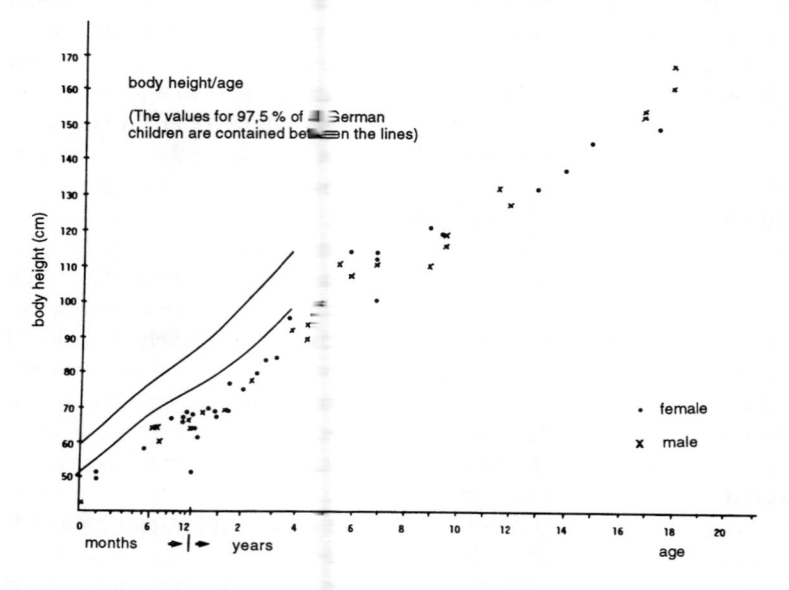

Figure 13.7 Height for Weight of Trobriand Children Compared to German Children

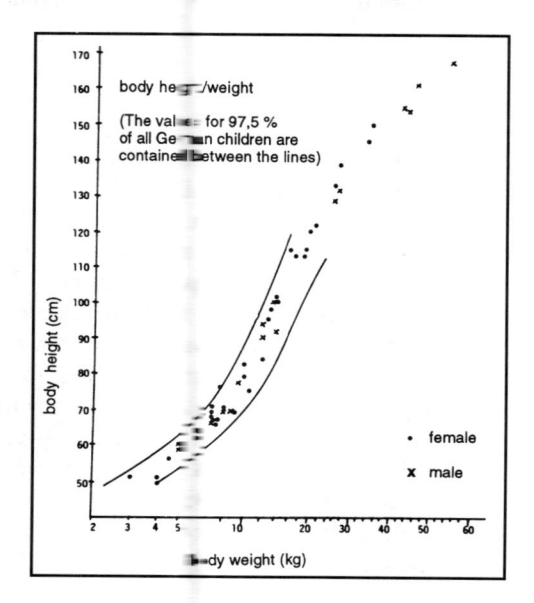

Whether this lag in body height and weight compared to Europeans indicates a genetic factor, or the lack of protein or other foods in the nutrition of infants and children, or a high parasite load, is uncertain at the present time. Malaria is endemic on the Trobriand Islands and most children have enlarged livers and spleens; some have mild-to-moderate forms of anemia due to chronic malaria. Intestinal worms are common, as are upper respiratory infections. But given the almost complete lack of modern medicine at times when our research station was unmanned, the general state of health of the Trobrianders is remarkably good. On average, menarche is around sixteen years of age. The two earliest pregnancies recorded by us since 1982 were of women at that age.

Obesity is virtually absent, and blood pressure values are very low compared to the standards of industrialized countries. A careful study by Lindeberg and Lundh (1993) on the Trobriand Island of Kitava has revealed that ischemic heart disease and stroke are absent on this island, which is slightly more isolated from the main island Kiriwina with its ongoing acculturation. The incidence of asthma in Tawema and the neighboring villages is the only unexpected finding. It is perhaps related to a marked increase of chewing betelnut (*Areca catechu*) with its slight narcotic and parasympathicomimetic properties. Generally speaking, however, no malnutrition or nutrition-related diseases were found in more than a decade of fieldwork. This seems to indicate that despite inequalities in individual and family success at gardening and exploiting marine resources, food sharing on the micro, meso, and macrolevels is functioning sufficiently well to neutralize effects on health. This finding is of importance also with regard to harvest gifts.

Uligubu – The Harvest Gifts

The Kilivila language of the Trobrianders has three terms to designate specific gardens (Bell-Krannhals 1990: 98). They are: (1) *kemugwa,* a garden for early harvest of various varieties of yam for consumption within the family, (2) *kemata,* a main garden with yam for the harvest gifts, (3) *tapopwa,* a garden for taro (*Colocasia esculenta*). The greatest effort is invested into the *kemata*. They are much larger than the other types and work done here is more conspicuous, more prestigious, and carried out with more extroverted behavior. In all gardens the different tasks are done by the nuclear family, that is, the wife, the husband, and their children as soon as they are old enough to take over some chores and are not among the few pupils who attend the village school in Kaduwaga. Occasionally, members of the extended family will participate regularly in the garden work, particularly unmarried persons who are not responsible for their own production unit.

Energy and time spent on the gardens, especially on the *kemata*, is surprising given the fact that the reef is nearby and marine resources can be used the whole year round. But carbohydrates are essential in human nutrition, and for the Trobrianders there is no food more important than yam. *Tetu* is the epitome of human existence, and if one does not have yam to eat, there is no enjoyment of the meal, no matter how precious or plentiful the other delicacies are.

We have calculated that each of the families who were tilling an average of 2.4 gardens of the above mentioned types had a total average plot of approximately 3,200 square meters. The land, by the way, belongs to only very few, mostly male, individuals who loan plots to members of the village community, and receive only little payment in the form of garden products.

The Trobrianders have a very ingenious method to estimate, in the course of a *kayasa* contest, the volume of the individual harvests of a family. As soon as the yams of the *kemata* gardens have been dug up from the ground, they are displayed in the respective gardens of the families. This is done by carefully placing them in such a way that they form a steep cone (see Figure 13.8). To impress bypassers, the biggest and most evenly grown yam tubers are placed at the outside of these heaps. Since the angle of these cones is more or less the same in all cases the Trobrianders are able to assess the volume by taking just one single measurement, namely that of the circumference of the cone on the ground. The length of this circumference is measured in fathoms and sub-units and then translated into a number of *peta*, the ordinary baskets used to carry the harvest into the village. The coefficient necessary to do this calculation was probably arrived at through a mixture of trial, error, and intuition. In a number of cases we have checked the Trobriand fig-

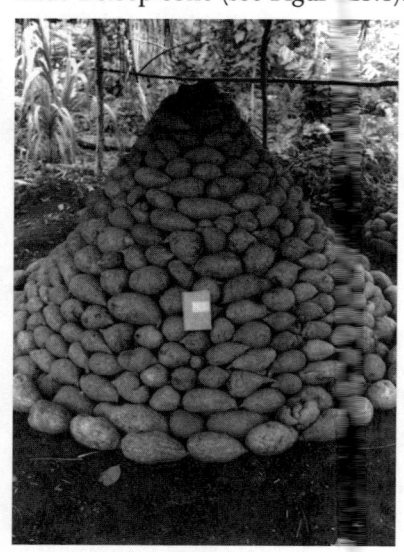

Figure 13.8 A Typical Conical Yam Heap Displayed During a Competitive Harvest (*Kayasa*)

ures and arrived at similar results. In 1983 and 1984 we took measurements of garden sizes and harvests and gathered information on the latter from various informants (Schiefenhövel and Bell-Krannhals 1986). Figure 13.9 represents the harvest in 1984 from the two main garden areas. The total amount of yams was close to seventy tons.

Figure 13.9 The 1984 Harvest from the Two Most Important Garden Areas of Tawema

	Size m²	Volume in baskets	Weight	Yield kg/ha	m²/kg
A	172,650	4,162	62,430	3,6	2.8
B	21,900	427	6,405	2,9	3.4
Total	194,500	4,589	68,835	3,5	2.8

In Figure 13.10, thirty-five men, each the male head of a family, are ranked according to the amount of yams they received. It is quite obvious that the men who receive the largest quantity of yams are not the ones with the biggest harvests and harvest gifts. As a matter of fact, rank positions one through six, with the exception of position number four, are well below the average amount of donated harvest gifts. Topiyesi, a very powerful man and successful gardener, harvested the largest single amount, at 390 baskets, but at the same time received 236 baskets. He clearly is a man who is rising in rank according to the typical Trobriand mechanism: you have to repeatedly give a lot to receive a lot later on. Vapalaguyau, who was also mentioned above was not quite as successful with his harvest, but he is one of those who received substantial amounts of yams from others.

Trobriand informants stress that the *liku* storage houses are not built by the potential recipient of large amounts of harvest gifts, but by those who plan to channel their yams toward this recipient. Most of the individuals who received large quantities of harvest gifts in 1984 are owners of such *liku* (see Figures 13.10. 13.1. 13.2, 13.3). Since the figures given here represent just one year in a series of annual harvests, mishaps can cause a normally well-endowed receiver to rank lower than in other years. This may have been the case with the *liku* owner Mwasei (rank position number 13). But the expectation of receiving a large amount of *uligubu* and the actual giving of yam by others seem to form a rather stable correlation. Over the years, there is probably little room for erratic developments. That is to say, this particular Trobriand tradition of harvest gifts has a stabilizing effect on the rank hierarchy in the village society. It must be mentioned that the often very large amounts of yam received by high-ranking men is used not only to feed their nuclear and extended families, but also to host guests at ceremonies important for the village society as a whole. In this respect the *uligubu*-yam can be seen as a kind of tax money that in part flows back to the community.

Figure 13.10 Donors and Recipients of Harvest Gifts *(Uligubu)* 1984

	Received yam (in baskets)	Number of donors	Male heads of households	Number of receivers	Given away yam (in baskets)
1	579	3	Mounaki	1	45
2	501	3	Kilagola (chief)	1	20
3	400	3	Bwegima	–	–
4	375	3	Tokunupei	1	150
5	257	1	Tomtawa	1	10
6	240	3	Motaesa	1	4
7	236	2	Topiyesi	1	390
8	207	3	Yaurabina	1	90
9	194	3	Vapalaguyau	1	150
10	160	2	Nusai	1	370
11	153	3	Bulasa (evangelist)	1	7
12	150	2	Mobiliuya	1	50
13	109	3	Mwasei	1	195
14	100	2	Sakau	–	–
15	79	2	Tosobu	1	257
16	55	1	Mogega	1	60
17	54	2	Tomalala	1	50
18	51	1	Taidyeri	1	20
19	50	1	Gerubara	1	100
20	49	2	Yoya	–	–
21	40	1	Tobwabwana	1	40
22	20	1	Mokelobu	1	40
23	10	1	Bwetadou	1	–
24	7	1	Bwemautila	–	–
25	2	1	Tosulala	1	2
26	–	–	Tokuyumila	–	–
27			Tovaula (+Simiya)	1	183
28	–	–	Mokiwola	1	100
29	–	–	Tolivalu	–	150
30	–	–	Dovana	1	100
31	–	–	Kalavatu	1	50
32	–	–	Tokobiyim	–	–
33	–	–	Kekitawa	1	100
34	–	–	Moyabvau	1	51
35	–	–	Moligogu	1	59

donors: 50;
households: 35;
donors per household: 1.4

The local people have given clear etic indications that the most efficient and socially acceptable way to gain status is to do so via gardening success and generous yam giving. This principle holds true for the ones who want to rise in rank, who are about or who have already managed to achieve status. But the most highly valued position is that of prime receivers of harvest gifts. A man who had a *liku* built for him and regularly filled with large amounts of yam stands in the climax of his life as a highly respected citizen. For all those who do not have the status of an ascribed chief with corresponding political powers, this position of high regard has to be achieved by climbing the ladder of the social hierarchy through earlier years of successful donorship. Figure 13.11 attempts to show the flow of a total of fifty-nine harvest gifts in the year 1984 by creating a fictitious ego comprised of all garden owners with harvests that year. The channels used by these combined owners of yam are symbolized as small or bold arrows indicating one, or respectively five, *uligubu* transactions.

Figure 13.11 The Channels of Harvest Gifts
The Fictitious Ego Combines All Donors

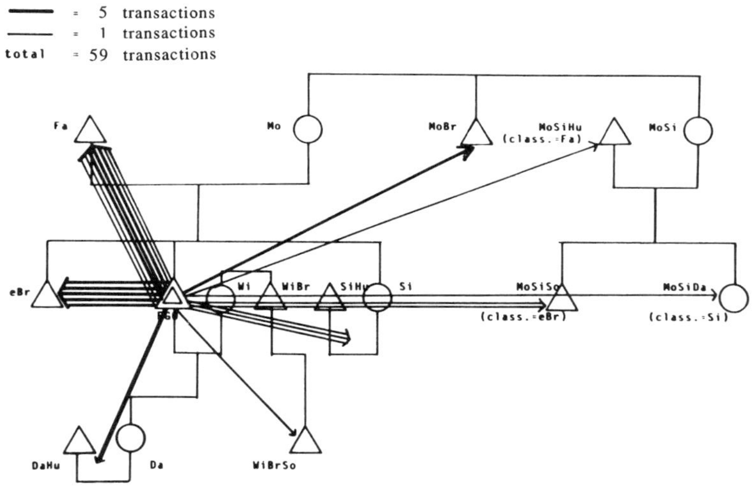

In contrast to Malinowski's statements (1935: 195), the most common channel was not that going to ego's sisters' husbands, but predominantly to ego's father or elder brother. This distribution pattern (as well as the one claimed by Malinowski) is basically congruent with the sociobiological paradigm of inclusive fitness. Malinowski himself, in the supplement of volume 1 of *Coral Gardens and their Magic* (1935) has presented data that contradict his statement in the book that sisters' husbands should be the main receivers of *uligubu*.

Weiner has also directed attention to the fact that the largest harvest gift exchanges take place between men, particularly between fathers and sons (1976: 141-47). Thus, it seems that the distribution pattern we observed represents normality rather than statistical exceptions. In Figure 13.12 we correlated fifty-nine transactions with degree of relatedness in the kinship system. It turns out that 83 percent of all harvest gifts were directed to very close genetic kin, such as parents, siblings or children; whereas 17 percent were divided between mother's brother and other relatives. Three percent of the receivers had no known genetic link with the donor.

Figure 13.12 Harvest Gifts 1984 According to Coefficient of Kinship

Genetic Relatedness	Receiver	n	Total	%
50%	eBr.	25		
	Fa	19		
	Da	2		
	Si	3	49	83
25%	MoBr	5	5	9
12.5%	MoSiHu	2		
	MoSiDa	1	3	5
"0"%	MoSiHu	1		
	WiBrSo	1	2	3

Discussion

The Trobrianders present an interesting case because their society combines various elements salient for the perspective of this book:

1. Food, often produced in surplus (in some years large quantities of stored yam rot unused), is one of the main "currencies" to gain high status.
2. Elements of strong but ritualized competition like the harvest contest (*kayasa*) and the *kula*-expeditions to obtain valuables are dominated by men by contrast to *sagali* post-mortuary ceremonies which are dominated by women.
3. Men achieve high status during their lifetime through success in gardening and prestige as generous bestowers of harvest gifts (*uligubu*); if all goes well their relatives build *liku* for them, the sign of influential male members of the society.
4. Men who owe their ascribed high rank to an institutionalized and matrilineally inherited position of political (and partly reli-

gious) leadership are the chiefs (*gweguyau*); they have *liku* of sometimes very large dimensions.

The Trobrianders thus have an interesting mix of ascribed chieftainship and men who achieve their rank and influence by merit. The latter position, as a rule, can not be transferred to the first position. But the male quest for status is channeled into a formalized procedure by which powerful, intelligent, and socially skillful men are allowed to rise to acknowledged rank.

The transition from an ordinary member of the village community to somebody who presents massive harvest gifts and later owns a *liku* may take place when a man is in his mid-thirties to fifties. The men usually marry at about twenty to twenty-five years of age. That means their acquired status of successful gardeners, harvest gift bestowers, and, later, *liku* owners comes too late to assist them in competing for spouses. It may coincide, however, with successful negotiation of marriages for their children. The same biographic-ontogenetic aspect is true for the other big Trobriand competition, the *kula*. Men who excel in this very complicated and risky status contest are also in the middle of their lives or older and can only indirectly influence their reproductive success, because tradition requires monogamy for all men except the few institutionalized chiefs, who can have fifteen or more wives. Marital separation, on the other hand, is possible and can be initiated by women or men. One could argue that a successful *kula* trader or *liku* owner would have better chances than other men to remarry a young woman. Statistics to test these hypotheses will be calculated when our demographic data for the period starting 1982 have been analyzed.

The women's impressive contest to produce and, in a very complicated process of bidding and exchanging, to barter skirts (*doba*) in the *lisaladabu* is carried out by women of virtually all age groups. A biological, i.e. reproductive, benefit of their success in this contest seems possible but remains to be shown. A number of factors are involved in this contest ceremony, as well as in the *kula* and *kayasa*, which are today more or less unconnected to reproduction. Another question is whether these ritualized contests originated in mechanisms fostering inclusive fitness.

As in other societies, the ground plan of settlements reveals important elements of the social structure of the society. In Tawema and other villages the *liku* are close to the center and therefore are well-situated to represent the power of their owners; the biggest, most important *liku* stand more toward or in the middle, while the other ones at some distance. The *liku* configuration therefore provides a good view into the rank hierarchy. The powerful chiefs, with their ascribed status and institutionalized political roles, have their often richly decorated and tall *liku* near or directly in the center of the village, where most of the important ceremonies have their nucleus and where the community is symbolically represented. The ethological concept of social rank as correlated to being the focus of attention (see Hold-Cavell, this volume) comes to mind immediately. In European villages or cities an important church or, after the onset of secularization the town hall would usually be located in such a spot.

It is interesting to speculate about ascribed and achieved status in Trobriand society. What was their origin; what was and is their function? The Trobrianders are well on the way to becoming a stratified society. Whether the mechanisms of *kayasa* and *uligubu* function as modifying and neutralizing inequalities for achieving status or whether clan membership also has a bearing on whether a man will have a *liku* or not remains unclear at the present time.

It appears possible that the institutionalized forms of contesting for top positions in *kayasa* and *uligubu* are mechanisms that limit the degree of competition. The male status quest, which can sometimes run out of control, is directed into highly ritualized competition based on yam. There is, by the way, another Trobriand form of conflict resolution: instead of drawing spears, knives or axes, two quarreling men will challenge each other to produce the longest and heaviest *kuvi*, a particular long variety of yam whose tubers often have enormous dimensions. Again, food is used in the struggle for status.

Ethnohistoric and comparative research may one day provide an answer to where the ritualized forms of status quest on the Trobriand islands came from. Is competing with yam in harvest contests a local development or was it introduced, perhaps by the Austronesian immigrants whose culture also had other attractive elements and whose language was adopted by the indigenous population? Was the ascribed role of political chiefs originally arrived at by successful gardening and generous giving or, in more general terms, is meritocracy the stepping-stone for institutionalized and inherited leadership? The English words for "chief" and "achieve" can be traced to Latin *caput* (French *chef*), and thereby to one common concept. For the Indoeuropean cultures this seems to suggest that inherited status did, in fact, grow out of achieved status. Possibly our forefathers have used ways as elegant as those of the Trobrianders to secure food and social position.

References

Bell-Krannhals, I. 1990. *Haben um zu geben. Eigentum und Besitz auf den Trobriand-Inseln, Papua New Guinea.* Ethnologisches Seminar der Universität und Museum f. Völkerkunde. Basel, Wepf und Co.

Bellwood, P.S. 1989. The colonization of the Pacific: Some current hypotheses. In *The Colonization of the Pacific. A Genetic Trail.*, eds. A.V. Hill and S.W. Serjeantson, 1-59. Oxford: Clarendon Press.

Lindeberg, S. and B. Lundh. 1993. Apparent absence of stroke and ischemic heart disease in a traditional melanesian population – a clinical study in Kitava. *Journal of Internal Medicine* 233: 269-75.

Malinowski, B. 1922. *Argonauts of the Western Pacific. An Account of Native Enterprise and Adventure in the Archipelagoes of Melanesian New Guinea.* London: Routledge and Kegan Paul.

Malinowski, B. 1929. *The Sexual Life of Savages in North-Western Melanesia. An Ethnographic Account of Courtship, Marriage, and Family Life Among the Natives of the Trobriand Islands, British New Guinea.* London: Routledge and Kegan Paul.

Malinowski, B. 1935. *Coral Gardens and Their Magic. A Study of the Methods of Tilling the Soil and of Agricultural Rites in the Trobriand Islands,* 2 vols. London: Allen and Unwin.

Schiefenhövel, W. and I. Bell-Krannhals. 1986. Wer teilt, hat Teil an der Macht: Systeme der Yams-Vergabe auf den Trobriand Inseln, Papua Neuguinea. Mitteilungen der Anthropologischen Gesellschaft in Wien 116: 19-39.

Serjeantson, S.W. and A.V. Hill. 1989. The Colonization of the Pacific: The Genetic Evidence. In *The Colonization of the Pacific. A Genetic Trail,* eds. A.V. Hill and S.W. Serjeantson, 286-94. Oxford: Clarendon Press.

Weiner, A.B. 1976. *Women of Value, Men of Renown: New Perspectives in Trobriand Exchange.* Austin: Univer. of Texas Press.

14. FOOD AND HOUSEHOLD STATUS IN NEPAL

Catherine Panter-Brick

The relationship between food proscriptions and caste status in the Indian subcontinent is very well known (Khare and Rao 1986; Vayda 1987). Indeed, Dumont's treatise (1966) on Indian caste ideology and structure was entitled *Homo hierarchicus*, and included a discussion of the rules governing caste relations with respect to potentially polluting food and drink. Similarly, Marriott (1968) examined the nature of food transactions that defined caste hierarchy and relations in one Indian village. In turn, Ferro-Luzzi (1975) detailed the types of food restrictions for as many as 260 animal and 130 vegetable species that served to mark the identity of particular human groups, whether tribes and castes, or vulnerable groups such as pregnant and lactating women.

This chapter examines the relationship between food and status at the level of individual households within and between castes, and the impact of status on food procurement, food consumption, and nutritional status, rather than conversely the use of food in the quest for status (see other contributors in this volume). It presents findings from rural Nepal to examine three main propositions: (1) low socioeconomic status compels a quest for food, (2) status affects food distribution within the household, and (3) status has an impact on nutritional well-being. Nepal is an appropriate setting for such an enquiry, since the caste hierarchy links many ethnic groups, broadly categorized into Tibeto-Burman and Indo-Aryan origin, which adopt very different subsistence strategies (Acharya and Bennett 1981).

Status and Food Procurement

The first proposition is that low socioeconomic status compels a quest for food. In overpopulated rural areas of Nepal, few households have sufficient land area to achieve food self-sufficiency. "Six months of eating one's food, six months of searching for food" is how one peasant hill farmer described his situation in the course of an interview. His harvests supplied the household with just six months of staple grains, and each year he had to "search" for extra supplies.

An anthropological study of household responses to food shortages shows that the particular strategies adopted are a marker of social and socioeconomic status (Panter-Brick and Eggerman, forthcoming). In-depth interviews of 120 randomly selected households were conducted in four villages of western Nepal (Gulmiuand Arghakhanchi districts), with proportional representation on the basis of land holdings and caste. These interviews uncovered the following five main courses of action and their specific social and economic contexts.

Emigration

Temporary emigration is widespread, prompted by extreme poverty or the desire for a better life. Cash from outside earnings enables a family to buy foodstuffs, hire labor and payoff loans. Some migrants will return without a penny, but in any event their absence has reduced the number of mouths to feed at home. Prolonged absence and employment can result in a steady income, but it leads to a shortage of manpower for female-headed households. In the words of one woman, "When the man is at home, it's easy work; when he is away, it's easy money" (Panter-Brick and Eggerman, forthcoming).

The type of work sought is tied to social factors, especially caste and educational level. Thus, men of Tibeto-Burman origin aspire to a military career and a regular pension. Most applicants find themselves rejected by the army, and turn to the "civil service", looking for employment as cooks, night watchmen, drivers or laborers, as far away as Bombay or Calcutta. In contrast, the high caste Bahun-Chetri seek high-status positions in government or finance, while the low-caste artisans restrict themselves to temporary or seasonal employment.

Wage labor

The opportunity for in-village wage labor varies enormously with the ecological and social circumstances of actual communities. In predominantly Tibeto-Burman localities, which tend to be in high-altitude areas with limited agricultural potential, each family cultivates its own terraces during the same season, and there is little possibility of working for another household. By contrast, in multi-caste localities, a pronounced economic disparity between high caste landowners and artisans creates a supply and demand for wage labor.

Other income

In rural areas, grain is bartered rather than sold, but few families produce a local surplus. However, the sale of livestock and other animals is a handy source of cash, and this strategy is encouraged by funding from organizations supporting a "Small Farmer Development Program". Again, different castes specialize in the sale of various products: some make straw or bamboo handicrafts, others sell alcohol (the avoidance of alcohol distinguishes pure castes from the (Nepali: *matwali)* alcohol-drinking castes, while artisans are sharply differentiated as blacksmiths, tailors, potters or musicians, each on an echelon in the caste hierarchy. Of course, the high castes and artisans are interdependent, and client-patron relationships eventually tie given households in a tight web of credit and labor obligations.

Loans

The volume of money changing hands through credit transactions is striking. Loans are taken out to purchase food for consumption, to invest in land and livestock, or to meet a crisis of some sort. Cassels et al. (1987) report that families in rural Nepal divide themselves into those that merely cope with an adverse situation, and those that are able to rise above it through judicious use of their resources ("coping" or "investing" strategies).

Moderate borrowing is a common strategy for poorer or female-headed households, actually preferred to complete financial independence because it establishes a credit line that can be drawn upon in an emergency. These loans can be repaid in labor during times of peak agricultural activity. But for very poor households, debt can become a dangerous whirlpool, swallowing up their land and animal resources. A Nepali proverb puts this quite simply: "Once an ear is lopped off, the other is soon to follow."

Change of diet

In periods of food shortages (Nepali: *anikal*), families change their staple diet, but among poor households the shift – paradoxically – is from boiled maize flour to prestigious white rice. Maize is nowhere available to buy, so rice is imported from nearby towns, a situation which underlines the dependence of these areas on a market economy. Intrahousehold food allocations can also change, although

Tibeto-Burmese households boast of no practices that discriminate against daughters-in-law or young children. Local people remark that the richest households (high caste) are those that tighten their belts to save or lend grain, while others (Tibeto-Burmese) consume all the grain and meat that come through their door.

In brief, rural households in these densely populated areas of western Nepal experience recurrent food shortages, but not a true "hungry season", in contrast to regions of West Africa (Sahn 1989). These Nepali households eat as much food as they can buy, and will buy food even if this means going into debt. Their true problem is not a shortage of grain, but a lack of solvency. This emphasizes the importance of external revenue and the credit and labor relationships between households. Villagers survive by adopting a whole range of strategies to assure them of income and food in times of difficulty. The particular strategy employed is closely related to a household's caste and socioeconomic status, and further reinforces its standing in the community (see Figure 14.1).

Figure 14.1 Status and Food Procurement

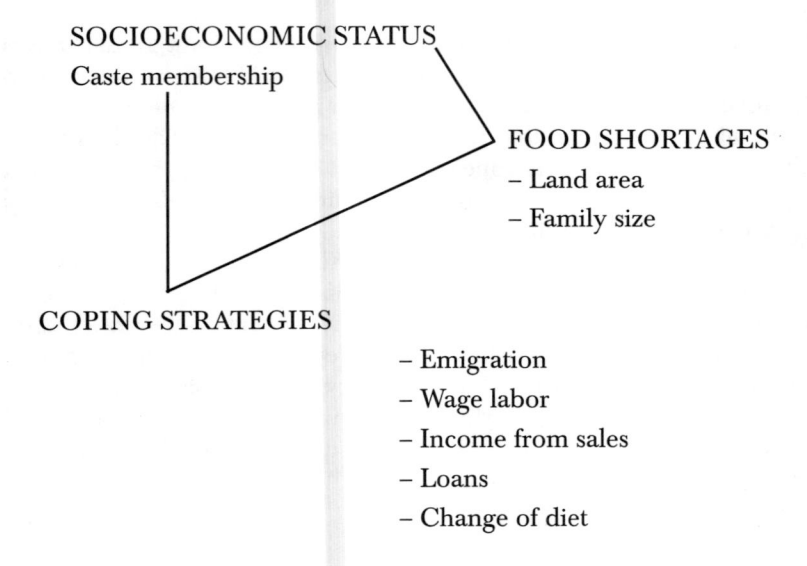

SOCIOECONOMIC STATUS
Caste membership

FOOD SHORTAGES
– Land area
– Family size

COPING STRATEGIES
– Emigration
– Wage labor
– Income from sales
– Loans
– Change of diet

Status and Intrahousehold Food Distribution

Food is rarely equally distributed within households: males are often favored over females (Chen et al. 1981, Basu et al. 1986, Harriss

1990), elders over adolescents or children (Dettwyler 1991), economically active members over housewives (Wheeler 1988), first-born over last-born children (Pelto 1991), stronger over weak or vulnerable children (Scheper-Hughes 1991), or those undergoing rites of passage to conform to ideal body type (Pagezy 1991, De Garine and Koppert 1991). In the words of Van Esterik (1985), "a bias in the distribution of food reflects the order and precedence and social value of the food consumers."

One anthropological study has recently emphasized *how* status preference is actually shown, rather than *who* receives preferential treatment. Gittelsohn (1991) undertook the direct observation of meals in 105 households of six villages in rural Nepal, recording the items and quantities of food consumed and the behaviour of participants at meal times. He developed a framework to examine meal behaviour explicitly, isolating six mechanisms of food allocation (see Figure 14.2): serving order, showing the priority given to each household member; serving method, such as automatic helpings, self-service, or specific requests; second helpings, which are especially relevant where food is scarce; serving refusals, since food requests (e.g. by children) may be ignored or denied; substitution quality, that is, serving less-desirable foods instead of high-status foods (rice); channeling quality, that is, whether high-quality foods (*ghee*) are served to high-status individuals (heads of household, guests); and food quantity, evaluated against recommended allowances for a given body weight.

Figure 14.2 Household Status and Food Distribution

FRAMEWORK	METHOD	RESULTS
Mechanisms of preferential food allocation	– Direct observation of meals	Data consists of scores for given age/sex groups
– serving order	– records of food items, quantity, and serving behavior	
– serving method		
– second helpings		
– serving refusals		
– substitution quality		
– chaneling quality		
– food quantity		

This framework provides valuable information on the social context of food distribution, which is necessary for explaining age and sex differences in food intake or nutritional status. Thus, Nepali children of both sexes are shown to receive top priority in serving order and food intake, contrary to the common assumption that working adults are always given priority. Yet their intakes are insufficient because they rarely receive second helpings. Adult women fare relatively worse than men, but they collude in this bias since they are responsible for food serving. Daughters-in-law, who have very low status in many Hindu (Indo-Aryan) households, are served last of all, eating low-status foods, proportionately less, and rarely asking for second helpings.

Status and nutritional well-being

The third proposition to examine is the impact of status on nutritional well-being. A documentation of how children are fed, for example, must amount to more than a mere record of actual food intakes. It must focus on the social, demographic, and ecological context of a household's food-related behaviors. Thus, Engle and Nieves (1993) have contrasted the rules of "need versus contribution," which determine different patterns of food allocation according to children's requirements for growth and development or perceived and future economic contribution. These represent two very different parental views in the West and in the Third World (Cassidy 1987).

In-depth anthropological fieldwork of household behaviors in a village of northwestern Nepal provides a case study to illustrate the relationship between status and child nutrition as mediated by women's lifestyle and child-care patterns. The village community is, by contrast to those in densely populated areas decribed above, isolated and self-sufficient in home-grown foods. There are two castes, Tamang agro-pastoralists of Tibeto-Burmese origin and low-caste blacksmith Kami of Indo-Aryan descent. The workloads of agro-pastoralist Tamang women double from the winter to the monsoon, even for those who are pregnant and lactating (Panter-Brick 1992). In contrast, the workloads of blacksmith Kami women are lower, affording more time for child care within the home.

Nursing patterns are related to the nature of women's work and the portability of children (Panter-Brick 1991). Tamang women invariably carry young infants to the fields, but increasingly leave older and heavier children behind. Kami women have fewer constraints on their time: they may nurse more extensively or prepare more supplementary foods. Thus Tamang children nurse less frequently as they get older, since they are increasingly separated from mothers who work away from home. Kami children nurse at irregular intervals irrespective of age, since their mothers offer supplementary foods.

Families eat two main meals and two snacks during the day. Mothers endeavor to cook special meals for young children, to allocate meat and milk generously, and to share snacks at the workplace with children who accompany them (Panter-Brick 1993). However, children mostly share the adult fare, which consists of a cereal gruel with a vegetable or plain chili sauce. Overall, children average very low intakes: 38 kcal a day, 328 kcal a day, 595 kcal a day, and 716 kcal a day in the first four years of life, eating only a limited amount due to the bulky cellulose content of the diet and the low frequency of meals. For this reason, children experience slow growth, especially three-to-six-year-olds who are the most vulnerable age groups in terms of height and weight for age (Koppert 1988).

The relationship between caste status and children's food intake is not what one might have expected. Low-caste Kami children average higher energy intakes and more animal protein per body weight than their Tamang counterparts (Panter-Brick 1993, Koppert 1988). Paradoxically, higher socioeconomic status does not necessarily entail better nutrition: Tamang women, who own more land and animals than the Kami blacksmiths, must work harder and longer hours outside the home. While they manage to nurse infants at the workplace, they have little time to prepare food for older children who remain at home. Thus, lifestyle constrains child-care patterns, which, in turn, have consequences for growth, morbidity, and nutritional well-being (see Figure 14.3). The particular regimen of prolonged nursing and supplementary feeding in combination with high workloads may also have an impact on women's resumption of ovulation after childbirth. Interestingly, Tamang mothers who spend a substantial time working away from home and rely more exclusively on lactation to feed their children experience long birth intervals, while the house-bound Kami who feed their children a mixed diet average higher fertility (Panter-Brick 1992).

Conclusions

This chapter has examined the relationship between household status and food as expressed in three ways. First, it illustrated the tight relationship between interhousehold status and the quest for food, identifying the strategies employed by households of different social and economic backgrounds to overcome shortages of food. Second, it discussed the processes whereby perceived social status is linked to intrahousehold food allocation. Third, it related caste status and subsistence lifestyle to mother-child relationships, feeding patterns and

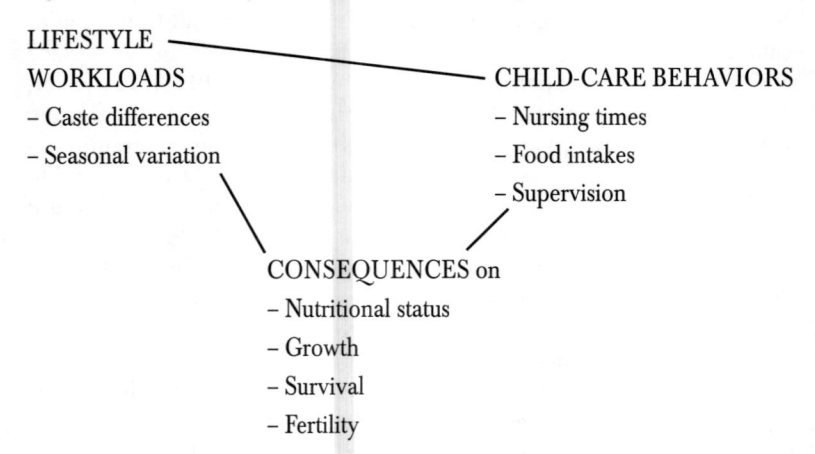

Figure 14.3 Status, Lifestyle and Nutritional Well-Being

LIFESTYLE
WORKLOADS
- Caste differences
- Seasonal variation

CHILD-CARE BEHAVIORS
- Nursing times
- Food intakes
- Supervision

CONSEQUENCES on
- Nutritional status
- Growth
- Survival
- Fertility

nutritional health. Thus, an anthropological focus on household status and food-related behaviors provides the context in which to establish the significance of these relationships. One might conclude with the tongue-in-cheek injunction attributed to Oscar Wilde: "Children, choose your parents carefully!"

References

Basu, A., S.K. Roy, B. Mukhopadhyay, P. Bharati, R. Guptua, and P.P. Majumder. 1986. Sex bias in interhousehold food distribution: roles of ethnicity and socioeconomic characteristics. *Current Anthropology* 27, no. 5: 536-39.
Cassels, C., A. Wijga, M. Pant, and D. Nabarro. 1987. Coping strategies of East Nepal farmers: can development initiatives help? Report of the impact of the Kosi Hill Area Rural Development Programme. Khardep, Kathmandu.
Cassidy, C.M. 1987. World-vew conflict and toddler malnutrition: change-agent dilemnas. In *Child Survival,* ed. by N. Scheper-Hughes, 293-324. Reidel: Dodretcht.
Chen, L.C., E. Huq, and S. D'Souza. 1981. Sex bias in the family allocation of food and health care in rural Bangladesh. *Population and Development Review* 7: 55-70.
De Garine, I. and G.J.A. Koppert. 1991. Guru-fattening sessions among the Massa. *Ecology of Food & Nutrition* 25: 1-28.

Dettwyler, K.A. 1991. Growth status of children in rural Mali: implications for nutrition education programs. *Ecology of Food & Nutrition* 3: 447-62.

Dumont, L. 1966. *Homo Hierarchicus: Le Systeme des Castes et ses Implications.* Paris: Editions Gallimard.

Engle, P.L. and I. Nieves. 1993. Intra-household food distribution among Guatemalan families in a supplementary feeding program: behavior patterns. *Soc. Sci. Med.*,36, no. 12: 1605-12.

Gittelsohn, J. 1991. Opening the box: intrahousehold food allocation in rural Nepal. *Soc. Sci. Med.* 33, no.10: 1141-54.

Ferro-Luzzi, G.E. 1975. Food avoidances of Indian tribes. *Anthropos,* 70: 385-427.

Harriss, B. 1990. Food distribution, death and disease in South Asia. In *Diet and Disease,* ed. G.A. Harrison and J.C. Waterlow,137-54, Cambridge Univer. Press, Cambridge.

Khare, R.S. and M.S.A. Rao.1986. *Food, Society and Culture: Aspects in South Asia Food Systems.* Carolina Academic Press.

Koppert, G.J.A. 1988. Alimentation et culture chez les Tamang, les Ghale et les Kami du Népal. Thèse, Faculté de Droit et de Science Politique, Aix-Marseille.

Marriott, McKim. 1968. Caste ranking and food transactions: a matrix analysis. In *Structure and Change in Indian Society,* ed. M. Singer and B. Cohen. New York: Aldine.

Panter-Brick, C. 1989. Motherhood and subsistence work – the Tamang of rural Nepal. *Human Ecology* 17, no. 2: 205-28.

Panter-Brick, C. 1991. Lactation, birth spacing and maternal work-loads among two castes in rural Nepal. *J. Biosoc. Sci.* 23: 137-54.

Panter-Brick, C. 1992. Women's working behaviour and maternal child health in rural Nepal. In *Physical Activity and Health,* ed. N. Norgan 190-206. Cambridge: Cambridge Univer. Press.

Panter-Brick, C. 1993. Mother-child food allocation and levels of subsistence activity in rural Nepal. *Ecology of Food and Nutrition* 29; 319-33.

Panter-Brick, C. and M. Eggerman (forthcoming). La soudure et ses solutions dans le Népal des collines. In *Fonctionnement des systèmes villageois dans les collines népalaises à Gulmi et Arghakhanchi,* ed. G. Toffin and P. Ramirez. Paris: C.N.R.S.

Pagezy, H. 1991. Fatness and culture among the southern Mongo (Zaire): the case of the primiparous nursing woman. *African Studies Monographs* 12: 149-60.

Pelto, G.H. et al. 1991. Household size, food intake and anthropometric status of school-age children in a Highland Mexican area. *Soc. Sci. Med.* 33 no.10: 1135-40.

Sahn, D.E 1989. Seasonal Variability in Third World Agriculture: the Consequences for Food Security. Baltimore: The Johns Hopkins Press.

Scheper-Hughes, N. 1991. Social indifference to child death. *The Lancet* 337: 1144-47.

Van Esterik, P. 1984. Intrafamily food distribution: its relevance for maternal and child nutrition. Cornell Nutritional Surveillance Program. Working Paper Series no. 31. Cornell University, Ithaca, N.Y.

Vayda, A.P. 1987. Explaining what people eat: a review article. *Human Ecology* 15, no. 1: 511.

Wheeler, E.F. 1988. Intra-household food allocation: a review of evidence. *Occasional Paper* no.12, London: London School of Hygiene and Tropical Medicine.

15. NUTRITIONAL SECURITY AND THE STATUS QUEST IN DEVELOPING COUNTRIES

Rainer Gross & Günter Dresrüsse

Der Mensch ist was er ißt (Ludwig Feuerbach)
(Man is what he eats)

Indisputably, humans eat for variety of reasons, and not solely to satisfy their nutrient requirements. Many other factors influence food intake, and one of them is the quest for personal or group status. This occurs in developed countries, where the main problem is overnutrition, as well as in developing countries, where many people suffer from malnutrition.

For the majority of the world's population, nutritional security is not granted. Nutritional security shall be understood in terms of ensuring that all people at all times have an adequate nutritional status to safeguard a physically and emotionally healthy life. This is analogous to the definition of food security of the Food and Agriculture Organization (FAO 1983). This chapter deals with the following questions: (1) What is the relationship between nutritional status, food intake, nutritional practices, and social status? (2) Which food and nutrition interventions are most effective in developing countries considering the role food plays in the status of an individual?

Factors Influencing the Consumption of Food

Nutritional problems have many roots. Figure 15.1 lists some of the problems that can cause poor nutrition in developing countries, due to inadequate nutrient intake and a high load of infectious and parasitic diseases. Inadequate intake of nutrients can be caused by a scarcity of available food at the household level, while a high prevalence of disease can be due to unfavorable environmental conditions and deficient health care. However, an ample supply of adequate food, effective health services, and good environmental conditions are insufficient to combat nutritional problems as long as foodstuffs are not used effectively. Therefore, all of these three factors must be taken into account in order to improve nutrition in a given culture or ethnic group.

Figure 15.1 Casual Model of Malnutrition

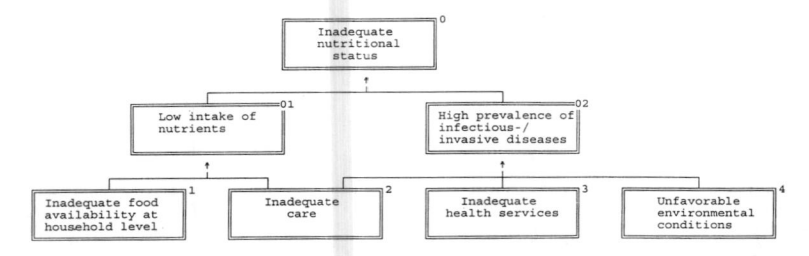

```
                          ┌─────────────┐ 0
                          │ Inadequate  │
                          │ nutritional │
                          │   status    │
                          └─────────────┘
                   ┌────────────┴────────────┐
          ┌────────┴────────┐ 01      02 ┌─────┴─────────────┐
          │ Low intake of   │            │ High prevalence of│
          │   nutrients     │            │ infectious-/      │
          │                 │            │ invasive diseases │
          └─────────────────┘            └───────────────────┘
     ┌─────────┴──────┐                 ┌────────┴───────────┐
┌────┴──────┐ 1  ┌────┴──────┐ 2  ┌─────┴─────┐ 3  ┌─────────┴──┐ 4
│Inadequate │    │Inadequate │    │Inadequate │    │Unfavorable │
│food       │    │   care    │    │  health   │    │environmental│
│availability│   │           │    │ services  │    │ conditions │
│at household│   │           │    │           │    │            │
│   level    │   │           │    │           │    │            │
└───────────┘    └───────────┘    └───────────┘    └────────────┘
```

If food is available at the macroeconomic level it is vital to ensure that it is also obtainable at the household level. Furthermore, it must trickle down and be accessible to each individual. Steering this distribution process requires several steps, from food production or purchase to food intake. As shown in Figure 15.2 food-related behavior can be broken down into food purchasing, food storage, food preparation, food distribution, and food consumption.

Food has physical and chemical properties that give the consumer a basis to characterize and value particular foodstuffs and dishes.

In addition to access to resources, including the money and time to purchase, store, prepare, and distribute food, food-related behavior is influenced by four consumer-related factors that are more or less interdependent (see Figure 15.3).

These factors are: (1) biological, i.e.,. metabolic needs, physiological constitution, and "organoleptic" or sensory acceptability related to age, gender, health status, and physical activity; (2) cognitive, i.e., formal and informal education, status of nutritional information, etc.; (3) emotional; (4) social.

With regard to the biological properties of food, the four sensory factors, taste, smell, color, and texture play an important role, influencing what we call "organoleptic acceptability". Even newborns are able to distinguish a variety of tastes. Steiner (1974) tested for the

Figure 15.2 Food Behavior Cascade

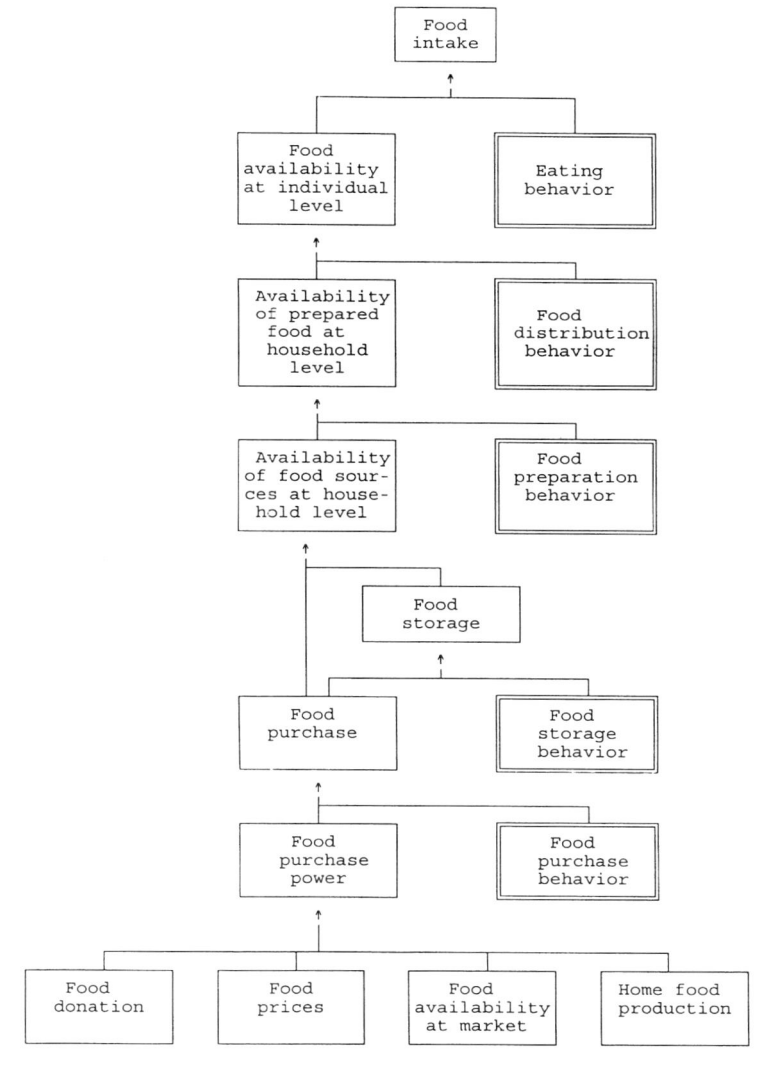

```
                        ┌──────────┐
                        │   Food   │
                        │  intake  │
                        └──────────┘
                             ↑
              ┌──────────────┴──────────────┐
     ┌─────────────────┐           ┌─────────────────┐
     │      Food       │           │                 │
     │  availability   │           │     Eating      │
     │  at individual  │           │    behavior     │
     │      level      │           │                 │
     └─────────────────┘           └─────────────────┘
              ↑
     ┌────────┴────────┐           ┌─────────────────┐
     │  Availability   │           │                 │
     │   of prepared   │           │      Food       │
     │     food at     │           │  distribution   │
     │    household    │           │    behavior     │
     │      level      │           │                 │
     └─────────────────┘           └─────────────────┘
              ↑
     ┌────────┴────────┐           ┌─────────────────┐
     │  Availability   │           │                 │
     │  of food sour-  │           │      Food       │
     │ ces at house-   │           │   preparation   │
     │   hold level    │           │    behavior     │
     └─────────────────┘           └─────────────────┘
              ↑
                        ┌──────────┐
                        │   Food   │
                        │  storage │
                        └──────────┘
                             ↑
              ┌──────────────┴──────────────┐
     ┌─────────────────┐           ┌─────────────────┐
     │      Food       │           │      Food       │
     │    purchase     │           │    storage      │
     │                 │           │    behavior     │
     └─────────────────┘           └─────────────────┘
              ↑
     ┌────────┴────────┐           ┌─────────────────┐
     │      Food       │           │      Food       │
     │    purchase     │           │    purchase     │
     │      power      │           │    behavior     │
     └─────────────────┘           └─────────────────┘
              ↑
   ┌──────────┬──────────┴─────────┬──────────┐
┌────────┐ ┌────────┐  ┌────────────────┐ ┌────────────┐
│  Food  │ │  Food  │  │      Food      │ │ Home food  │
│donation│ │ prices │  │  availability  │ │ production │
│        │ │        │  │   at market    │ │            │
└────────┘ └────────┘  └────────────────┘ └────────────┘
```

effect of sweet, sour, and salty substances before the first feeding after birth; newborns reacted by smiling and making sucking movements or by making signs of disgust and rejection. By the age of about four years, children have developed a stable association between taste and color, for instance, from this age on they expect chocolate to be brown and not green. About at the same time they have specific expectations with regard to the texture of particular foods.

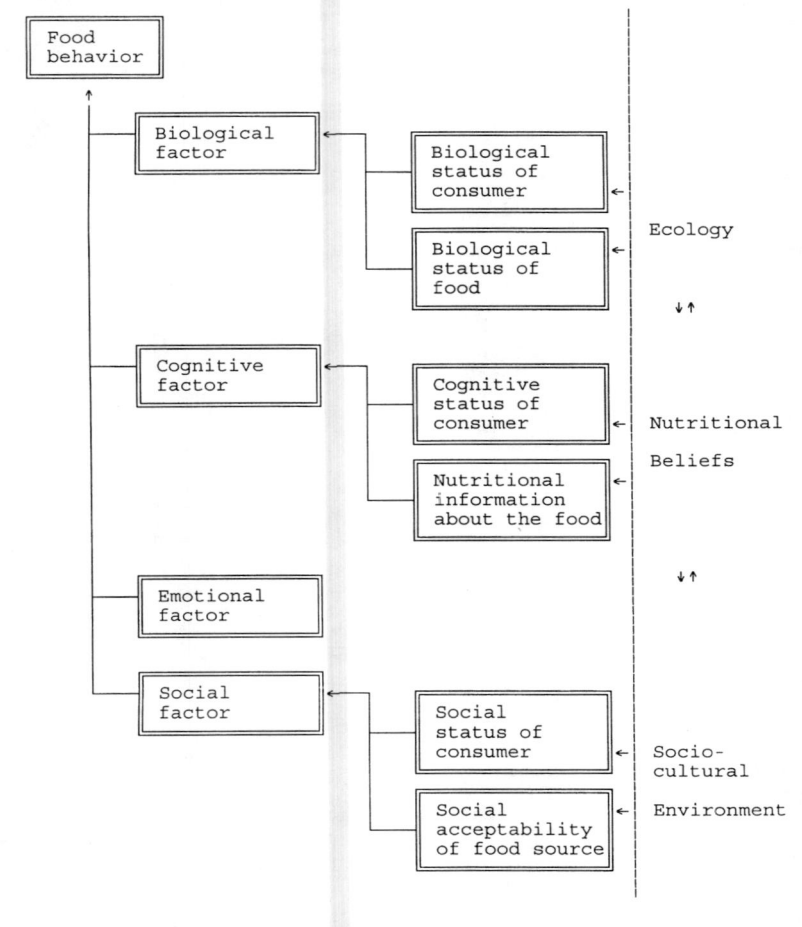

Figure 15.3 Factors Influencing Food Behavior and Practices

```
Food
behavior
  ↑
  ├── Biological ←──┬── Biological status of consumer ←┐
  │   factor        │                                   │
  │                 └── Biological status of food    ←──┤  Ecology
  │                                                     │
  │                                                     ↓↑
  ├── Cognitive  ←──┬── Cognitive status of consumer ←──┤
  │   factor        │                                   │  Nutritional
  │                 └── Nutritional information      ←──┤  Beliefs
  │                     about the food                  │
  │                                                     ↓↑
  ├── Emotional
  │   factor
  │
  └── Social     ←──┬── Social status of consumer   ←───┤  Socio-
      factor        │                                   │  cultural
                    └── Social acceptability        ←───┤  Environment
                        of food source                  │
```

More complex is the identification of biological food behaviors related to the nutrient requirements of individuals, because it is difficult to distinguish the various levels of consciousness in cognitive food behavior. Many animals not only rely on biologically programmed behaviors for finding appropriate food, but, through learning, they find about the edibility of some foodstuffs and dangers of others. In humans, cognitive processes in choosing food are much more developed, resulting in the extraordinarily wide spectrum of human foods and sophisticated techniques used to detoxify or to make palatable foodstuffs that could otherwise not be used. In Peru, for example, the majority of traditional staple foods come from plants. The lack of certain amino acids in plant protein is overcome by combining different foods in the diet. However, most of the plant food sources lack B vitamins, specifically vitamin B-12. The use of *chicha*, a fermented alcoholic maize drink, prevents vitamin B deficiencies. Iodine deficiencies, which are very common in mountainous regions all over the world, are prevented in traditional Peruvian nutrition by the incorporation of *chocallullu*, which are macro algae brought to the Andean region from the coast.

Age, gender, health status, and physiological activity must be taken into account, because at various life stages or in different physiological situations specific nutrients are required. In all cultures infants have a very different diet than adults, and in many societies pregnant and/or breastfeeding women consume different foods than nonpregnant or nonlactating women. Furthermore, individuals who are ill may receive a special diet, often according to the perceived needs of their disease.

The physical constitution may furthermore dictate food-related behavior independent of the required nutrients. For example, small children or elderly persons may lack teeth, necessitating different eating patterns than those of persons with a functioning set of teeth. Individuals who run a high fever often suffer from anorexia, although the body would need more energy at this time. However, the biocybernetical mechanisms influencing human food-related behavior are not fully understood at the present time. It is likely that the perception of processes in one's body and specific behavior patterns have been shaped in the course of our evolutionary history. More often than not, they are likely to have adaptive functions.

Food habits not only depend on the biological constitution of the individual but also on the biological status of food, its physical and chemical properties. Lupines *(Fabaceae),* which grow under poor soil conditions, have seeds with high protein content, but bitter and toxic chinolicidin alkaloids prevent the consumption of this grain without prior modification. To overcome this obstacle, human inhabitants of the Old and the New World apparently discovered independently that Lupine alkaloids can be washed out by soaking the seed for several days in water. Many other such interesting techniques are found throughout the world.

In addition to biological need and nutritional awareness, food-related behavior is influenced by the emotional state of individuals, and these behaviors strengthen networks within and among the social groups, as demonstrated by many chapters in this volume. For instance, guests are offered snacks or beverages, and official meetings are opened or closed with meals to confirm relationships. The social status of food is often determined by the upper echelon when such stratification exists.

The Status of Food and Individuals

As seen in Figure 15.3, the social status of individuals is an important factor in the formation of respective food behaviors, and it is interconnected with ecological, environmental, and cultural parameters. To improve one's own ranking in a given society, for instance by food sharing, one has to make sure that the right food has been selected, properly prepared, and served. Therefore, the contribution of food to the status quest can not be discussed without considering the status of food itself. The status of food is influenced by four factors.

The Eco-Religious Factor

The agricultural food production of early societies depended upon local ecological conditions and usually served the physiological needs of the individuals in the various populations. The corresponding food-related behaviors were encoded and maintained by socioreligious traditions.

In ancient Peru, for example, more than 90 percent of energy and protein sources for the highland population was derived from plant foods (Gross and von Baer 1976). The Andean region is characterized by extremely harsh topographic conditions: wide variations of altitude are present within short overland distances and suitable areas for agricultural production are scarce. Therefore extensive animal production, through which plant carbohydrates are converted to animal protein, with a high loss of energy and protein, was not possible within the limits of the food chain. Furthermore, the difficulties presented by the rugged topography hindered widespread trade of food. To counteract these constraints as well as population pressure, the highlanders developed an extraordinary system of food production largely based on plants. Little is known about the social status of certain foods or how they were used in the status quest of pre-Columbian society.

Among Indo-European populations, on the other hand, animal food sources played an important role. The large, fertile plains of their regions allowed extensive animal food production, and plants could be converted easily to animal protein. In these areas, too, an increase of population occurred, giving rise to many waves of migrations throughout the millennia. The high prestige of animal protein in present-day Western societies still reflects the food behavior of the Indo-European cultures, although physiologically there is no justification for the value attached to meat. In the Indo-European cultures of the Old World, cattle, often the bull or a corresponding symbolic representation, were integrated into religious beliefs and practices, while in the New World maize was at the center of religious life.

For millenniums, Bali farmers have produced specific rice varieties that are not used for human consumption, but only for ceremonial activities. All governmental efforts to entice people to use these non-food production areas for growing new high-yield varieties have failed. As a result, Bali still is the home of a rich gene pool of traditional rice varieties that otherwise would have been lost. Co-evolutionary processes intertwining ecology and tradition, particularly religious tradition, can be found in various other societies as well.

The Colonial Factor

When one society invaded and colonized another, it often introduced or imposed production systems and food-related behavior that did not necessarily suit the ecological conditions of the conquered area nor the nutritional and social traditions of the local inhabitants. For example, the food practices of Indo-European populations have influenced food policy and food supply until the present day. Legumes, which played an important role as protein source in ancient Europe, were replaced by animal protein and relegated the socially determined stigma of "poor people's food". The history of the lupine provides an interesting case. First, Indo-European invaders essentially obliterated the production and consumption of the lupine in European areas (Gross 1987), but later nonIndo-European Arabs reintroduced it into Europe, interestingly, under its old Greek name. However, with the fall of the Arabic empire in the Iberian peninsula, the production and consumption of lupines declined once again. The descendants of Indo-European invaders, mostly coming from the Iberian peninsula after the Conquest, discouraged the production and consumption of lupines in the Andean region to the extent that only traditional communities still produce and consume their grains today.

The Urban Factor

Since urban societies purchase their food with money, they are less dependent on ecology and on internal food production. The development of natural sciences since the Renaissance as well as increasing trade made purchased food less dependent upon local ecological conditions. It is interesting to note this is also the period in which the urban elites became more and more secularized. It seems possible that the detachment of food productions from local ecology and religious traditions was one factor in this development.

Several studies have demonstrated that the duration of breastfeeding is related to the desire of the mother to achieve high social status. After World War II, with its severe food shortages, more educated mothers living in good socioeconomic conditions breast-fed their children for increasingly shorter periods of time. This trend can also be observed in many developing countries that are now undergoing the process of urbanization (Schürch and Favre 1985). However, in the past ten or twenty years elite urban mothers from developed countries have started to breast-feed their children for longer periods of time, thereby reversing the pattern of breast-feeding. Existing reports show that the same process of women preferring to nurse their babies for longer periods is now occurring in urban areas of developing countries (Gross et al. 1987; Monteiro et al. 1987). Once again this trend started with mothers from high-income groups, as shown in the case of Sao Paulo (Monteiro et al. 1988) of Kuala Lumpur (Khor 1992).

The International Factor

Whereas the colonizing powers often introduced new foodstuffs and food habits into invaded cultures through dominance and administrative control, international society is now experiencing an almost cosmopolitan process of acculturation by which international companies, local business people, and other local elites are successfully marketing new foods using worldwide advertisement. Such advertisements play on status images, often ones of being modern, affluent, "with the times". Fast-food chains and certain beverages, usually originating in the United States, can now be found on all five continents. Apart from that, there is a general trend in the food industry to separate the food components from their biologically given compound by recombining these components into a new market-tailored product. These "designer foods" and certain stereotypic lifestyles connected to them by effective public relations and advertising machineries have changed food habits in many parts of the world.

The list of factors that influence food behavior as summed up in Figure 15.3 may not be complete. However, it is important to note that several other factors in addition to the social aspects of food which determine food behavior. Figures 15.1 and 15.2 show that the quest for social status is only one of many elements that influence food intake and the nutritional status of the individual. However, there is no doubt that the status quest has to be taken into consideration if measures for improvement of nutrition are to be planned and implemented.

Food-related behavior plays an important role in maintaining and establishing a healthy life. It is influenced by and, in turn, influences food production systems; energy expenditure; expenditure of natural resources; climatic conditions; macroeconomic conditions, international trade and national debts; human rights and social security. The consumption of particular foods to improve or maintain the social status of the consumers may have significant side effects that, in turn, influence important areas of life, conditions that again affect the nutritional situation.

Food and Nutrition Intervention Related to the Social Status of Food

The many possible causes of nutritional problems create a wide range of possible interventions. The following is an overview over the most commonly found programs.

Through feeding programs, food is delivered to population groups living in specific circumstances that are unable to produce or acquire enough food for a healthy life. By contrast, food aid assists people of all age groups suffering from natural or man-made catastrophies that make it impossible to purchase food. School feeding programs are implemented in low-income communities to improve school attendance and performance of children. Soup kitchen programs and public dining room programs (*comedores publicos*) are set up mainly in Latin America to improve the food supply of the urban poor. Food-for-work can be an important tool for communities that lack basic infrastructures such as terraces or irrigation canals to make land arable or wells useable. Food-for-learning compensates for time spent learning. This program is specifically geared toward helping women who lack formal or informal education, and who have to drop activities in the household to participate in educational programs.

Food supplementation programs mainly target preschool children and pregnant or lactating women. The major objective of these health programs is to prevent stunted growth and ensure adequate lactation. Nutrient supplementation programs usually deliver vitamin A pills and iron supplements to pregnant women and young children. In nontargeted food supplementation programs, vitamin A, iron, and iodine are mixed with food components such as salt, sugar, glutamine, and vegetable oil. Many governments use price policy to improve access to basic foods for poor sectors of the population through price control and food subsidies. Food subsidies can be targeted to the consumers through the use of food stamps, vouchers, coupons, etc.

Through nutrition education programs people receive information about the nutritional value of food and its proper use, as well as knowledge about what their own contribution toward good health should be. Social marketing uses commercial advertisement strategies to convince consumers to eat nutritious food. As in commercial advertising, the status of particular foods is elevated to make it seem more desirable to purchase and consume them. The programs of governmental and nongovernmental organizations are not the only agents spreading information about food. Commercial advertisement also influences food behavior and practices. Advertising may work against sound nutrition by promoting foods that have low nutritional value and by providing misleading information, particularly when it suggests that one food is better than another (Musgaier 1983).

The social status of individuals or groups may help to positively influence food behavior and the success of nutritional intervention programs. A project in Peru assisted by the German Agency of Technical Cooperation (GTZ) provided an interesting example. The objective was to increase consumption of indigenous food. In the beginning of the 1970s the prestige of local food sources was low and was associated with uneducated, poor Indians of the highlands. By producing new foods and connecting these products with high-ranking people, the image of pre-Columbian food sources was elevated. Today in Peru, indigenous food sources are very popular, and there is not a single day when local foods are not mentioned in the mass media.

The following aspects should be considered in food programs with a special emphasis on the status of the consumer and the status of food:

1. According to the United Nations declaration "Food as a Human Right", food is accepted as one of the most essential basic needs to secure a healthy life (United Nations 1989). Furthermore, it is the right of human beings to be supplied with food adequate in quantity, quality, safety, social function, and cultural acceptance.
2. Food with a high social and cultural acceptance may be of low physiological value, not meeting the needs of the malnourished segment of the population; of external and nonlocal or national production which may in turn, alter the international trade balance; based on food production systems that require a great amount of energy and natural resources or create environmental hazards.
3. Food intervention programs have as their objective to reestablish or maintain adequate consumption of food for communities, so that they are able to supply themselves with nutritious food. Such programs, however, can run the risk of making individuals and communities dependent upon certain foods to a greater extent than before the food intervention program began.
4. Up to now, study of the social function of food as a means of communication and expression of social status has been widely

neglected. Given the important social aspect of food, humans must have the right to acquire food sufficient in quantity and quality to satisfy the physiological needs as well as the social ones.
5. Food intervention programs must not burden the beneficiaries with a social stigma. Therefore, before the food is delivered, the prestige of potential food sources should be assessed; no food should be distributed that is determined to be low in a social context. This also applies to food price subsidies and food stamp programs.
6. Food for work programs should be implemented locally only to stimulate local food production; improve the social relationships and development within households and communities; increase the economic purchasing power of the rural food producer; promote and support local food-related behavior that does not violate the ecological conditions, but helps to safeguard the environment.

As recommended by ACC/SCN (1988), food commodities placed at the disposal of the German government are sold by GTZ-assisted projects in urban areas to generate cash that, in turn, is used to purchase local food items from local production.

Research Questions on the Improvement of Nutritional Status

The following questions which require further research, pertain primarily to developing societies and fall into three categories: (1) possible informational deficits, (2) methodology for research and planning, and (3) implications of food and nutrition intervention programs. Some questions for future research are:

1. What is the causal relationship between the nutritional status of people and the status of different foods within the society?
2. How can the social status of individuals influence food-related behavior, and how does food-related behavior influence the social status of the consumer?
3. Which environmental and cultural conditions exert important influences upon choice of food and perception of that food's value?
4. Which simple indicators measure the social function of food and could be used in research, program planning, and monitoring?
5. Which qualitative methods can be used in research on the social functions of food, particularly those related to the quest for status?

6. How can social status be used to increase the consumption of adequate food?
7. The effect of exposure to advertisement on food choices has not been studied beyond the topic of infant formula (Atkinson 1991). What is the role of commercial advertisements in creating social pressure to consume certain products or to prefer one food over another?

Summary

The quest for status and the use of food to accomplish this objective plays an important role within the domain of food-related behavior. It appears that in all societies individuals and groups use food production, food distribution, and food consumption as important means to achieve high status. Furthermore, as has been shown above, certain foods can acquire associated social values that often are derived from the preferences and values of the elite. The high status attributed to colonial powers that successfully conquered other regions has, in the history of humankind, created various problems because the foods introduced by force or by persuasion were not compatible with the pre-existing ecological or social conditions. For efficient planning and implementation of food intervention programs in developing societies, it is necessary to gain more information about the role of food in the quest for status.

References

ACC/SCN. (United Nations Administrative Committee on Coordination/Subcommittee on Nutrition). 1988. *Nutrition in Times of Disaster*. Geneva.

Atkinson, S.J. 1991. Nutrition in urban programmes and planning. Urban Health Programme, Health Policy Unit, London School of Hygiene and Tropical Medicine.

Food and Agriculture Organization (FAO). 1983. Director-general's report on world food security: a reappraisal of the concepts and approaches. Rome: Committee on World Food Security.

Gross, R. 1987. First Reinhold von Sengbusch memorial lecture: lupines in the old and new world - a biological-cultural coevolution. Proceedings of the 4th International Lupin Conference, 244-77, Geraldton.

Gross, R. and E. von Baer. 1976. Eiweißproduktion, aber wie? *Umschau aus Wissenschaft und Forschung,* 76: 305-08.

Gross, R., M. Stange, N.W. Solomons, U. Oltersdorf and I. Rios Esquivel. 1987. The influence of economic deterioration in Brazil on the nutritional status of children in Rio de Janeiro, Brazil. *Ecol. Food Nutr.* 19: 265-79.

Khor, G.L. 1992. The nutritional situation in metropolotan Kuala Lumpur, with focus on squatters. Proceedings of the Asian Workshop on Nutrition in the Metropolitan Area. *Southeast Asian Journal of Tropical Medicine and Public Health* 23.

Monteiro, C.A., H.P.P. Ziga, M.H.D´A Benicio, M.F. Rea, E.S. Tudisco, and D.M. Sigulem. 1987. The recent revival of breast-feeding in the city of Sao Paulo, Brazil. *Am.J.Public Health* 77:964-66.

Monteiro, C.A., H.P.P. Ziga, M.H.D´A Benicio, and M.F. Rea. 1988. Breast-feeding patterns and socio-economic status in the city of Sao Paulo. *J.Trop. Pediat.* 34: 186-92.

Musaiger, A.O. 1983. The impact of television food advertisements on dietary behavior of Bahraini housewives. *Ecol. Food Nutr.* 13: 109-14.

Schürch, B. and A.-M. Favre. 1985. *Urbanization and nutrition in the third world.* Nestlé Foundation, Lausanne, Switzerland.

Steiner, J. 1974. Innate discriminative human facial expressions to taste and smell stimulation. *Annals of the New York Academy of Science* 237: 229-33.

United Nations. 1989. *Right to adequate food as a human right.* Geneva, New York: Centre for Human Rights.

NOTES ON CONTRIBUTORS

Ingrid Nina Bell-Krannhals Ph.D. studied anthropology and linguistics at the University of Basel in Switzerland. She has conducted fieldwork with the Lummi Indians, State of Washington, in 1980, resulting in M.A. thesis on traditional and modern fishing technology. As of 1982, she has been doing fieldwork in the Trobriand Islands, Papua New Guinea, resulting in a Ph.D. thesis on property and possession. Between 1982-1987 she worked at the Research Group for Human Ethology in the Max-Planck-Society. Since 1987 she has been a lecturer at the Institute of Anthropology at the University of Basel, Switzerland.

Peter Damerow studied mathematics and philosophy at the Free University of Berlin. He now works as a senior scientist for the Max Planck Institute for Human Development and Education in Berlin conducting research on culture and cognition with a focus on the history of number concepts.

Michael Dietler is Associate Professor of Anthropology at the University of Chicago. His graduate education was at the University of California, Berkeley (PhD. 1990). His primary archaeological research focus is the colonial encounter in Iron Age southern France, particularly the role of consumption in the political economy. He has also conducted ethnoarchaeological research on material culture and economic history in western Kenya and is engaged in a study of the manipulation of Celtic identity in modern Europe.

Günter Dresrüsse is currently a Director at the FAO Agricultural Services Division in Rome. He has an academic background in tropical agriculture and social, agricultural and political economics. Before joining FAO, he spent fourteen years working for the GTZ,

Deutsche Gesellschaft für Technische Zusammenarbeit, in both Germany and Benin. He built up and headed the Food Security Division in the GTZ, developing and implementing household food security, food reserve and food aid programs.

Irenäus Eibl-Eibesfeldt, Ph.D. is Prof. of Zoology at the University of Munich. From 1951-1970 he was a research associate of Konrad Lorenz. Since 1970 he has been Director of the Research Institute for Human Ethology in the Max-Planck-Society and has conducted long-term cross-cultural research in several different cultures: San, Himba, Yanomami, Eipo and Trobriands amongst others. In 1992 he founded the Ludwig-Boltzmann-Institute for Urban Ethology in Vienna.

Barbara Fruth studied Zoology at the University of Munich. In 1988-1989 she conducted field research on the Ivory Coast in the project "Tradition in West African Chimpanzees" by Ch. & H. Boesch.

Since then she has been doing field research on ecological and social aspects of bonobos behavior at Lomako/Zaire. In 1992 she became attached to the Research Group for Human Ethology in the Max-Planck-Society, Andechs. She obtained her Doctorate from Munich University in 1995 on bonobos nest-building behavior and is now a researcher at the Max-Planck-Institut fur Verhaltensphysiologie in Seewiesen, Germany and a post-doctoral fellow at the Dept. of Zoology, Miami University, Oxford Ohio.

Igor de Garine (Ph.D. Paris Sorbonne 1962) is Director of Research in the Centre National de la Recherche Scientifique (CNRS) and leader of the team *Ecology and Anthropology of Food*. A former head of the section on food habits and nutrition of the FAO (1967-1970), he is currently chairman of the International Chairman for the Anthropology of Food (IUAES). His research interests are the economic, social and religious organization of African populations and the anthropology of food. His main long-term field work has been in Sahelian Africa (Tchad, Cameroon) among the Massa and Mussey, but he also conducted field studies in Anthropology of food in the African rain forest (CAR and Cameroon) as well as in Senegal, Pacific Islands and Nepal.

Karl Grammer received his Doctorate from the University of Munich in 1983 and his Habilitation from the University of Vienna in 1991. Between 1978 and 1991 he worked in the Research Group for Human Ethology in the Max-Planck-Society. He is currently is the scientific director of the Ludwig-Boltzmann-Institute for Urban Ethology in Vienna/Austria. His main field of research was coalitional politics in children, and his interest has now turned to the biology of sexual strategies and the urban environment.

Rainer Gross is a staff member of the Deutsche Gesellschaft für Technische Zusammenarbeit (GTZ) which implements assistance for projects of developing countries for the Ministry of Economic Cooperation of the German Government. He has an academic background in the fields of nutrition and agriculture and has worked in developing countries for many years. Currently he is the team leader and advisor for the implementation of the Regional Centre in Community Nutrition at the University of Indonesia, Jakarta.

Brian Hayden is a Full Professor in the Archaeology Department of Simon Fraser University in British Columbia, Canada. He has done extensive ethnoarchaeological research in Australia, Guatemala, and British Columbia. He has used an ecological perspective to address questions of the origins of food production, socioeconomic inequalities, and prestige technologies. The ecological analysis of feasting is his main research focus at present.

Gottfried Hohmann studied Biology at the Ludwig-Maximilians University of Munich. Following two years of experimental research on captive primates at the Max-Planck-Institute for Psychiatry, Munich, he became a research fellow at the Centre for Ecological Sciences, Indian Instutite of Science Bangalore. There he completed more than two years of fieldwork, focusing on comparative studies of primate behavior and vocal communication. After obtaining his Doctorate from the University of Munich in 1988, he joined the Research Group for Human Ethology in the Max-Planck-Society, Andechs. Since 1989 he has been collecting behavioral and ecological data on wild bonobos in Lomako, Zaire. He is currently employed as researcher at the Max-Planck-Institut für Verhaltensphysiologie, Seewiesen, Germany.

Barbara Hold-Cavell received her Doctorate from the University of Munich. Between 1971 and 1979 was attached to the Research Group for Human Ethology in the Max-Planck Society, conducting research on children's groups. In 1976 she undertook fieldwork among the !Ko-Bushmen of Botswana and in 1977 in Japan. Between 1979-1983 she was a scientific member of the Institute for Developmental Psychology at the University of Regensburg.

Pierre Lemonnier holds a Doctorat de troisième cycle (1975) from University Paris V (René Descartes). He has done fieldwork since 1978 among the Anga people of Papua New Guinea on numerous topics including war and peace-making and the anthropology of technology. He is a Director of Research at the Centre National de la Recherche Scientifique (Cemtre de Recherche et de Documentation sue l'océanie, Marseilles) and teaches at Université de Provence at Aix-en-Provence.

William C. McGrew is Professor of Anthropology and Zoology at Miami University, Oxford, Ohio. He holds a D. Phil in Psychology from the University of Oxford and a Ph.D. in Anthropology from the University of Stirling. He has spent over five years in the field studying wild chimpanzees across Africa, in Gabon, Senegal and Tanzania. His book, *Chimpanzee Material Culture: Implications for Human Evolution,* won the 1995 W.W. Howells Book Prize.

Catherine Panter-Brick received her PhD. from Oxford in Biological Anthropology (1987) and is currently a lecturer at the University of Durham. She has undertaken fieldwork in Nepal since 1982 as well as in India and Saudi Arabia in the area of maternal and child health, energy balance, nutrition and fertility. She now is involved in researching the lives and health of street children.

Wulf Schiefenhövel, M.D. studied medicine at the University of Munich and Erlangen. In 1970 he received his M.D. and in 1984 his Habilitation in medical psychology and ethnomedicine from the University of Munich, where he was subsequently appointed Professor. Since 1977 he has been a research associate of Prof. Dr. I. Eibl-Eibesfeldt at the Research Group for Human Ethology in the Max-Planck-Society, Andechs. Since 1965, he has carried out long-term field research in Papua New Guinea and Irian Jaya on a wide variety of topics including ethnomedicine, birth behavior, early infancy, non-verbal communication, chronobiology and Austronesian migrations.

Polly Wiessner received her PhD. from the University of Michigan, Ann Arbor in 1977 and is currently a research associate at the Research Group for Human Ethology in the Max-Planck-Society, Andechs. Between 1973 and 1977 she worked on reciprocity, exchange networks and style in artifacts among the !Kung San. Since 1985 she has been doing ethnohistorical work on environment, exchange networks, warfare and cults among the Enga of Papua New Guinea.

INDEX

Abelam 90, 120
Abramovitch, R. 24, 29
absence of malnutrition 240
abutu 90
ACC/SCN 272f
accumulator 103, 112, 130f
Ache 66, 82, 84, 172, 174, 176, 180, 182, 188
acquisator 130
Adams, R.M. 150, 166
adaptation 79, 83, 101, 192
Adick, W. 84
administration 160, 167, 235
administrative document 150f
Adrian, J. 214f
advertisement 96, 105, 269, 270f, 273f
Africa 12, 57, 65, 93, 120f, 123, 172, 184, 187f, 190, 193, 201, 213f, 216, 255, 260, 277, 279
aggression 2, 6, 21, 25, 28, 30, 33ff, 38, 71, 73ff, 77f, 84
aggression ritualized 37
agonistic interactions 20, 49, 55
agriculture 9, 94, 102f, 208, 228, 260, 262, 273, 276, 278
Agta 172ff, 176, 180, 182, 188
Akkadian 152, 159
Alantika range 206
alcohol/compare 'beer', 'wine' 8, 12, 15, 18, 90, 102, 112, 119, 121f, 124, 194, 203f, 206, 210, 212-215, 254, 266
Alexander, R.D. 83
Algaze, G. 150, 166
alpha position 7, 20ff, 41,ff, 45
alpha rank 45
alpine lake dwelling 103
Altman, J. 172, 179, 187
Amazonia 139
Amelsvoort, V.F.P.M. van 232

Amerindian 27, 187f, 189, 276
Ammassalik Inuit 172, 174, 176f, 180, 182
Amphlett Island 239
amphora 107ff, 113f
Andamanese 172, 174, 176, 180, 182
Anderson, J.L. 80, 83
Anga 223, 230, 279
animal protein 197, 267
Anonidium mannii 53
antagonistic drinking 209
Apfelbaum, M. 196, 216
Appadurai, A. 88f, 98, 110f, 116
Arcelin-Pradelle, C. 108, 116
archaeology 8, 17f, 87ff, 98, 101f, 105, 111, 115, 117-120, 126, 136f, 139, 140, 142, 144f, 187f, 190, 232, 276, 278
Areca catechu 242
Arensberg, C. 122
Arnold, B. 119
Asia 172
aspect of possession 36
Atkinson, S.J. 273
atole 137f
attention center of 6, 10, 19, 24-28
attention seeking 25ff
attention structure 3, 19, 21f, 24, 26, 29ff, 73ff, 83f, 188
Attic 109
attitude toward body shape 199
Atzwanger, K. 74, 76, 78f, 83f
Australia 144, 172, 188, 232, 278
Australian aborigines 148
Australian hunter-gatherer 144, 187
Austria 106, 278
Austronesian 234f, 249, 279
Avebury 123, 140
Axelrod, R. 47, 65
aye-aye 39

Ayoréode 172, 174, 176, 180, 182
Azande 97

Baal, J. van 227, 232
baboon 20, 29, 31, 39, 45, 66, 192, 215
Babylonia 149, 159
Badrian, A. 48f, 65
Badrian, N. 48f, 65
Baer, E. von 274
Baganda 97
Baghats 194
Bahuchet, S. 65, 172, 177f, 185ff
Bailey, G.N. 120, 122
Bailey, K. 33, 38
Bailey, R. 187
Bali 172, 187, 268
Balkan 103
banana 10, 41f, 44, 48, 210ff
Bandkeramik culture 103
Bard, D. 196, 216
Barker, G. 103, 116
Barlett, P.f. 99, 117
barley 103, 156, 160
Barnard, A. 172, 178, 185, 187
Barth, F. 95, 117, 230
Baruya 223f, 231
Basu, A. 255, 259
Batek 172, 174, 176, 179, 180, 182, 187
Bateson, P.P.G. 84
Bats, M. 88, 108, 117, 119, 121
Bavaria 2, 106
beauty 77, 80, 81, 85, 196f, 200f
Beek, W.E.A. van 207, 216
beer 94f, 97, 112, 120, 122, 137, 152, 154, 156, 167, 203f, 207f, 210, 212, 214
begging 54
behavioral predisposition 1, 48
Bell-Krannhals, I. 10, 234, 237, 250, 276
Bellwood, P.S. 250
Bender, B. 88, 103, 117
Benedict, R. 130, 143
Benicio, M.H.D'A 274
Benoit, F. 109, 113, 117
Bernstein, I.S. 71, 83
Bertucchi, G. 108, 117, 119, 121
betelnut 37, 242
Betzig, L.L. 82, 85
Bharati, P. 255, 259
Bicchieri, M.G. 187, 189
Biel, J. 109, 117
Biers, W. B. 117
Big-man (compare 'Great-Man') 6, 11, 13, 37, 96, 112, 119, 123, 128, 134f, 139, 144, 218, 220-228, 231f
Bihor 172, 174, 176, 180, 182

Binford, L.R. 100f, 117, 171, 187, 190
biological adaptation, counter examples 200, 206, 214, 246
biological theory 17
Bird-David, N. 184, 187
Blake, M. 130, 138, 143, 144
Bloch, M. 119, 232
Blurton Jones, N.G. 47, 65
Boas, F. 9, 17, 132, 143
body shape 83, 199, 215
Boelaars, J.H.M.C. 227, 230, 233
Boesch, C. 40f, 43f, 48, 63, 65, 277
Boesch, H. 40f, 43f, 48, 63, 65
Bonfante, L. 107, 117
Bonnemère, P. 230
bonobo/pygmy chimpanzee 7, 40, 47-53, 58-67, 277f
Bonsall, C. 122, 124
Bontamba-Lokuli, J.P. 64
Bonzenza, P. 64
Borgerhoff Mulder, M. 82f
Borsu.i.attention seeking 26
Borsutzky, D. 23, 27, 30, 74, 76, 84
Bouloumié, B. 107, 109, 111, 117
Bouly de Lesdain, S. 210, 215
Bourdieu, P. 4, 17, 89f, 92f, 95, 98, 110, 117, 193f, 215
Boyd, D.J. 221, 230
Bradley, R. 105f, 118, 123
Brahmin 193
bread 152, 154, 156, 213
breadfruit 211, 213
breast-feeding 16, 266, 268, 274
Bremen, V. von 172, 186, 190
bridewealth 11, 91, 94f, 179, 186, 195, 200, 220, 222-225
Brigant, L. 196, 216
Brillat-Savarin, A. 193, 215
Bronze Age 106, 111, 118
Brothwell, D. 102, 118
Brothwell, P. 102, 118
Brown, J.A. 117, 121, 122
Brown, P. 227, 230, 231
Brumfiel, E. 144
bucket 106, 111, 119
Bulmer, R. 231
bulrush millet 202
bureaucracy 148
Burger, R. 105, 118
Burgess, C. 105, 118
Burgundy 109
burial 99, 104, 106, 109, 111, 139, 207, 209
Buss, D.M. 80, 83

cacao 137
Calabria 193, 216

Callicebus spp. 39
Callitrichidae 39
Calusa 136, 141, 145
Cameroon 9, 119, 194f, 197, 203f, 209f, 213, 277
Campbell, B. 85
Campo 209
Cancian, F. 93, 118
cannibalism 44, 227, 232
caribou 141
Carlsmith, J.F. 23, 29
Carnac 104
Caro, T.M. 81, 83
Carpenter, C.R. 20, 29
Carthage 108
Cary, M.S. 23, 29
Casati 97, 118
cash economy 206, 209
Cashdan, E. 187
cassava 209-212
Cassels, C. 254, 259
Cassidy, C.M. 257, 259
caste 16, 194, 252-255, 257, 259f
caste distinction viii
cattle 10, 90, 94f, 103, 137, 140, 163, 195ff, 200ff, 204-207, 209, 267
cattle-lending system 196
causewayed enclosure 105, 140
Cavigneaux, A. 162f, 166
Cebidae 39
Central Europe 123f
Cephalophus sp. 52
Cercopithecidae 39
cereal 103, 152, 154, 195, 200, 202, 209, 258
ceremonial axes 140
Chad 195, 204
Chagnon, N.A. 82ff
Chalcolithic 104
Chance, M.R.A. 20, 22, 29ff, 83f, 188
Charlesworth, W. 24, 30
Chen, L.C. 255, 259
Cheney, D.L. 39, 65, 216
Cheney, R.M. 45
Chhabra, K.B. 214f
chicha 266
chief 93, 97, 99, 105, 123, 128, 134f, 139, 156, 193, 199, 205f, 209, 235, 237-240, 246, 248f
children 3, 12ff, 16, 19, 21, 23-31, 35, 37f, 70, 72-76, 78ff, 82, 84f, 135, 173, 181, 188, 200ff, 225, 228f, 235, 240ff, 247f, 255-258, 260, 264, 266, 269f, 278f
chimpanzee 7, 21, 29f, 34f, 38-42, 44f, 47ff, 62-67, 101, 118, 277, 279
China 145, 148

Chipewyan 172, 174, 176, 180ff, 189
Chisholm, B. 119
Choiseul Island 91, 123
Christiaans F. & L., 64
Claessen, H. 123
Clarke, D.L. 102, 118
Clarke, J. 130, 138, 143f
Clastres, P. 172, 178, 182, 187
Clough, T.H.M. 105, 118
Clutton-Brock, T.H. 83
co-evolutionary process 268
coconut 219, 225, 228
Codere, H. 9, 17, 91, 118, 126, 132, 144
cognac 210
Cohen, A. 89, 118
Cohen, B. 260
Cole, K.J. 30
Coles, J.M. 106, 118
collector 77, 100, 171
Colocasia esculenta 242
colonial interaction 8, 107, 114, 118
commensal politics 88, 90ff, 97, 99-102, 106ff, 110, 112f
competition 3f, 9ff, 14f, 28, 37, 41, 63f, 67, 80, 98, 105, 111, 113, 119, 127ff, 135, 140f, 184, 186, 203f, 218f, 221, 226, 231, 238, 240, 249
competition ritualized 247
competition status 3, 28, 39
competitive harvest 234, 243
competitive hospitality 99
complex hunter-gatherer (compare 'hunter-gatherer')102f, 136, 141f, 171, 184
Congès, G. 119, 121
Congleton, R.D. 76f, 83
control 6, 18, 22, 25, 41, 70, 102, 110, 112, 124, 128-131, 133, 140, 160, 166, 185, 192, 201, 205, 216, 218, 238, 270
Copper Inuit 172, 174, 176, 180, 182
corvée 93, 97, 105
Cosmides, L. 3, 18
Cosnier, J. 84
Coula edulis 48
Crawford, C.B. 83
credit 4f, 96, 112, 132f, 152, 175, 184, 197, 254f
Cree 172, 174, 176, 180, 182, 189
Cristofani, M. 122
culinary labor 90, 102
Cummins, W.A. 105, 118
Czechoslovakia 106

D'Souza, S. 255, 259
DAAD 64

Dahlberg, F. 189
Dalton, G. 111, 118
Damas, D. 172, 180f, 187ff
Damerow, P. 14f, 150, 156, 163, 166f, 276
Daubentonia madagascarensis 39
Dawkins, R. 83
debts 8, 126, 131-134, 136, 138, 179, 222, 269
deer 100, 102, 140
delicacy 8, 9, 129, 133, 136, 141
Dennell, R. 100, 102f, 118
Dentzer, J.M. 88, 98, 107, 118
Désy, P. 4, 17
Dettmann, H. 64
Dettwyler, K.A. 256, 260
developing country 16, 262, 269, 278
development program viii
DeVore, I. 64, 67
DFG 64
Diakonoff, I.M. 167
Dietler, M. 8, 12, 88, 90, 94f, 105, 107-110, 118f, 127, 137, 144, 276
Dimbleby, G.W. 144
Dioscorea alata 211, 234
distinction 4, 15, 63, 91, 98f, 104, 111, 117, 171, 177, 193f, 215
distribution 15, 42, 66, 90f, 93, 122, 128, 145, 148ff, 154, 163, 166, 170, 175ff, 179-183, 188, 212, 220, 263
distribution attention 73
distribution ceremonial 225
distribution mortuary 10
distribution pattern 246f
distribution roles 49, 63
distribution *sagali* 13
dominance 2, 7, 18-22, 24, 30f, 33, 37ff, 41f, 69, 71, 76, 79, 82, 118, 183-186, 192, 269
dominance dyadic 20, 69
dominance female 45
dominance hierarchy 20f, 69, 72, 74, 83
dominance male 40
dominance nurturant 33, 35, 37f
dominance political 205
dominance preschool children 29
dominance rank 43
dominance relationship 71-77, 82
dominance repressive 8ff, 33, 37, 38
dominance social 41
dominance status 22, 73
dominance structure 28
dominance submission pattern 34
Douglas, M. 6, 9, 12, 17f, 89, 110, 119, 122
Dowling, J. 176, 187

Downs, J.F. 172, 178, 187
Dresrüsse, G. 16, 276
drinking 8, 17f, 98f, 106, 108f, 111, 113f, 118, 122, 124, 128, 144, 199, 202ff, 206, 208ff, 213f, 254
Duala 209, 213
duiker 52
Dumont, L. 252, 260
Dunbar, R.I.M. 39, 44
dwarf humpless cow 207

Early Iron Age 100
earth oven 137
earthenware pots 239
Eastern Europe 123
economic self-interest 131
Edmonds, M. 105, 118
egalitarianism 5, 127, 173, 184
Eggerman, M. 253, 260
Egypt 148
Ehara, A. 45, 66
Eibl-Eibesfeldt, I. 1, 7, 11f, 15, 17, 23f, 29, 33ff, 38, 48, 64f, 184, 187, 277, 279
Elam 149
elderly person 266
Elias, N. 98, 119
elite 98, 106, 110f, 114, 128, 142f, 150, 268f, 273
Elkin, A.P. 231
Ellsworth, P.C. 23, 29
Ellyson, S.L. 23, 30
Emory, G.R. 22, 29
Endicott, K. 172, 187
Enga 119f, 226, 231ff
Engle, P.L. 257, 260
Englund, R.K. 149ff, 156, 159, 163, 166f
Epple, G. 39, 44
éprouvettes gastronomiques 193
equality 2, 37, 175, 184, 186
Erasmus, C.J. 93f, 119
Esser, A.H. 70, 83
Essock-Vitale, S.M. 82f
Esterik, P. van 256, 261
ethology 1-4, 17f, 30f, 69, 83f, 184, 249, 276
Etkin, W. 64f
Etruscan 107f, 113, 117
Europe 1, 8, 94, 101-104, 106, 111, 116, 118ff, 122f, 140, 142, 203, 235, 240, 242, 249, 268, 276f
European Commission on the Anthropology of Food and Nutrition vii
European prehistory 89, 100, 107, 114, 118

Everett, M. 120
evolutionary biology 3, 13, 84
evolutionary function viii
exchange/exchange system 5, 11, 37, 48, 89ff, 93ff, 105, 112f, 118f, 121, 127ff, 136, 221, 223f, 226f, 231f, 247
exchange ceremonial 11, 13, 123, 218, 220f, 223, 225f, 228
exchange competitive 10, 129, 138, 221, 225
exchange dyad 92
exchange intergroup 222, 224f
exchange *kayasa* 10
exchange *kula* 10, 119
exchange network 90, 103-106, 139ff, 177, 181, 183
exchange partnership 4, 173, 179f, 219, 222
exchange pattern 91, 139
exchange reciprocal 135
exchange sister 223, 225
Exline, R.V. 22f, 30

Fabaceae 266
Falkenstein, A. 150, 167
Fallon, A.E. 199, 215
Fang 210
FAO 262, 273, 276f
fat 6, 80, 83, 137, 180, 193, 195, 197, 199f, 202, 216, 221, 227
fatness 80, 194, 199f, 215, 260
Favre, A.M. 269, 274
feast 99, 110, 127, 133, 146, 206
feast cargo 131
feast celebratory 8, 127, 134
feast ceremonial exchanges 219
feast commensal politics 87, 89
feast competitive viii, 9, 93, 126-131, 133-143, 173, 227
feast diacritical 8, 98f, 104, 106, 114, 128
feast entrepreneurial 8, 92, 95, 99, 105, 112
feast equipment 106, 109, 111
feast initiated men 181
feast *kelo* 91
feast large 96
feast Marind-Anim 227
feast monthly 210f
feast Ndambu 232
feast New Guinea 137
feast organizer 219, 226
feast political economy 104
feast prehistoric competitive 140
feast redistributive 8, 128
feast religious 95, 134
feast ritual 104, 106, 205

feast surplus 8
feast work-party 93-97, 105, 118, 127f
feasting 8-11, 18f, 91ff, 98, 105ff, 111-114, 126f, 130, 136f, 140, 143, 278
feasting facility 139
feasting food 129, 136f, 142, 212
feasting gear 106, 111
feasting structure 139
feasting support group 134
feather 219
feeding program 16, 270
Feierman, J. 38
Feil, D.K. 90, 119, 228, 231
Feistner, A.T.C. 62, 65
Ferro-Luzzi, G.E. 252, 260
fertility rites 227f
Finkbeiner, U. 162f, 166
Firth, R. 93, 119
Fischer, F. 109, 119
Fischer, H. 231
Flannery, K 139, 144
Flinn, M.V. 82
Florida 136, 145
flour 90, 152, 156, 209, 254
flying squirrel 62
focus of attention 2, 11, 22, 173f, 175, 181, 183, 249
Foley, R.A. 67
food abundance 6
food acquired 52
food aid 270
food allocation 254, 256-261
food anxiety 195
food artificial 57
food as a human right 271, 274
food as currency 247
food behavior 264f, 267, 269, 271
food chain 269
food competition 128
food component 270
food consumption 6, 52, 59, 89, 98, 104, 204, 206, 212, 215, 252, 262f, 271, 273
food contribution 267
food designer 16, 269
food distribution 6ff, 13, 15, 47, 59, 152, 184, 216, 218, 226, 252, 255f, 259ff, 263, 273
food division 55, 60-63
food exchange 11, 51, 56f, 63, 90, 218, 220, 224f, 229
food habits 16, 213, 216, 269, 277
food intake 35, 81, 256f
food intake children 258
food interaction unit 57
food introduction. 119
food item 51f, 59, 61, 63f, 195, 210, 272

food leadership 124
food low status 16, 257
food manipulation 103
food marketing 269
food pattern 89
food plant 41, 48f, 52-55, 58f, 62-64, 100, 102, 267
food practice 98, 268
food preference 59, 63, 203
food privilege 202
food procurement 252f, 255
food production 11, 15f, 18, 102f, 119, 126f, 144, 148ff, 166, 188, 195, 263, 267ff, 271ff, 278
food related behavior 10, 15f, 257, 259, 263, 266-269, 272f
food resource 60f, 100
food security 97
food self-sufficiency 253
food sharing 6f, 12, 18, 34f, 37f, 39f, 42f, 45, 47-66, 101, 118, 120f, 127, 145, 187f, 190, 219, 242, 267
food shortage 15, 200, 204, 253ff, 268
food social status 47, 270
food source 266f, 271f
food staple 173, 234, 265
food supplementation 257, 270
food supply 6, 15, 20, 166, 268, 270
food surplus 126, 130, 136, 138, 219
food transfer 34f, 52, 56, 59, 61f, 260
food-for-learning 270
food-for-work 270
forager (compare 'hunter-gatherer') 10ff, 14, 28, 84, 100, 102, 170f, 173, 175f, 178, 181, 183f, 186, 188, 189, 215
forager affluent 122
Fox, J. 144
France 10, 18, 103, 106-109, 117ff, 121, 144, 189, 194, 216, 276
Frankenstein, S. 109f, 119
Freedman, D.G. 31
Fried, M. 5, 18
Friedman, J. 91, 93, 96f, 119
Frisch, R.E. 80, 83
Froment, A. 196, 216
fruit 26, 40, 50, 52ff, 61-64, 103, 210f
Fruth, B. 7, 277
Fulani 202ff, 209, 213
funeral 89, 144, 201, 204f, 210
funerary ritual 104
Fürstensitze 109, 121
Furuichi, T. 60, 65

!G/wi San 24, 28ff, 172-176, 179-182, 188
Gamble, C. 100, 119

game 100, 177, 178, 179, 180, 187, 204, 207, 210, 213, 226
game. 210
Gantes, L.F. 108, 119
Gargett, R. 97, 119, 130, 144
Garine, I. de vii, 9f, 12, 14f, 65, 196f, 199f, 215f, 256, 259, 277
Garnsey, P. 123
Geertz, C. 17
Gelb, I.J. 160, 167
generosity 44, 97, 144, 173ff, 181, 219
Germany 24, 28, 79, 103, 109, 119, 277
Geschire, P. 96, 119
Ghiglieri, M.P. 65
gibbon 39, 47, 66
Gibson, D.B. 119
gimaiye 90
Gittelsohn, J. 256, 260
Gluck, C.M. 196, 216
goats 103, 162, 195, 204ff
Godelier, M. 220, 223, 231
gold 106, 109
Goldizen, A.W. 47, 65
Goldman, R.F. 196, 216
golla 196
Gombe 30, 38, 40, 42-45, 48, 66f
Goodall, J. 21, 30, 34, 38, 40f, 43ff, 47f, 65, 67
Goodenough Island 90
Goodenough, W. 4, 18
Goody, J. 6, 18, 98, 111, 119
Gopaldas, T. 194, 215
Gordon, R. 190
Gosden, Ch. 134, 144
gossip 185
Gould, R. 130, 144, 172, 179, 183, 187f
grain 95, 103, 112, 142, 152, 156, 163, 253ff, 266, 268
Grammer, K. 2, 12, 14, 22, 24, 26f, 30, 73f, 76, 78-81, 84, 174, 184, 277
Gras, M. 107, 119
Graslund, B. 144
great apes 40, 45
Great-man (compare 'Big-Man') 13, 222-225
Greece 2, 98, 103, 107ff, 111, 113, 268
Green, M.W. 162, 167
Griffin, P.B. 172, 180, 186, 188
Grinker, R.R. 213, 215
Gross, R. 16, 269, 273f, 278
GTZ 64, 271f, 276ff
Guayaki 172, 174, 176, 178ff, 182, 187
Guemple, L. 187
Guillaumet, J.P. 106, 123
Gujarat 194, 215
Gunwinggu 172, 174, 176, 180, 182

Gupta, A. 194, 215
Guptua, R. 255, 259
gurna 197-200, 204, 215
guru 152, 196ff, 200, 259
guru fattening institution 14, 15, 201f, 206, 213ff
guru walla 9, 196, 199ff, 215f
Gusinde, M. 172, 175, 181, 188
Guttman L. 4
Guttman, R. 4

Hadza 172, 174, 176ff, 180, 180ff
Halls, W. 17
Hallstatt 106, 109f, 114, 119, 121
Hamburg, D.A. 45
Hamilton, W.D. 47, 65
Hanfman, E. 70, 84
Harako, R. 172, 178f, 188
Harcourt, A. 84
Harding, A.F. 106, 118
Harding, R. 188
Harris, M. 127, 144
Harrison, G.A. 260
Harriss, B. 255, 260
Hart an der Alz 106
Hartman, L.F 152, 167
harvest 11, 127, 141, 201, 208, 234, 238, 240, 242ff, 246f, 249, 253
harvest gift 10, 234, 242, 244-248
Hasegawa, T. 42, 45
Hawkes, C.F.C. 106, 119
Hawkes, K. 188
Hayden, B. 8f, 18, 88, 93, 97, 100, 103, 119, 127, 130, 136, 141f, 144, 171, 173, 184, 188, 278
health problem 81, 240
Heath, D.B. 12, 18, 90, 119f
Heinz, H.J. 172, 179, 188
Heltne, P.G. 66
Henry, J. 172, 178, 188
Henson, A. 23, 29
Herdt, G. 231f
high regard 1, 24, 26f, 29f, 35, 84, 173f, 201, 246
Highland Maya 137
Hill, A.V. 250
Hill, K. 82, 84, 188
Hinde, R.A. 74, 84
Hinduism 193
Hiraiwa-Hasegawa, M. 42, 45
Hladik, A. 53, 65
Hladik, C.M. 53, 65, 192, 215
Hocart, A.M. 93, 120
Hochdorf 109, 117
Hofer, H. 64
Hogbin, I. 90, 120
Hohmann, G. 7, 278

Hold-Cavell, B.C.L. 2, 21, 23f, 26ff, 30, 73-76, 84, 173, 184, 188, 249, 278
Homo hierarchicus 252, 260
honey 102, 137
horticulturist 235
Horton, E.S. 196, 216
hospitality 8, 37, 64, 91-95, 97f, 112, 114f, 204
hospitality commensal 89ff, 93, 96, 99, 114
Hrozny, F. 152, 167
Hudson, J. 121
Hudson, P.T. 24, 30
human ethology vii, 3, 17, 38, 187, 277ff
human life cycle 78f
Humfries, S. 232
Hunn, E. 144
Hunter, M. 97, 120
hunter-gatherer (compare 'forager') 10, 12, 66, 100f, 103, 117, 120ff, 127, 130, 136f, 141, 144, 148, 170f, 173f, 184, 187f, 190, 235
hunting success 42, 178
Huq, E. 255, 259
Hurtado, A. 188
Hylobates spp. 39

Ifaluk 82
Iglilik 180
Iglulik Inuit 172, 174, 176, 181
Ihobe, H. 48, 62, 65
Ikala-Lokuli, M. 64
inclusive fitness (compare 'reproductive success') 13, 61, 69, 194, 214, 246, 248
Indian 2, 27, 193, 252, 260, 271, 278
Indian subcontinent 15, 252
Indo-Aryan 252, 257
Indo-European 2, 249, 267f
Indri indri 39
inequality 18, 35, 69, 94f, 98, 121, 123, 141, 215, 232
Ingold, T. 187, 189f
interest 70, 102, 126f, 129, 132, 134, 148, 224, 278
Inuit of Quebec 172, 174, 176, 180ff, 189
Inuit of West Greenland 180
investment 4, 80, 112, 131ff, 135, 136f, 142
investment parental 12, 85
invulnerable resource 136, 140f
Iron Age 8, 12, 106f, 118f, 123f, 144, 276
Irons, W. 82, 84

Iroquois 139
Irvingia gabonensis 54
Isaac, G. 48, 65, 101, 120
Isherwood, B. 6, 17, 89, 110, 119
Italy 107, 193
Ivory Coast 40, 277

Jacobsthal, P. 109, 120
Jacomet, S. 103, 120
jade axe 138
Jahai 172, 174, 176, 178ff, 182, 190
Japan 24, 28f, 136, 138, 141, 192, 278
Jaqaj 225, 227
Jelliffe, D.B. 202, 216
Jochim, M. 100ff, 120
Joffroy, R. 109, 120
Jolly, C. 22, 29
Jomon 136, 138, 141
Jonaitis, A. 123

Kaberry, P.M. 91, 120
Kaenel, G. 107, 120
Kaileuna 235f, 237ff
Kaingáng 172, 174, 176, 180, 182, 188
Kalbermatten, U. 24, 30
Kambayi Bwatshia 64
Kami 257, 258, 260
Kande Muamba 64
Kano, T. 48, 51, 60, 62, 65ff
Kaplan, D. 18
Kaplan, H. 47, 66, 82, 84, 172, 181, 188
Katz, V. 39, 44
Kavanagh, M. 47, 64, 66
Kawabe, M. 48, 66
Kawai, M. 45, 66
Kawanaka, K. 63, 66
kayasa 10, 13, 234, 238ff, 243, 247ff
Kazadi, N. 213, 216
Kelleher, P.C. 196, 216
Kelly, R.C. 231
kelo 91
Kennard, R.C. 123
Kennedy, J. G. 93f, 120
Kenya 82, 94, 276
Keraki 226
Khare, R.S. 252, 260
Khor, G.L. 269, 274
Kimam 226, 232
Kimmig, W. 109, 120
kin selection 47, 60
kindergarten 21
king 151, 160
King, H. 232
Kinzey, W.G. 67
Kipsigisis 82
Kiriwina 235, 237, 239, 242

kiss-feeding 34
Kiwai 226, 231
Kleivan, I. 172, 188
!Ko San 172, 174, 180
Koma 10, 14f, 194, 206-209, 214
Kondo, S. 45, 66
Koppert, G. 196f, 200, 215, 256, 258ff, 260
Krebs, U., 84
Kühn, C. 64
kula 10, 13, 119, 234, 247f
Kummer, H. 76, 84
!Kung San 172ff, 176f, 179f, 182, 188ff
Kuroda, S. 47f, 51, 57f, 60, 62, 66
kuvi contest 249
Kwakiutl 17, 91, 118, 123, 132, 143
Kyangali, A. 227, 232

La Tène 107, 120
labor 4ff, 11, 13, 15, 39, 48, 91, 93-97, 102, 104f, 112f, 118, 122, 128ff, 133ff, 137, 142, 150ff, 166ff, 219, 220, 229, 253ff
LaFrenière, P. 24, 30
Lagrand, C. 108, 120
Lamb, Th.A. 33, 38
Landtman, G. 226, 231
Landy, D. 81, 85
Langdon, S. 150, 167
langur 47, 192
Larsen, R.R. 29ff, 84, 188
Laschan, P. 64
Latin America 270
Le Berre, S. 214, 216
Le Tensorer, J.M. 101, 121
Leach, E. 119
Leach, J.W. 119
Leacock, E. 190
leader 4, 7, 11, 14, 21, 25, 27, 38, 70, 73, 91, 96, 100, 112f, 123, 163, 184, 186, 205, 207, 219, 221, 226, 237, 277f
leadership 5, 9, 11, 18, 21, 24, 71, 74, 92, 100, 101, 113, 172, 184, 186, 216, 231, 248f
Lederman, R. 231
Lee, R. 127, 144, 172, 178f, 188ff
Leeuw, S. van der. 113, 123
legume 103
Lemonnier, P. 9, 11, 37, 92, 96, 112, 121, 218, 220f, 228, 231, 278
Leupold, K.H. 24, 30
Levant 141
Lévi-Strauss, C. 6, 18, 192, 216
life-crisis ceremonies 89
liku 10, 237f, 240, 244, 246-249
Lindberg, T. 83

Lindeberg, S. 242, 250
Linton, R. 3f, 18
loan 127, 131-136, 139, 177, 227, 243, 253ff
Locke, J. 2, 18
Lomako 59
Lombeya Bosongo Likundelio 64
Long, B. 23, 30
Longworth, I.H. 118
Loots, G.M.P. 27, 30
Lorenz, K. 12, 18
Lorimer, B. 30
losing face 212
Lothrop, S.K. 172, 178, 189
Lundh, B. 242, 250
luxury goods 109

Maddison, M. 118
Mahale Mountains 40, 45, 66
Mair, L.P. 97, 121
maize 137, 254, 266f
Majumder, P.P. 255, 259
Malenky, R.K. 47ff, 62, 64ff
Malinowski, B. 250
malnutrition 216, 240, 242, 259, 262f
malt 156, 160
manager 96, 112
Mandelbaum, D. 90, 121
Manihot 211
Manners, R. 18
Marler, P. 45
marmosets 39, 47, 65
Marquard, L. 66
Marriott, M. 252, 260
Marseille 108, 117, 119, 121, 123, 260
Marshall, F. 101, 121
Marshall, L. 172, 179, 189f
Mary-Rousseliere, G. 172, 189
Massa 9, 13ff, 194-204, 206, 213ff, 259, 277
Massim 18, 119, 124, 216, 235
matrilineality 237
Mauss, M. 7, 17f, 35, 38, 90f, 97, 121, 131, 144, 179, 183, 189
Max-Planck-Society, vii, viii2, 64, 276ff
Mazur, A. 33, 38
McCown, E.R. 45
McGovern, P.E. 117
McGrew, P.L. 24, 30
McGrew, W.C. 7, 21, 24, 30, 39f, 42, 44f 47f, 62-66, 70, 84, 279
meat 11f, 42ff, 48, 52f, 59, 62-65, 90, 97, 100f, 105, 141, 170, 172-184, 188f, 194, 201f, 204-207, 210-215, 255, 258, 267
meat distribution 11, 172, 174f, 177ff, 181, 183

meat sharing 43, 45, 48f, 52, 54f, 59, 62f, 100, 102, 179ff, 184f
Mediterranean 8, 35, 103, 106f, 109-114, 121, 123f
megalithic tomb 104, 140
Meggitt, M. 189, 222, 231f
Melanesia 93, 138
Mellars, P. 100f, 121
Melpa 90, 220, 226
Mercer, R.J. 137, 144
Merhart, G. von 106, 121
meritocracy 10
Mesoamerica 119, 144, 148
Mesolithic 8, 101, 118, 122ff, 126, 140ff
Mesopotamia 15, 148ff, 163, 167
Metha, U. 214f
Mexico 137ff, 143
milk 163, 195-200, 202, 204, 258
Miller, D. 99, 121
Mimica, J. 232
Misasi, N. 193, 216
Mitra, A. 193, 216
modesty 177f
Modjeska, N. 92, 121, 220, 232
Mohen, J.P. 101, 121
moka 90, 132, 220, 231
monopolization 61, 98
Monteiro, C.A. 274
Moore, J. 47, 66
Mordant, C. 118
Morel, J.P. 107f, 121
Moscati, P. 122
Mukhopadhyay, B. 255, 259
Müller-Karpe, H. 106, 121
Munini, P. 227, 232
Murray, O. 88, 98, 107, 121
Musaiger, A.O. 271, 274
Mussey 14f, 194, 198, 200, 202-206, 213f
Mvae 14f, 194, 209-215
Mycenaean 106, 123
Myers, F. 172, 189

Nabarro, D. 254, 259
Nadeau, J. 83
Nahoum, V. 193, 216
Nardi, G. 122
Nash, L.T. 47, 66
Natufian 141
Near East 148, 150, 167f
Neolithic 103ff, 118, 122, 124, 139f, 142, 144, 231
Nepal 252-257, 259f, 277, 279
Netsilik Inuit 172, 174, 176, 179f, 182
Neuffer, E. 109, 120
Neuweiler, G. 64

New Guinea 9, 11, 13, 121ff, 132, 135f, 139, 216, 218-222, 228-232, 234f
New Guinea British 250
New Guinea Highland 6, 24, 71, 122, 219, 221, 224, 227, 229, 231ff
New Guinea Melanesia 250
New Guinea Papua 119, 218, 220, 250, 276, 279
New Guinea South 223-228, 232f
Nieves, I. 257, 260
Nishida, T. 40-43, 45, 47f, 63, 66
Nissen, H.J. 149f, 152, 156, 159, 162, 166f
nonhuman primates 6f, 19f, 39, 76, 192, 212
Norgan, N. 260
North America 144, 172, 184, 187ff
North Cameroon 206, 213, 215
Northwest Coast cultures 136, 140
nutritional health 257, 259
nutritional security 262

Oates, J.F. 192, 216
Ockov 106
officials 159f, 168
olive 66, 103
Oltersdorf, U. 269, 274
Omark, D.T. 31
Omolulu, A. 213, 216
Ona 172, 174ff, 178, 180, 182
Oppenheim, A.L. 152, 167
orangutan 39
ostracism 185
Ott, E., 64
ownership 35, 52, 56, 60f, 127, 131, 141, 152, 175ff, 179, 183, 187, 195

Pagezy, H. 256, 260
Paleolithic 8, 100f, 119ff, 126, 141
Pan species 62f
pan-European 104
Panda oleosa 48
Pandolfini, M. 122
Pant, M. 254, 259
Panter-Brick, C. 14f, 253, 257f, 260, 279
Papio spp. 39
parasite load 242, 263
Pare, C. 109, 121
Parish, A. 49, 60, 66
Parry, J. 232
Parry, W. 138, 144
Pasquet, P. 196, 216
patron-role 8f, 90f, 94ff, 99, 101, 105ff, 111f, 114, 122f, 126-129, 133f, 136-139
Paulik, J. 106, 121

peace ceremony 218, 220f, 224f
Peacock, D.P.S. 113, 121
Pearson, H. 122
pecking order 19
Pele, J. 214, 216
Pelto, G.H. 256
Pelto, G.H. et al. 260
Pennisetum sp. 202
Perinari fruit 41
Persia 82, 150, 163
Peru 105, 265, 267, 271
Peruvian 266
Peterson, N. 172, 179, 187
Philippines 173
physical fitness 197, 200
Pickford, M. 45
pig 9, 11, 90, 103, 132, 136f, 144, 163, 182, 213, 216, 218-232, 234
pig-as-life-substitute. 221
Pintupi 172, 174, 176, 180, 182
Pires-Ferreira, J. 139, 144
Planck, D., 117
plate 111
Ploog, D. 64
Polanyi, K. 97, 122
politicosymbolic drama 104
Pollock, J.I. 39, 45
Pollock, N.J. 215f
polygyny 96, 135
polythetic typology, 140
Pongo pygmaeus 39
pony 204
popolo grosso 193
popolo magro 193
pork 137, 204, 218, 221, 223, 225f
potlatch 91, 118, 123, 131f, 193f, 212
pots 104, 108, 113f, 121, 123, 145, 208f
Powdermaker, H. 93, 122
Powell, M. 168
power 5, 8f, 12, 15, 17, 19, 30, 69ff, 74f, 82, 85, 87, 90, 92f, 101, 103, 110, 112-115, 118, 129ff, 134, 139, 144, 148, 173, 186f, 189f, 193, 200f, 205, 223, 231, 248, 253, 272
pre-Columbian 267, 271
prehistoric Europe 88, 99
prehistoric society 96
prestige 4f, 8, 14, 92, 94ff, 100ff, 105, 112, 129, 135, 173, 175, 183, 200, 212ff, 219f, 226, 247, 267, 271f, 278
prestige container 138
prestige food 211 ff
prestige goods 95, 106, 109 f, 132, 136, 138 f, 141, 143
prestige value 77
Price, J.A. 172, 189
Price, T.D. 102, 117, 121 f

Index

Pritchard, A.C. 123
prosimian species 39
prosperity 193, 197, 209
prosperity magic 201
protein 144, 190, 200, 204, 214, 242, 258, 265-268
proto-cuneiform 15, 148, 150, 163
proto-elamite 15, 149 f, 163, 166
proto-elite 135
Pryor, F. 97, 122
Py, M. 107 f, 122
Pygmy 182, 187, 190, 213, 216
Pygmy Aka 172, 174, 176, 178, 180, 182
Pygmy Mbuti 172, 174, 176, 179 f, 182f, 188

R.H. Tuttle, R.H. 215
Radcliffe-Brown, A. 172, 189
Rai, N.K. 180, 189
Ramesh, P. 214f
Ramirez, P 260
rank aggressive behavior 76
rank concept 98
rank dominance 44
rank hierarchy 2-9, 11, 14, 16, 19f, 22, 26, 28f, 37f, 45, 69, 73ff, 83, 128, 160, 173, 184, 237, 244, 249
rank high 2f, 5, 7, 10, 16, 19f, 22-28, 34, 40, 42, 73-78, 80, 144, 160, 205, 207, 213, 235, 237f, 240, 244, 247, 271
rank inherited 3, 40
rank low 2, 19f, 22-25, 27f, 42, 73ff, 77f, 80, 160, 244
rank middle 24f
rank preschool group 74
rank repression 11
rank society 5, 10, 144
rank specific behavior 30, 84, 188
Rao, M.S.A. 252, 260
Rappaport, R. 139, 144, 214, 216
Rathwakoli 194
Rea, M.F. 274
reciprocity 7, 9, 35, 37, 60, 76, 117, 179, 187, 190, 223
redistribution 8, 97, 110
Rehfisch, F. 93, 122
relief operation viii
Renfrew, C. 103, 105, 122
reproductive success (compare 'inclusive fitness') 3, 7, 13f, 39f, 42ff, 62f, 78ff, 82-85, 188, 248
reputation 5, 12, 94f, 112, 133, 181
respect 1, 10, 24f, 128, 134, 207, 240, 246
returns on investment 129
rhesus monkey 22, 31

Rhône 108-111, 118, 120
Richards, A 97, 122
Riches, D. 187, 189f
Riches, J. 189
ridicule 183, 185, 239
Rios Esquivel, I. 269, 274
risk sharing 171, 185
Riss, D.C. 45
Riss, E. 63, 67
rites of passage 89, 256
ritualization 89, 212, 219, 232, 238, 248f
Robbe, B. 18
Robbe, P. 4, 172, 178, 181, 186, 189
Robbins, R.H. 111, 122
Roberts, C. 64
Rogers, E.S. 172, 189
role of wives 111
Rolley, C. 109, 122
Röllig, W. 152, 167
Roman 24, 107, 121
Rosman, A. 9, 18
Rouillard, P. 108, 122
Rousseau, J. 2, 18
Rowe, D.W. 196, 216
Rowell, T. 20
Rowlands, M.J. 109f, 119
Rowley-Conwy, P 102, 122
Roy, S.K. 255, 259
Rozin, P. 199, 215
Rubel, P. 9, 18
Rubenstein, D. 67
Ruoff, U. 107, 122

Sadu 193
sagali 10, 240, 247
Sahlins, M. 37f, 97, 122, 185, 189
Sahn, D.E. 255, 260
Saint-Romain-de-Jalionas 106
Saladin d'Anglure, B. 172, 178, 183, 189
Salisbury, R. 90, 92, 111f, 122
salt 211, 224
Salter, F. 8, 18
Samia 94, 118
sanskritisation 194, 215
Sardinia 108
Savin-Williams, R. 28
Saxena, K. 194, 215
Sayerse, C. 214f
scarce commodity 192
Schapera, I. 97, 122
Schebesta, P. 172, 189
Scheffler, H.W. 91, 93, 112, 123
Scheil, V. 149, 163, 167
Scheper-Hughes, N. 256, 259f
Schernthaner, U. 74, 84

Schessler, T. 47, 66
Schibler, J. 103, 120
Schiefenhövel, W. 10, 115,250, 279
Schjelderupp-Ebbe, T. 19, 31, 69, 84
Schropp, R. 27, 31, 72, 75, 78, 84
Schürch, B. 269, 274
Schwarcz, H.P. 119
Schwarz, K. 79, 84
Scott, C. 172, 189
sea mammal 140
Seidel, U. 162f, 166
self-aggrandizement 128, 143
Sellen, D.W. 83
Semang 172
Sept, P.K. 65
Sept, S. 65
Serjeantson, S.W. 250
Serpenti, L. 232
Seyfarth, R.M. 39, 45, 65, 216
sharing practice 183
sharing system 186, 192
Sharp, H.S. 172, 178, 181, 189
sheep 103, 162, 195, 206, 210
shell 111, 138, 219f, 222, 224f
Shennan, S.J. 106, 123
Sherratt, A. 104, 123
Shibasaka, H. 23, 31, 78, 84
Siani 90
Sieveking, G. 118
Siewert, H.H. 162f, 166
Sigall, H. 81, 85
Sigulem, D.M. 274
Silberbauer, G. 172, 175, 179, 181, 189f
Silk, J.B. 48, 63, 66
Sims, E.A.H. 196, 216
Singer, M. 260
Singh, D. 81, 85
Sluys, C. van der 172, 178f, 181, 186, 190
Smith, E.A. 190
Smith, I.F. 105, 123
Smith, M.A. 106, 119, 123
Smuts, B.B. 39, 45, 65, 216
snack food 204, 206
social structure 4, 22, 29ff, 39, 41, 67, 69, 84, 123, 167, 188, 192, 232, 248
socioeconomic factor 193
Soffer, O. 119
Solomon Sea. 234
Solomons, N.W. 269, 274
Sommer, V. 64
Sorenson, E.R. 221, 232
sorghum 15, 195ff, 199-204, 207, 209, 214
South Africa 188
South America 172, 178, 184

South Cameroon 204, 209
South-East Europe 124
Spain 108
Speth, J. 6, 18, 137, 144, 190
Spielmann, K. 137, 144, 190
Standen, V. 67
Stange, M. 269, 274
Stanjek, K. 26f
Startin, W. 105, 123
starvation 185, 193
status achieved/aquired 3f, 7, 11, 14, 139, 193, 201, 203, 207, 212, 219, 246, 248f
status ascribed 3, 10, 193, 212, 246, 249
status caste 252, 258
status children 274
status competition 80, 114
status concept 2ff, 73f, 173, 183
status difference 2, 5, 7, 12, 29, 97, 106, 149, 186, 192, 193
status distinction 93, 170, 184
status food 15, 218, 266f, 271f
status group 262
status hierarchy 19, 21, 27, 160
status high 3, 14, 16, 21, 26, 76-82, 138, 160, 174f, 184, 247, 253, 256, 273
status household 256
status inherited 249
status item 138, 140
status low 16, 77, 257
status nutritional 15f, 190, 193, 252, 256, 259, 262, 269, 272
status relation 3, 6, 8, 16
status seeking 2f, 7, 9f, 12f, 15f, 19, 26, 82f, 170, 184, 213
status social 8, 15f, 30, 39, 41f, 50, 60, 69, 74, 79-82, 98, 131, 148f, 160, 166, 193, 258, 262, 266-273
status socioeconomic 4, 213, 252f, 255, 258, 274
steel ax 111
Steiner, J. 263, 274
Stent, G.S. 84
Stevenson-Hinde, J 74, 84
Stiles, E.W. 49, 66
Stol, M. 152, 167
Stonehenge 104
storage 11, 103, 112ff, 141, 171, 185f, 190, 237f, 240, 244, 263
Strathern, A. 90, 111f, 121, 123, 126, 132, 144, 220f, 227, 231f
stratification 5, 8, 14, 98f, 110, 150, 166, 266
Strayer, F.F. 31, 72, 85
Strayer, J. 72, 85

Struhsaker, T.T. 39, 45, 65, 216
Strum, S.C. 47, 66
Struve, V.V. 160
stunting 242
submission 33, 38, 41, 71, 82
success 7, 11, 134, 137, 143, 174, 183ff, 201, 218f, 222f, 235, 246ff, 271
success biological 84, 192
success family 242
success military 128
success social 195, 207
Sumerian 156, 159
surplus 14, 96, 112, 129-136, 140f, 143, 177, 183, 210, 247, 254
Susa 149, 163
Süsskind, G. 117
Sussman, R.L. 65f
Suttles, W. 91, 123
Switzerland 103, 109, 274, 276

Tai 40, 43f, 63, 65
Tai Forest 40, 48
Tamang 257f, 260
tamarins 39, 44, 65
Tanaka, J. 172, 190
Tanzania 40, 45, 66, 279
Tassa 14
Taylour, W. 106, 123
Tchernia, A. 107, 123
tee 119f, 231f
Teleki, G. 40, 45, 48, 63, 67, 188, 190
Teleki, R.H. 188
Testart, A. 171, 190
testosterone 33, 74
Teti, V. 193, 216
Thompson, P.R. 48, 67
Thompson-Handler, N. 64
Thornhill, R. 81, 84
Tibeto-Burman 252f
Tinkle, D.W. 83
titi monkey 39
Toffin, G 260
toli kayasa 239f
Tooby, J. 3, 18, 64, 67
Topping, P. 118
Tosh, J. 93, 123
Treculia africana 50, 53, 57
Trenkenschuh, F. 232
Tréziny, H. 119, 121
Tringham, R. 102ff, 123, 144
Trinidadians 82
Triple A individual 8, 130f, 133-136, 138ff, 142f
Trivers, R.L. 7, 18, 35, 38, 47, 60, 67, 80, 85
Trobriand 10, 13, 37, 234-239, 241-244, 247-250, 276f

Tudisco, E.S. 274
Tumu, A. 227, 232
tumulus 106, 109, 111, 123
Turke, P.W. 82, 85
Turnbull, C.M. 172, 190
Tutin, C.E.G. 42, 44f
Tuttle, R.H. 215

Ucko, P. 144
Uehara, S. 40, 45
umiak 183
Underhill, A.P. 138, 145
Unger, B. 64
United Nations 271, 274
urban civilization 148, 150, 277
Urnfield 106
Uromastyx sp. 62
Uruk 148, 150, 163, 166f

Vaughn, B. 24, 31
Vayda, A.P. 252, 261
vegetable 103, 172f, 201f, 209ff, 213, 252, 258, 270
Velde, P. van de 110, 123
Verger, S. 106, 123
Vertenten, P. 233
vervet 192
vessel 98f, 104, 106, 110f, 117, 136ff, 140f
vessel bronze 106, 109, 114
vessel burial 110
vessel Maya 138
vessel wine 8, 109
Villard, F. 108f, 123
Virgo, H.B. 31
vitamin B deficiency 266
Vix 109, 111, 120
Voandzeia 211
Volkman, T.A. 93, 123
Voytek, B. 103, 123

Waal, F. de 21, 29, 45, 47, 51, 65, 84, 101, 118
Waddell, J. 120
Waetzoldt, H. 160
wage labor 111, 143, 253ff
Wais, A. 117
Waldren, W.H. 123
Wamba 48f, 57f, 60, 62, 65f
Washburne, C. 97, 124
Waterhouse, H.B. 31
Waterhouse, M.J. 31
Waterlow, J.C. 260
Waters, E. 24, 31
Watts, E.S. 83
Wawra, M. 31
Weber, M. 4, 18

Weiner, A.B. 13, 18, 237, 247, 250
Weiner, J.F. 231
Wells, P. 109f, 124
West Greenland Inuit 172, 174, 182
Western countries, 13
Western culture 19
Western Desert 172, 174, 176, 180, 182f
Western Europe 8, 12, 103f, 107f, 114, 118
Western Hallstatt Culture 106, 108, 121
Westernization 15, 214
wheat 103, 140, 209
Wheeler, E.F. 256, 261
White, F.J. 49, 60ff, 67
Whittaker, C.R. 123
Whittle, A. 103f, 106, 123f
Widmer, R. 141, 145
Wiessner, P. 1, 11, 28, 35, 38, 64, 100ff, 115, 171f, 185, 190, 227, 232f
Wijga, A. 254, 259
Williams, B.J. 172, 190
Williams, F.E. 225, 227, 233
Williams, N. 144
Wilmsen, E. 190
Wilson, D. 137, 145
Wilson, E. 75, 85
Wilson, K.E. 118
wine 8, 98, 103, 107-113, 123, 210, 212
Winterhalder, B. 127, 145, 190
women's contest 248
Woodburn, J. 171f, 178, 185, 187, 189f
worker 152, 200
Wrangham, R.W. 39ff, 44f, 49, 61, 63, 65, 67, 216

Xanthosoma 211

yam 10, 91, 137, 207, 211, 219, 223, 225, 234, 238, 243f
Yanomami/Yanomamö 82f, 277
Yassa 15, 194, 209-214
Yomut Turkmen 82
Young, M. 9, 18, 90, 93, 111, 124, 126, 129, 145, 194, 216
Yudkin, J. 214, 216

Zaire 49, 65f, 187f, 215, 260, 277f
Zana Ndontoni 64
zebu 207
Zegwaard, G. 233
Ziga, H.P.P. 274